Osteoarthritis: The Complete Guide

Osteoarthritis: The Complete Guide

Edited by Willard Leopold

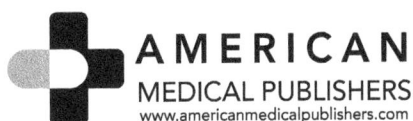

AMERICAN
MEDICAL PUBLISHERS
www.americanmedicalpublishers.com

American Medical Publishers,
41 Flatbush Avenue,
1st Floor, New York,
NY 11217, USA

Visit us on the World Wide Web at:
www.americanmedicalpublishers.com

ISBN: 978-1-63927-402-4

Cataloging-in-Publication Data

Osteoarthritis : the complete guide / edited by Willard Leopold.
     p. cm.
   Includes bibliographical references and index.
   ISBN 978-1-63927-402-4
 1. Osteoarthritis. 2. Osteoarthritis--Diagnosis. 3. Osteoarthritis--Treatment.
 4. Osteoarthritis--Prevention. 5. Arthritis. I. Leopold, Willard.
RC931.O67 O78 2022
616.722 3--dc23

Table of Contents

Preface..IX

Chapter 1   Inhomogeneity of immune cell composition in the synovial sublining: linear
            mixed modelling indicates differences in distribution and spatial decline
            of CD68+ macrophages in osteoarthritis and rheumatoid arthritis.............................1
            Johanna Mucke, Annika Hoyer, Ralph Brinks, Ellen Bleck, Thomas Pauly,
            Matthias Schneider and Stefan Vordenbäumen

Chapter 2   Concurrent validity of different functional and neuroproteomic pain
            assessment methods in the rat osteoarthritis monosodium iodoacetate
            (MIA) model...11
            Colombe Otis, Julie Gervais, Martin Guillot, Julie-Anne Gervais,
            Dominique Gauvin, Catherine Péthel, Simon Authier, Marc-André Dansereau,
            Philippe Sarret, Johanne Martel-Pelletier, Jean-Pierre Pelletier, Francis Beaudry
            and Eric Troncy

Chapter 3   Integrating genome-wide DNA methylation and mRNA expression profiles
            identified different molecular features between Kashin-Beck disease and
            primary osteoarthritis...27
            Yan Wen, Ping Li, Jingcan Hao, Chen Duan, Jing Han, Awen He, Yanan Du,
            Li Liu, Xiao Liang, Feng Zhang and Xiong Guo

Chapter 4   Association between general joint hypermobility and knee, hip, and lumbar
            spine osteoarthritis by race..35
            Portia P. E. Flowers, Rebecca J. Cleveland, Todd A. Schwartz, Amanda E. Nelson,
            Virginia B. Kraus, Howard J. Hillstrom, Adam P. Goode, Marian T. Hannan,
            Jordan B. Renner, Joanne M. Jordan and Yvonne M. Golightly

Chapter 5   From osteoarthritic synovium to synovial-derived cells
            characterization: synovial macrophages are key effector cells...............................42
            Cristina Manferdini, Francesca Paolella, Elena Gabusi, Ylenia Silvestri,
            Laura Gambari, Luca Cattini, Giuseppe Filardo, Sandrine Fleury-Cappellesso
            and Gina Lisignoli

Chapter 6   S100A8/A9 increases the mobilization of pro-inflammatory Ly6C^{high}
            monocytes to the synovium during experimental osteoarthritis.............................54
            Niels A. J. Cremers, Martijn H. J. van den Bosch, Stephanie van Dalen,
            Irene Di Ceglie, Giuliana Ascone, Fons van de Loo, Marije Koenders,
            Peter van der Kraan, Annet Sloetjes, Thomas Vogl, Johannes Roth,
            Edwin J. W. Geven, Arjen B. Blom and Peter L. E. M. van Lent

Chapter 7   The effects of resistance training on muscle strength, joint pain, and hand
            function in individuals with hand osteoarthritis..69
            Nicoló Edoardo Magni, Peter John McNair and David Andrew Rice

Chapter 8   **CX3CL1 promotes MMP-3 production via the CX3CR1, c-Raf, MEK, ERK, and NF-κB signaling pathway in osteoarthritis synovial fibroblasts**................80
Sheng-Mou Hou, Chun-Han Hou and Ju-Fang Liu

Chapter 9   **New insights on the MMP-13 regulatory network in the pathogenesis of early osteoarthritis**....................92
Heng Li, Dan Wang, Yongjian Yuan and Jikang Min

Chapter 10   **Are estrogen-related drugs new alternatives for the management of osteoarthritis?**....................104
Ya-Ping Xiao, Fa-Ming Tian, Mu-Wei Dai, Wen-Ya Wang, Li-Tao Shao and Liu Zhang

Chapter 11   **Is the relationship between increased knee muscle strength and improved physical function following exercise dependent on baseline physical function status?**....................113
Michelle Hall, Rana S. Hinman, Martin van der Esch, Marike van der Leeden, Jessica Kasza, Tim V. Wrigley, Ben R. Metcalf, Fiona Dobson and Kim L. Bennell

Chapter 12   **Glucocorticoid-induced leucine zipper (GILZ) is involved in glucocorticoid-induced and mineralocorticoid-induced leptin production by osteoarthritis synovial fibroblasts**....................122
Olivier Malaise, Biserka Relic, Edith Charlier, Mustapha Zeddou, Sophie Neuville, Céline Deroyer, Philippe Gillet, Edouard Louis, Michel G. Malaise and Dominique de Seny

Chapter 13   **CCL17 blockade as a therapy for osteoarthritis pain and disease**....................137
Ming-Chin Lee, Reem Saleh, Adrian Achuthan, Andrew J. Fleetwood, Irmgard Förster, John A. Hamilton and Andrew D. Cook

Chapter 14   **Accuracy of magnetic resonance imaging to detect cartilage loss in severe osteoarthritis of the first carpometacarpal joint: comparison with histological evaluation**....................147
Michael S. Saltzherr, J. Henk Coert, Ruud W. Selles, Johan W. van Neck, Jean-Bart Jaquet, Gerjo J. V. M. van Osch, Edwin H. G. Oei, Jolanda J. Luime and Galied S. R. Muradin

Chapter 15   **Curcumin slows osteoarthritis progression and relieves osteoarthritis-associated pain symptoms in a post-traumatic osteoarthritis mouse model**....................155
Zhuo Zhang, Daniel J. Leong, Lin Xu, Zhiyong He, Angela Wang, Mahantesh Navati, Sun J. Kim, David M. Hirsh, John A. Hardin, Neil J. Cobelli, Joel M. Friedman and Hui B. Sun

Chapter 16   **Proximal tibial trabecular bone mineral density is related to pain in patients with osteoarthritis**....................167
Wadena D. Burnett, Saija A. Kontulainen, Christine E. McLennan, Diane Hazel, Carl Talmo, David R. Wilson, David J. Hunter and James D. Johnston

Chapter 17   **Progranulin derivative Atsttrin protects against early osteoarthritis in mouse and rat models** 176
Jian-lu Wei, Wenyu Fu, Yuan-jing Ding, Aubryanna Hettinghouse,
Matin Lendhey, Ran Schwarzkopf, Oran D. Kennedy and Chuan-ju Liu

Permissions

List of Contributors

Index

Preface

Every book is initially just a concept; it takes months of research and hard work to give it the final shape in which the readers receive it. In its early stages, this book also went through rigorous reviewing. The notable contributions made by experts from across the globe were first molded into patterned chapters and then arranged in a sensibly sequential manner to bring out the best results.

Osteoarthritis is a clinical condition which leads to a breakdown of joint cartilage and the underlying bone. It commonly causes joint pain and stiffness. Symptoms usually occur after exercise initially, but with time, they become constant. Commonly, the joints at the base of the thumb, near the ends of the fingers, lower back, knee and hips are affected. Osteoarthritis can occur due to genetic factors or due to abnormal joint or limb development, or joint injury. The mainstay of treatment for osteoarthritis is exercise and weight loss. Medications consisting of acetaminophen along with NSAIDs are given for pain relief. Balance, gait and functional therapies are used to manage impairments of strength, balance and position sense in individuals who have lower extremity arthritis. This book contains some path-breaking studies in osteoarthritis. Also included herein is a detailed explanation of the various treatment and prevention strategies of osteoarthritis. The topics covered in this book offer the readers new insights in this medical condition.

It has been my immense pleasure to be a part of this project and to contribute my years of learning in such a meaningful form. I would like to take this opportunity to thank all the people who have been associated with the completion of this book at any step.

Editor

Inhomogeneity of immune cell composition in the synovial sublining: linear mixed modelling indicates differences in distribution and spatial decline of CD68+ macrophages in osteoarthritis and rheumatoid arthritis

Johanna Mucke[1], Annika Hoyer[2], Ralph Brinks[1], Ellen Bleck[1], Thomas Pauly[3], Matthias Schneider[1] and Stefan Vordenbäumen[1*]

Abstract

Background: Inhomogeneity of immune cell distribution in the synovial sublining layer was analyzed in order to improve our mechanistic understanding of synovial inflammation and explore potential refinements for histological biomarkers in rheumatoid arthritis (RA) and osteoarthritis (OA).

Methods: Synovial tissue of 20 patients (11 RA, 9 OA) was immunohistochemically stained for macrophages (CD68), synovial fibroblasts (CD55), T cells (CD3), plasma cells (CD38), endothelial cells (vWF) and mast cells (MCT). The synovial sublining layer was divided into predefined adjacent zones and fractions of the stained area (SA) were determined by digital image analysis for each cell marker.

Results: Distribution of CD68, CD55, CD38 and MCT staining of the sublining area was heterogeneous (Friedman ANOVA $p < 0.05$). The highest expression for all markers was observed in the upper layer close to the lining layer with a decrease in the middle and lower sublining. The SA of CD68, CD55 and CD38 was significantly higher in all layers of RA tissue compared to OA ($p < 0.05$), except the CD38 fraction of the lower sublining. Based on receiver operating characteristics analysis, CD68 SA of the total sublining resulted in the highest area under the curve (AUC 0.944, CI 95 % 0.844–1.0, $p = 0.001$) followed by CD68 in the upper and middle layer respectively (both AUC 0.933, CI 95 % 0.816–1.0, $p = 0.001$) in both RA and OA. Linear mixed modelling confirmed significant differences in the SA of sublining CD68 between OA and RA ($p = 0.0042$) with a higher concentration of CD68+ towards the lining layer and more rapid decline towards the periphery of the sublining in RA compared to OA ($p = 0.0022$).

Conclusions: Immune cells are inhomogeneously distributed within the sublining layer. RA and OA tissue display differences in the number of CD68 macrophages and differences in CD68 decline within the synovial sublining.

Keywords: Rheumatoid arthritis, Osteoarthritis, Sublining layer, Macrophages, CD68, Synovitis score

* Correspondence: stefan.vordenbaeumen@med.uni-duesseldorf
[1]Hiller Research Center Rheumatology at University Hospital Düsseldorf,
Medical Faculty, Heinrich-Heine-University, Merowingerplatz 1a, 40225
Düsseldorf, Germany
Full list of author information is available at the end of the article

Background

Histological analysis of the synovial membrane is a powerful tool for the investigation of pathological changes in rheumatoid arthritis (RA) in order to elucidate the pathogenic mechanisms involved in the disease [1]. In addition, the assessment of synovial biomarkers is quite useful in dose-finding studies, for the stratification of patient groups, and to identify new therapeutic targets [2]. Although not part of the clinical daily routine, the use of synovial biopsies in certain clinical situations is unquestioned [3–5]. For instance, CD68-positive macrophages in the sublining layer have repeatedly been shown to be one of the best activity markers for RA [6, 7]. Besides macrophages, further cells are of major interest in synovial biopsies: synovial fibroblasts are considered key players in the pathogenesis of rheumatoid arthritis [8]. T cells are major components of inflammatory infiltrates and trigger autoimmunity in cooperation with antibody-producing plasma cells [9–11]. Mast cells have been identified to modulate B cells and produce proinflammatory cytokines in RA [12, 13] whereas endothelial cells function as a marker for increased angiogenesis in inflamed tissue [14].

Although the synovial sublining is generally considered as a whole, we consistently noted inhomogeneous distribution of immune cells, particularly prominent under pathological conditions within this particular compartment of the synovium. A more precise definition of the relevant areas within the sublining layer might improve our pathophysiologic understanding of inflammatory joint diseases and potentially lead to improved diagnostic usage of synovial biopsies. Thus, we set out to analyze histological features and the cellular composition of the sublining layer in more detail.

Methods
Patients and synovial sampling

Synovial tissue was obtained from a total of 20 patients (11 RA, 9 OA) who underwent synovectomy (elbow ($n = 1$), wrist (1), shoulder (1) or total joint replacement (11 hips, 6 knees)) at the Department of Orthopaedics at the River Rhein Center for Rheumatology, St. Elisabeth Hospital, Meerbusch-Lank, Germany. All patients diagnosed with RA fulfilled the 2010 American College of Rheumatology criteria for RA. Osteoarthritis (OA) was diagnosed based on the ACR criteria for knee or hip OA [15, 16]. All patients gave their full informed consent. The samples were taken under visual control from macroscopically inflamed areas, were immediately snap frozen in tissue-TEK (Sakura Finetek Germany, Staufen, Germany) and stored at −80° until further processing.

Histology and immunohistochemistry

Seven-micron sections were obtained from the snap-frozen tissue and fixed for 10 minutes in 3 % paraformaldehyde in phosphate-buffered saline (PBS). After conventional hematoxylin and eosin (H&E) staining (Merck, Darmstadt, Germany), synovial morphology was evaluated for tissue quality and the presence of a continuous lining layer. The sections were used for the determination of the synovitis score according to Krenn [17], which is a semi-quantitative 4-point sum score assessing the synovial lining layer hypertrophy, inflammatory infiltrate and cellular density of resident cells. For immunohistochemistry, parallel sections were incubated with primary monoclonal mouse antibodies against CD68, mast cell tryptase (MCT), CD15, CD19, CD56 (all Dako, Glostrup, Denmark), CD55 (Southern-Biotech, Birmingham, AL, USA), CD3, CD38, von Willebrand factor (vWF), CD83 (all BD Biosciences, San Jose, CA, USA), IgG1 as isotype control (Dako, Glostrup, Denmark) and secondary antibody of the Dako Real Detection System (Dako, Glostrup, Denmark), according to the manufacturer's instructions. In three cases tissue quantity was insufficient for sublining layer analysis of single antibodies (1 × CD68 (RA), 2 × MCT (RA, OA)).

Imaging and calculation of stained areas

Sections were photographed at × 200 magnification (Axioskop 2 plus: Carl Zeiss, Jena, Germany; Nikon DS Vi 1: Nikon, Düsseldorf, Germany) and stored in TIF format (resolution of 1600 × 1200, 96 dpi) (Image acquisition software: NIS-Elements F, Nikon). Rectangular regions of interest (ROI) of 500 × 250 pixels (661.5 μm × 330.5 μm) size were created using ImageJ [18] and the upper sublining ROI was placed adjacent to the lining layer with the lower layer at greatest distance from the synovial surface. ROIs for the middle and lower layer were set contiguously in a row. Visual inspection of all tissues preceded the definition of the ROIs' size of 500 × 250 pixels, which was considered suitable to delineate each layer separately without including parts of the opposite sublining area, especially critical in villous formations of RA tissue. The lumina of blood vessels within the selected regions were delineated and subtracted from the respective layer area still including respective endothelial cells in the analysis. Images were then thresholded to highlight the stained areas but not the respective isotype controls. After converting the image into a binary image, the highlighted section was measured and presented as a fraction of the selected region. For linear mixed model analysis the three ROIs were divided in half to create six equally sized ROIs. To obtain representative results, measurements were made from three different regions of each sample and mean values were used for statistical analysis.

Statistical analyses

For continuous scales data are given as mean ± standard deviation (SD), ordinal data such as the synovitis score is presented as median and 1st quartile to 3rd quartile (interquartile range, IQR). Student's t test for independent samples and Mann–Whitney U test were used to compare the two groups as appropriate. Analysis of the different layers was carried out with Friedman's two-way analysis of variance (ANOVA) and Dunn's post hoc test. Correlations between the synovitis score and the stained areas were calculated according to Spearman. Receiver operating characteristics (ROC) analysis with calculation of the area under the cure (AUC) was used to examine the diagnostic value of the evaluated cell markers. Aforementioned statistical analyses were carried out using IBM SPSS statistics (IBM Corp., Armonk, NY, USA) at a significance level of $\alpha = 0.05$. For comparison of the decline in CD68+ staining between OA and RA, we applied a linear mixed model (LMM) with random intercept for the CD68+ concentration with following independent variables: distance of the ROI, disease status and interaction between distance and disease status. For the LMM we used the function PROC MIXED of SAS 9.3 (SAS Institute Inc., Cary, NC, USA).

Results

Patients' demographics and clinical features

Eleven patients with RA (nine female, aged 63.5 ± 10.6 years) and nine with OA (six female, aged 69.4 ± 11.1 years) were included in this study. Of the RA patients three had synovectomy of shoulder, hand and elbow, respectively. Five underwent total hip replacement and three had a total knee replacement. OA tissue was obtained from six patients undergoing total hip replacement and three cases of total knee replacement. Demographic and clinical data is summarized in Table 1.

Synovitis score (H&E staining)

On histological analysis of H&E-stained sections, the median synovitis score was 6 (interquartile range (IQR) 5–7) in RA patients and 3 (IQR 1.5–5) in the OA group

($p = 0.002$). The RA group showed significantly higher numbers for all three subscores, e.g. lining layer, inflammatory infiltrate, and cellular density (Table 2).

Next, we were interested to determine if the synovitis score as a measure of inflammatory activity in the entire synovial layer is reflected by individual cellular markers within the sublining layer. Correlation analyses revealed a moderate to high correlation for the total stained area of CD68, CD3 and CD55 and the total synovitis score with its subscores in all patients (RA and OA) except CD55 and the cellular density. CD38 and MCT total stained area did not correlate with the synovitis score, and vWF showed moderate correlation only with the subscore cellular density (Table 3). Typical histological findings of RA and OA are exemplified in Fig. 1.

Immune cells are inhomogeneously distributed within the sublining layer

In order to assess cellular distribution within the sublining layer, immunohistochemistry was applied to stain for macrophages (CD68), synovial fibroblasts (CD55), T cells (CD3), plasma cells (CD38), endothelial cells (vWF) and mast cells (MCT) (Fig. 1). The fraction of stained area was determined by digital image analysis in three predefined zones of the sublining layer with the upper layer closest to the lining layer and the lower layer representing the deeper sublining. While expression of CD68, CD3, CD55, vWF and CD38 could be visualized in all cases, MCT was abundant in three tissues (two RA, one OA). Analysis revealed an inhomogeneous distribution of CD68-, CD55-, CD38-, and MCT-positive cells ($p < 0.05$ according to Friedman two-way ANOVA). Staining of CD19+ B cells, CD15+ granulocytes, CD56+ natural killer cells and CD83+ dendritic cells was discontinued due to very low expression in both RA and OA tissue. Details on inhomogeneity of distinct immune cells within the sublining layer are given in Fig. 2.

The percentage of stained area of CD68, CD3, CD55 and MCT differs significantly between RA and OA

We then set out to compare cell marker expression between RA and OA. These analyses revealed significant

Table 1 Demographic and clinical features

	All patients	RA	OA	RA vs. OA
	$n = 20$	$n = 11$	$n = 9$	p values
Age at surgery, yrs (±SD)	66.2 (±10.9)	63.5 (±10.6)	69.4 (±11.1)	0.233
Female, n (%)	14 (75.0)	9 (81.8)	6 (66.7)	
CRP, mg/dl (±SD)	2.5 (±2.7)	3.7 (±3.2)	1.2 (±1.0)	**0.001**
Leucocytes,/µl (±SD)	8570.0 (±4784.4)	10,654.5 (±5639.0)	6022.2 (±1157.3)	**0.001**
RF, IU/ml (±SD)	71.5 (±156.9)	126.3 (±198.5)	4.4 (2.4)	**<0.001**
ESR, mm/h, (±SD)	22.2 (±20.9)	29.4 (±23.3)	14.1 (15.3)	0.079

Comparison by Student's t test, significant results are printed in bold
RA rheumatoid arthritis, *OA* osteoarthritis, *SD* standard deviation, *CRP* C-reactive protein, *RF* rheumatoid factor, *ESR* erythrocyte sedimentation rate

Table 2 Synovitis score

	All patients	RA	OA	RA vs. OA
	$n = 20$	$n = 11$	$n = 9$	p values
Synovitis score[a], median (IQR)	5 (3–6)	6 (5–7)	3 (1.5–5)	**0.002**
Lining layer hypertrophy	1.5 (1–2)	2 (1–3)	1 (0–1.5)	0.025
Inflammatory infiltrate	1.5 (1–3)	3 (1–3)	1 (0.5–1.5)	**0.007**
Cellular density	2 (1–2)	2 (2–2)	1 (0.5–1.5)	**0.002**

Comparison by Student's t test, significant results are printed in bold
RA rheumatoid arthritis, *OA* osteoarthritis, *IQR* interquartile range
[a]Synovitis score according to Krenn and colleagues [17]

differences between all sublining layers with consistently higher percentages of staining in RA tissue for the three parameters CD68, CD55 and CD38. Typical staining patterns in RA and OA are shown in Fig. 2. Results of the comparison of RA and OA are summarized in Table 4.

CD68 remains the best parameter to distinguish RA from OA

In order to estimate the most reliable parameter for differentiation between RA and OA in the current study, receiver operating characteristics (ROC) analyses with determination of the area under the curve (AUC) were performed. CD68 total stained area within the sublining was identified as the most reliable marker to discriminate between RA and OA (AUC 0.94, CI 95 % 0.84–1.00, $p = 0.001$) followed by the CD68-stained area in the upper and middle sublining (both AUC 0.93, CI 95 % 0.82–1.00, $p = 0.001$). Furthermore, staining of CD3 upper layer (AUC 0.86, CI 95 % 0.69–1.00, $p = 0.07$) and CD55 middle layer (AUC 0.89, CI 95 % 0.71–1.00, $p = 0.03$) and the total stained area (CD3: AUC 0.83, CI 95 % 0.64–1.00, $p = 0.014$; CD55: AUC 0.89, CI 95 % 0.74–1.00, $p = 0.03$) provided considerable accuracy for RA tissue, whereas no difference was observed for CD38, vWF or MCT.

Linear mixed modelling indicates significant differences in decline of CD68 staining within the synovial sublining between OA and RA

We set out to further specify the differences in CD68 expression between OA and RA by modelling the distribution of CD68-positive cells within the sublining layer. Three observations can be made: (1) in RA, the number of positive cells starts on higher level than in OA ($p < 0.0001$). (2) For both diseases, the number of positive cells decreases with growing distance from the lining layer ($p < 0.0001$). (3) The decrease is significantly stronger in RA compared to OA ($p = 0.003$). Details of the linear mixed model are outlined in Fig. 3 and Table 5.

Discussion

The synovial membrane in patients with RA and OA has been subject to a broad variety of studies, which have substantially contributed to the elucidation of pathogenic mechanisms. So far, the lining layer has been intensively studied and histological features in RA such as hypertrophy and the accumulation of macrophages, fibroblasts and giant cells within the lining have been well described [19]. In this study, we focused on the sublining layer and the ongoing pathophysiological changes in this area since important observations have been made in this zone. In particular, CD68-positive sublining macrophages have been identified as a very potent biomarker: they reflect disease activity [20] and synovial inflammation in refined magnetic resonance imaging (MRI) procedures [21]. Most strikingly, changes in sublining CD68 macrophages are a potent biomarker for response to therapy across academic centres [6], and they are likely not liable to placebo effects [7]. This renders synovial biopsies a powerful tool in early- phase clinical studies

Table 3 Correlation between the total stained area of the synovial sublining and the synovitis score

	Synovitis score[a]	Lining layer hypertrophy	Inflammatory infiltrate	Cellular density
CD68	**0.706 ($p = 0.001$)**	**0.554 ($p = 0.014$)**	**0.604 ($p = 0.006$)**	**0.576 ($p = 0.010$)**
CD3	**0.852 ($p < 0.001$)**	**0.798 ($p < 0.001$)**	**0.757 ($p < 0.001$)**	**0.601 ($p = 0.005$)**
CD55	**0.651 ($p = 0.002$)**	**0.622 ($p = 0.003$)**	**0.668 ($p = 0.001$)**	0.428 ($p = 0.060$)
CD38	0.245 ($p = 0.298$)	0.122 ($p = 0.608$)	0.154 ($p = 0.518$)	0.419 ($p = 0.066$)
vWF	0.437 ($p = 0.054$)	0.302 ($p = 0.195$)	0.344 ($p = 0.138$)	**0.576 ($p = 0.008$)**
MCT	0.083 ($p = 0.743$)	0.362 ($p = 0.140$)	−0.071 ($p = 0.780$)	0.008 ($p = 0.974$)

Correlations according to Spearman, significant correlations are printed in bold
CD68 macrophages, *CD3* T cells, *CD55* synovial fibroblasts, *CD38* plasma cells, *vWF* von Willebrand factor, *MCT* mast cell tryptase
[a]Synovitis score according to Krenn and colleagues [17]

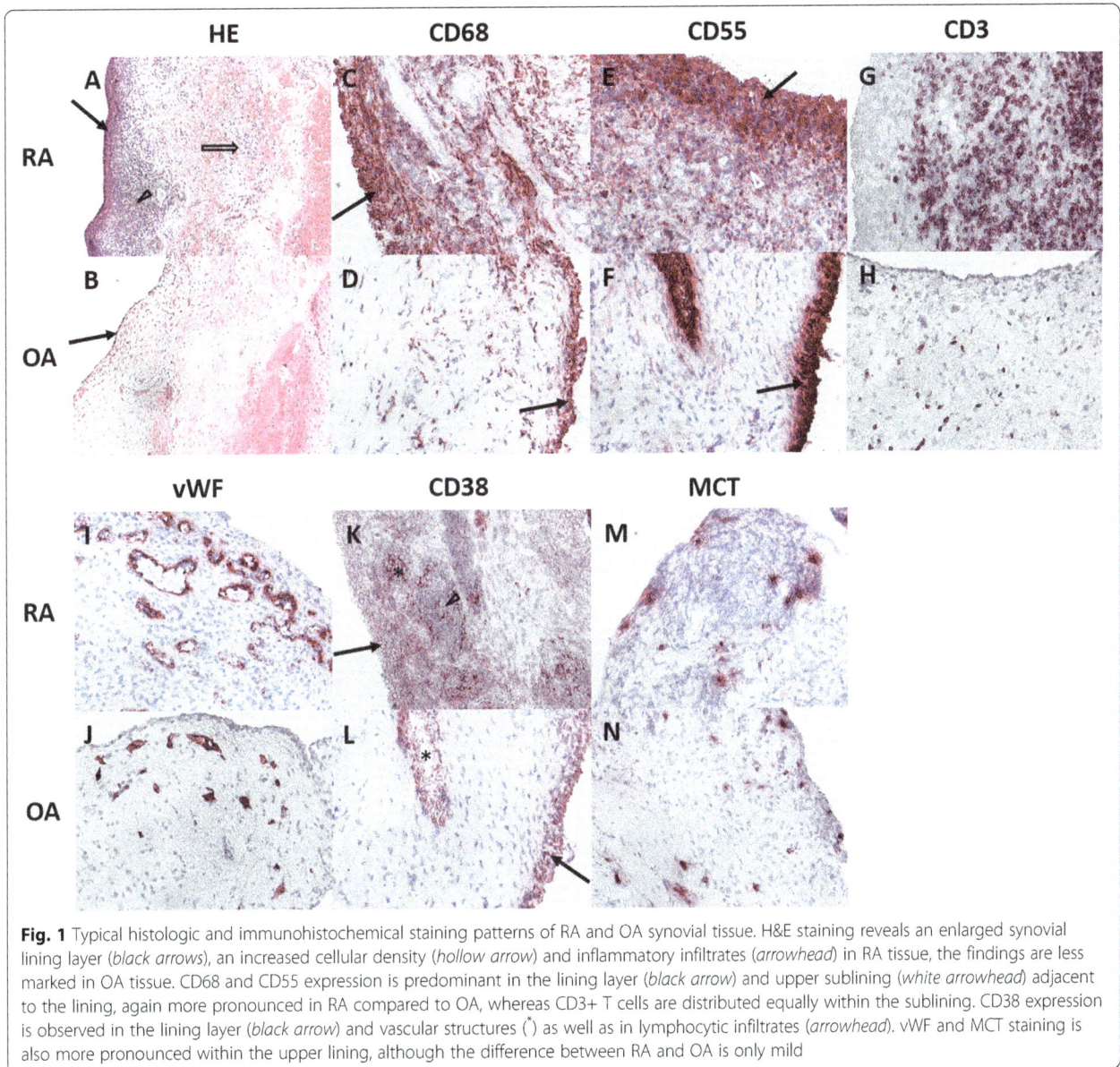

Fig. 1 Typical histologic and immunohistochemical staining patterns of RA and OA synovial tissue. H&E staining reveals an enlarged synovial lining layer (*black arrows*), an increased cellular density (*hollow arrow*) and inflammatory infiltrates (*arrowhead*) in RA tissue, the findings are less marked in OA tissue. CD68 and CD55 expression is predominant in the lining layer (*black arrow*) and upper sublining (*white arrowhead*) adjacent to the lining, again more pronounced in RA compared to OA, whereas CD3+ T cells are distributed equally within the sublining. CD38 expression is observed in the lining layer (*black arrow*) and vascular structures (*) as well as in lymphocytic infiltrates (*arrowhead*). vWF and MCT staining is also more pronounced within the upper lining, although the difference between RA and OA is only mild

[22]. These findings suggest that the synovial sublining may also play a substantial role in disease mechanisms of RA. However, the synovial sublining is ill-defined and our own circumstantial observations suggested that cellular distribution within this area may be inhomogeneous. In the present study, we partitioned the sublining layer and comprehensively analyzed immune cellular composition as this might lead to an improved understanding of disease mechanisms and potential future refinements in its use as a biomarker. We demonstrate a strikingly inhomogeneous distribution of most immune cells and fibroblasts within the sublining layer of both RA and OA tissue with a clear tendency of macrophages (CD68), synovial fibroblasts (CD55), plasma cells (CD38) and mast cells (MCT) and endothelial cells (vWF)

to accumulate in the upper sublining. Of note, we refrained from adjusting for multiple testing, because a low to moderate amount of statistical hypothesis was tested for the above markers, and because of concerns for overemphasizing the sensibility of p values [23]. However, as outlined in the tables, some borderline statistically significant findings would probably not have crossed the 5 % threshold in case of adjustments. Furthermore, we applied linear mixed modelling to the distribution of sublining CD68 cells in order to assess potential regularities in the distribution of macrophages with distance to the lining layer being the independent variable. The advantage of this particular model was a precise and accurate analysis of macrophage allocation since special focus was set on the distance to the lining

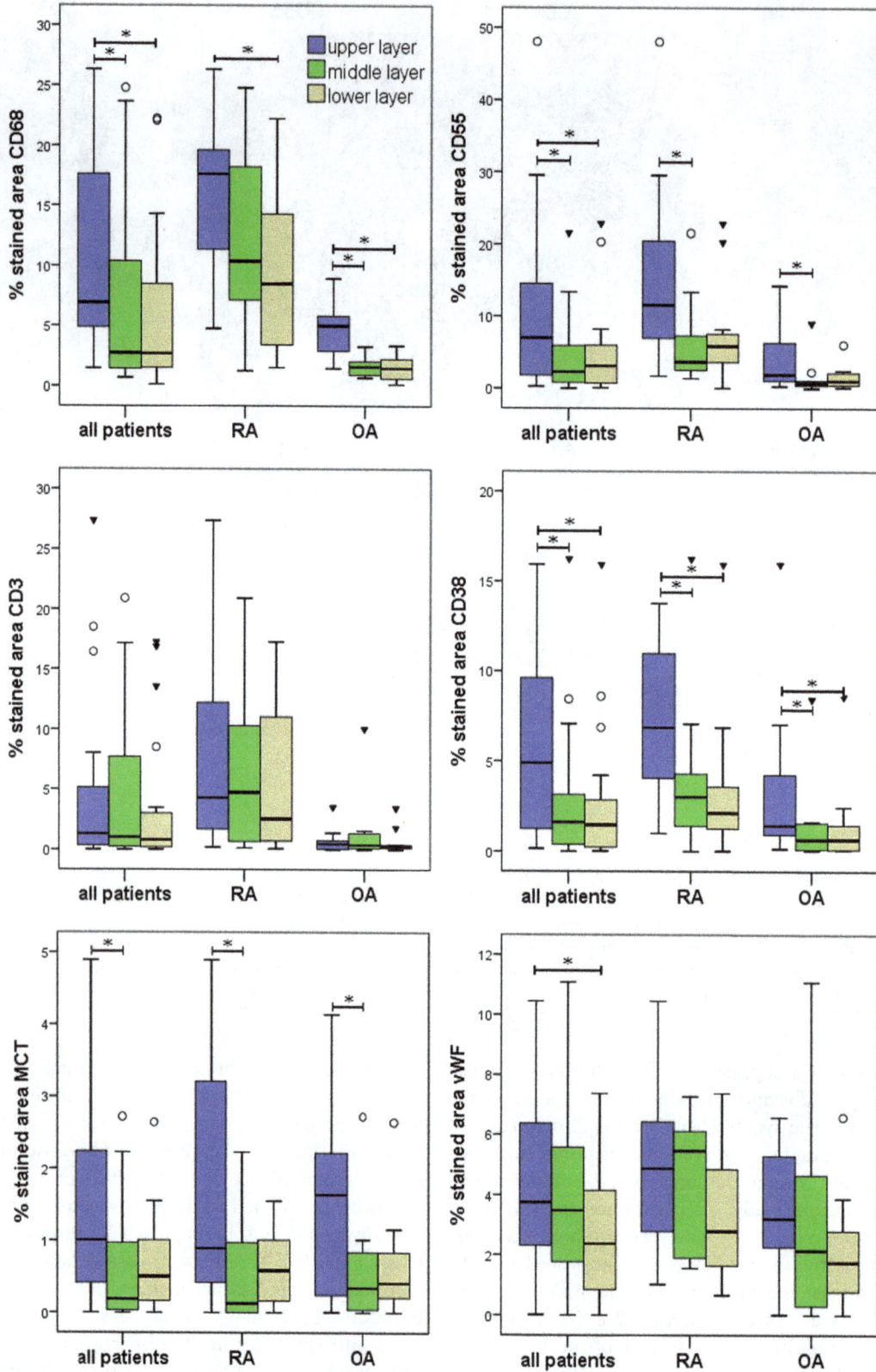

Fig. 2 Differences within the sublining layer for expression of CD68, CD55, CD3, CD38 and MCT in all patients and patients with RA and OA respectively. Expression of cellular markers was highest in the upper sublining adjacent to the lining layer (*blue*), with a decrease towards the middle (*green*) and lower (*fawn*) layers within the deeper synovium (except CD3). *Statistically significant; °outliers; ▼extremes

Table 4 Mean percentage of stained area in the synovial sublining

		All patients (mean ± SD)	RA (mean ± SD)	OA (mean ± SD)	Mann–Whitney U (p value)
CD68	Upper	10.52 (±7.75)	15.89 (±6.88)	4.55 (±2.42)	**0.001**
	Middle	7.12 (±7.82)	12.04 (±8.05)	1.66 (±0.89)	**0.001**
	Lower	5.92 (±6.92)	9.85 (±7.66)	1.56 (±1.06)	**0.001**
	Total area	7.85 (±7.33)	12.59 (±7.30)	2.59 (±1.34)	**<0.001**
CD3	Upper	4.79 (±7.74)	8.06 (±8.88)	0.79 (±1.11)	**0.006**
	Middle	4.38 (±6.27)	6.68 (±7.32)	1.58 (±3.22)	0.056
	Lower	3.56 (±5.70)	5.86 (±6.91)	0.75 (±1.15)	0.095
	Total area	4.24 (±6.05)	6.86 (±7.09)	1.04 (±1.78)	**0.012**
CD55	Upper	10.80 (±11.93)	15.81 (±13.61)	4.67 (±5.45)	**0.012**
	Middle	4.29 (±5.40)	6.46 (±6.11)	1.64 (±2.86)	**0.002**
	Lower	5.00 (±6.20)	7.73 (±7.21)	1.66 (±1.88)	**0.007**
	Total area	6.70 (±6.59)	10.00 (±7.00)	2.66 (2.92)	**0.002**
CD38	Upper	5.75 (±4.95)	7.43 (±4.34)	3.68 (±5.10)	**0.046**
	Middle	2.86 (±3.94)	3.97 (±4.55)	1.50 (±2.68)	**0.038**
	Lower	2.74 (±3.85)	3.60 (±4.52)	1.69 (±2.73)	0.175
	Total area	3.78 (±4.01)	5.00 (±4.16)	2.29 (±3.47)	**0.046**
vWF	Upper	4.19 (±2.67)	4.87 (±2.77)	3.37 (±2.43)	0.295
	Middle	3.84 (±2.92)	4.52 (±2.29)	3.02 (±3.51)	0.175
	Lower	2.88 (±2.28)	3.46 (±2.39)	2.18 (±2.06)	0.175
	Total area	3.64 (±2.17)	4.28 (±1.94)	2.86 (±2.30)	0.152
MCT	Upper	1.53 (±1.53)	1.53 (±1.68)	1.54 (±1.42)	0.897
	Middle	0.58 (±0.79)	0.53 (±0.73)	0.64 (±0.91)	0.696
	Lower	0.67 (±0.70)	0.66 (±0.59)	0.69 (±0.86)	0.897
	Total area	0.93 (±0.90)	0.90 (±0.85)	0.96 (±1.01)	0.829

Comparison of rheumatoid arthritis (RA) and osteoarthritis (OA) by Mann–Whitney U, significant results are shown in bold. Upper layer adjacent to lining layer; lower layer with greatest distance from lining layer within the deeper synovium

RA rheumatoid arthritis, *OA* osteoarthritis, *SD* standard deviation, *CD68* macrophages, *CD3* T cells, *CD55* synovial fibroblasts, *CD38* plasma cells, *vWF* von Willebrand factor, *MCT* mast cell tryptase

taking into account the intra-patient correlations which were integrated into the statistical calculations [24]. We found a high accumulation of macrophages towards the lining layer and a fast decline in RA compared to OA. Since the lining layer faces the joint cavity, we assume that rather than the total CD68+ cells within the whole sublining layer, those in close proximity to the joint cavity are of foremost importance for the inflammatory joint reaction [25]. This is further supported by looking at the pathophysiological implications of CD68 homing: the increase of vWF expression reflects the early dysregulation of angiogenesis that occurs in inflammatory disorders [26] and is considered to be a prerequisite for immune cells to enter the synovial membrane [14, 26]. In RA, the process of angiogenesis and the subsequent recruitment of immune cells and synovial fibroblasts further results in the formation of pannus tissue producing inflammatory cytokines that lead to cartilage and bone destruction [27]. The close proximity of the respective immune cells to the lining layer and thus the surface of the synovial membrane may be an essential step towards fast pannus formation and consecutive destruction of adjacent cartilage. We hypothesize that the preferential presence of CD68+ cells towards the lining layer and the joint cavity with a rapid decline in the lower layers is due to an increase in extravasation of precursor cells from the blood, with more rapid homing towards the lining layer. Further evidence for this hypothesis is provided by the significantly higher expression of CD68, CD55, CD38 and CD3 in RA compared to OA which is in accordance with destructive pannus formation of RA being composed of macrophages, synovial fibroblasts, plasma cells, leucocytes and mast cells [28, 29].

In contrast to all other evaluated immune cells, CD3+ T cells did not have the tendency to accumulate in the upper sublining, but were distributed homogeneously. Depending on the inflammatory activity, CD3+ T cells were either absent, randomly distributed or clustered in

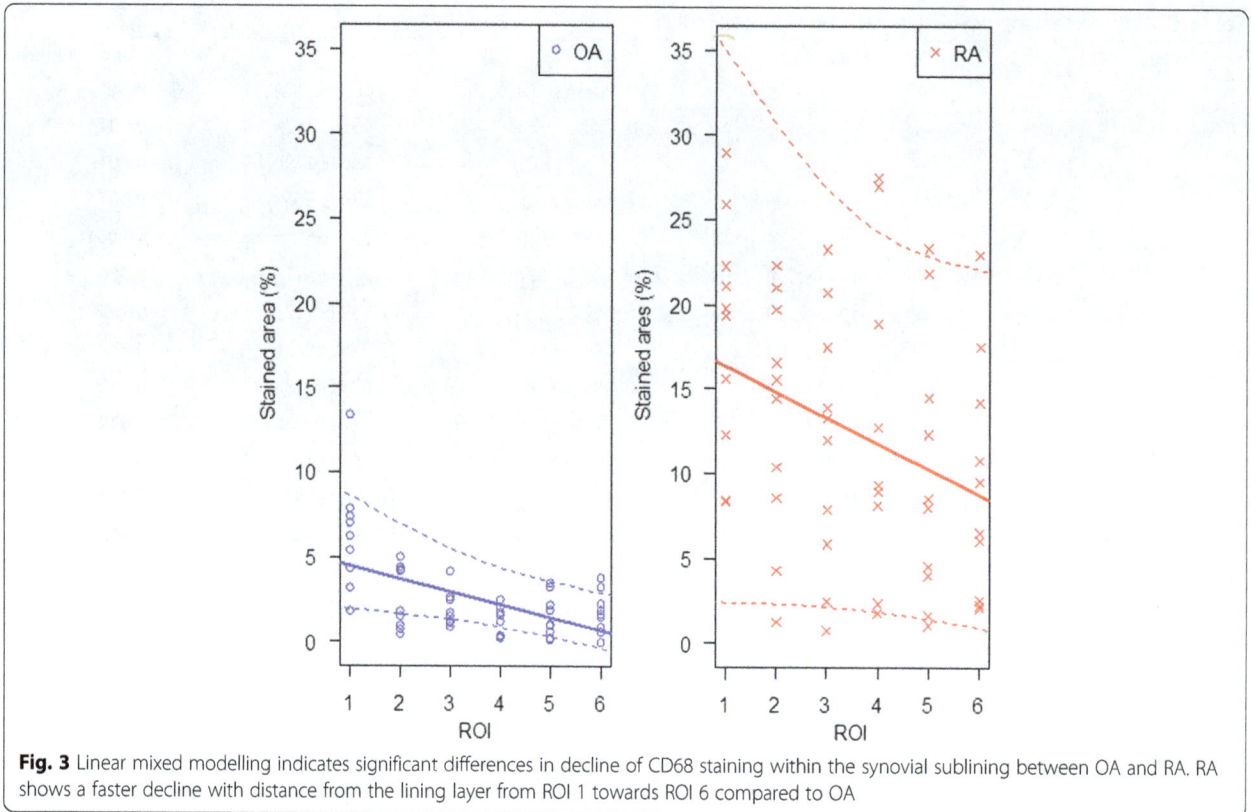

Fig. 3 Linear mixed modelling indicates significant differences in decline of CD68 staining within the synovial sublining between OA and RA. RA shows a faster decline with distance from the lining layer from ROI 1 towards ROI 6 compared to OA

follicle-like structures. These follicles, predominant in RA, spanned the entire sublining resulting in an intensive, but homogeneous staining pattern across all layers. Our description of different patterns is consistent with previous studies identifying and defining these histomorphological features in RA synovitis as 'follicular', 'diffuse' and 'pauci-immune' [30, 31].

Despite their inhomogeneous distribution patterns, we observed a moderate to high correlation of total CD68-, CD3- and CD55- staining in the entire sublining (i.e. not

Table 5 Linear mixed model of CD68+ macrophages spatial distribution within the synovial sublining: progressive decline in CD68+ macrophages with distance from the lining layer in OA and in RA

Effect	Disease	Estimate	Standard error	p value
Intercept		5.23	1.91	0.003
ROI distance		−0.75	0.20	<0.0001
Disease	OA	0		
Disease	RA	12.6	2.6	<0.0001
Interaction: ROI and disease	OA	0		
Interaction: ROI and disease	RA	−0.77	0.27	0.003

Estimates without standard error refer to the reference category
ROI region of interest, OA osteoarthritis, RA rheumatoid arthritis

partitioned into different layers) and the synovitis score and its components, which has been established as a valuable tool to assess synovitis activity and to discriminate between low- and high-grade synovitis [17]. These data on one hand confirm CD68- expression as a valuable disease activity parameter and on the other hand prove the amount of sublining T cells and synovial fibroblasts to reflect the grade of synovitis and estimate disease activity. This again is supported by our finding of significantly higher expression of immune cell markers in RA, representing a more inflammatory phenotype [32] compared to OA.

There are some limitations to this study. Owing to the lack of any histological criteria clearly defining each layer, we divided the sublining into three zones of the same diameter which allowed us to directly compare results but did not consider interindividual differences regarding the extent of the sublining. We considered potential measurement inaccuracies rather minimal since ROIs were defined based on extensive study of all tissues and were set in similar areas adjacent to a straight lining layer with a sublining area of good tissue quality. To reduce intraindividual variations, three loci of each sample were analyzed. Since the patient selection was made according to clinical diagnosis only, without regarding other parameters like disease activity, duration of disease and medication due to ethical restrictions, the patient population was rather heterogeneous. In spite of that, results were consistent. Owing to our relatively small sample size, we did not further subclassify RA synovitis according to the aforementioned histological patterns [31, 33]. Furthermore, tissue obtained from either joint replacement or synovectomy implies a chronic or advanced state of disease. Future studies can assess cellular distribution within the synovial sublining employing linear mixed modelling in early disease states and its sensitivity to change following treatment. Hence, it has to be stressed that CD68 modelling is not yet fit for reliable diagnostic decision making until further diagnostic studies in early undifferentiated arthritis, including various inflammatory joint conditions, confirm our results in established RA. Moreover, although immune cell distribution is generally considered to be comparable between affected joints in polyarticular disease [34], we cannot fully exclude that differences observed reflect sample site rather than disease state.

Another limitation is that the semi-quantitative digital image analysis we applied, allowed a selection or deselection of single cells only to a limited extent through the thresholding step. CD38 can be present at low density in cells other than plasma cells like NK cells, B cells, T cells and macrophages so that in non-automated analyses usually only strong positive cells with the typical plasma cell morphology are counted [25]. We adjusted the threshold accordingly; nonetheless CD38 staining might be overestimated. Moreover, antibodies for immunohistochemistry typically represent the designated target cell, and are widely used for these purposes [35–37]. However, it should be noted that neither CD55 nor CD38 or CD68 are exclusively expressed by synovial fibroblasts, plasma cells, and macrophages [25, 38].

Conclusions
Macrophages, synovial fibroblasts, plasma cells and mast cells show an inhomogeneous distribution within the synovial tissue in both RA and OA with highest concentrations in the upper sublining layer. Linear mixed modelling revealed a significantly higher concentration close to the lining layer with a more rapid decline in RA compared to OA. The model should be further analyzed for its performance as a biomarker and has pathophysiological implications.

Abbreviations
ANOVA, analysis of variance; AUC, area under the curve; IQR, interquartile range; LMM, linear mixed model; MCT, mast cell tryptase; OA, osteoarthritis; RA, rheumatoid arthritis; ROC, receiver operating characteristics; SD, standard deviation; vWF, von Willebrand factor

Acknowledgements
Not applicable.

Funding
The authors gratefully acknowledge financial support of this study by an unconditional grant from the "Hiller-Stiftung", Erkrath.

Authors' contributions
JM participated in the conception of the study, prepared and stained synovial tissue, read synovial histologies, analyzed and interpreted data, and drafted the manuscript. AH participated in data interpretation and statistical analysis. RB interpreted data and carried out statistical analyses. EB prepared and stained synovial tissue, and participated in data interpretation. TP carried out synovial biopsies. MS participated in the conception of the study and data interpretation. SV conceived the study, read synovial histologies, analyzed and interpreted data, and drafted the manuscript. All authors read, revised and approved the final manuscript.

Authors' information
Not applicable.

Competing interests
The authors declare that they have no competing interests.

Consent for publication
Not applicable.

Author details
[1]Hiller Research Center Rheumatology at University Hospital Düsseldorf, Medical Faculty, Heinrich-Heine-University, Merowingerplatz 1a, 40225 Düsseldorf, Germany. [2]German Diabetes Center, Institute for Biometry and Epidemiology, Düsseldorf, Germany. [3]Department Orthopaedics, River Rhein Center for Rheumatology at St. Elisabeth Hospital, Meerbusch-Lank, Germany.

References
1. Gerlag DM, Tak PP. How to perform and analyse synovial biopsies. Best Pract Res Clin Rheumatol. 2013;27:195–207.
2. van de Sande MGH, Gerlag DM, Lodde BM, van Baarsen LGM, Alivernini S, Codullo V, et al. Evaluating antirheumatic treatments using synovial biopsy: a recommendation for standardisation to be used in clinical trials. Ann Rheum Dis. 2011;70:423–7.
3. Vordenbäumen S, Joosten LA, Friemann J, Schneider M, Ostendorf B. Utility of synovial biopsy. Arthritis Res Ther. 2009;11:256.
4. Gerlag DM, Tak PP. How useful are synovial biopsies for the diagnosis of rheumatic diseases? Nat Clin Pract Rheumatol. 2007;3:248–9.
5. Saaibi DL, Schumacher HR. Percutaneous needle biopsy and synovial histology. Baillieres Clin Rheumatol. 1996;10:535–54.
6. Bresnihan B, Pontifex E, Thurlings RM, Vinkenoog M, El-Gabalawy H, Fearon U, et al. Synovial tissue sublining CD68 expression is a biomarker of therapeutic response in rheumatoid arthritis clinical trials: consistency across centers. J Rheumatol. 2009;36:1800–2.
7. Haringman JJ, Gerlag DM, Zwinderman AH, Smeets TJM, Kraan MC, Baeten D, et al. Synovial tissue macrophages: a sensitive biomarker for response to treatment in patients with rheumatoid arthritis. Ann Rheum Dis. 2005;64:834–8.
8. Huber LC, Distler O, Tarner I, Gay RE, Gay S, Pap T. Synovial fibroblasts: key players in rheumatoid arthritis. Rheumatol Oxf Engl. 2006;45:669–75.
9. Mellado M, Martínez-Muñoz L, Cascio G, Lucas P, Pablos JL, Rodríguez-Frade JM. T Cell migration in rheumatoid arthritis. Front Immunol. 2015;6:384. Available from: http://www.ncbi.nlm.nih.gov/pmc/articles/PMC4515597/. Accessed 12 Oct 2015.
10. Alunno A, Manetti M, Caterbi S, Ibba-Manneschi L, Bistoni O, Bartoloni E, et al. Altered immunoregulation in rheumatoid arthritis: the role of regulatory

T cells and proinflammatory Th17 cells and therapeutic implications. Mediators Inflamm. 2015;2015:751793.

11. Humby F, Bombardieri M, Manzo A, Kelly S, Blades MC, Kirkham B, et al. Ectopic lymphoid structures support ongoing production of class-switched autoantibodies in rheumatoid synovium. PLoS Med. 2009;6(1):e1. Available from: http://www.ncbi.nlm.nih.gov/pmc/articles/PMC2621263/. Accessed 26 May 2016.

12. Hueber AJ, Asquith DL, Miller AM, Reilly J, Kerr S, Leipe J, et al. Mast cells express IL-17A in rheumatoid arthritis synovium. J Immunol Baltim Md 1950. 2010;184:3336–40.

13. Palm A-KE, Garcia-Faroldi G, Lundberg M, Pejler G, Kleinau S. Activated mast cells promote differentiation of B cells into effector cells. Sci Rep. 2016;6:20531.

14. Colville-Nash PR, Scott DL. Angiogenesis and rheumatoid arthritis: pathogenic and therapeutic implications. Ann Rheum Dis. 1992;51:919–25.

15. Altman R, Alarcón G, Appelrouth D, Bloch D, Borenstein D, Brandt K, et al. The American College of Rheumatology criteria for the classification and reporting of osteoarthritis of the hip. Arthritis Rheum. 1991;34:505–14.

16. Altman R, Asch E, Bloch D, Bole G, Borenstein D, Brandt K, et al. Development of criteria for the classification and reporting of osteoarthritis. Classification of osteoarthritis of the knee. Diagnostic and Therapeutic Criteria Committee of the American Rheumatism Association. Arthritis Rheum. 1986;29:1039–49.

17. Krenn V, Morawietz L, Burmester G-R, Kinne RW, Mueller-Ladner U, Muller B, et al. Synovitis score: discrimination between chronic low-grade and high-grade synovitis. Histopathology. 2006;49:358–64.

18. Schneider CA, Rasband WS, Eliceiri KW. NIH Image to ImageJ: 25 years of image analysis. Nat Methods. 2012;9:671–5.

19. Fassbender HG. Pathology and pathobiology of rheumatic diseases. Berlin: Springer Science+Business Media; 2013.

20. Vordenbäumen S, Sewerin P, Lögters T, Miese F, Schleich C, Bleck E, et al. Inflammation and vascularisation markers of arthroscopically-guided finger joint synovial biospies reflect global disease activity in rheumatoid arthritis. Clin Exp Rheumatol. 2014;32:117–20.

21. Vordenbäumen S, Schleich C, Lögters T, Sewerin P, Bleck E, Pauly T, et al. Dynamic contrast-enhanced magnetic resonance imaging of metacarpophalangeal joints reflects histological signs of synovitis in rheumatoid arthritis. Arthritis Res Ther. 2014;16:452.

22. de Hair MJH, Harty LC, Gerlag DM, Pitzalis C, Veale DJ, Tak PP. Synovial tissue analysis for the discovery of diagnostic and prognostic biomarkers in patients with early arthritis. J Rheumatol. 2011;38:2068–72.

23. Baker M. Statisticians issue warning over misuse of P values. Nature. 2016; 531:151–1.

24. Verbeke G, Molenberghs G. Linear mixed models for longitudinal data. Berlin: Springer Science +Business Media; 2009.

25. Tak PP, Smeets TJ, Daha MR, Kluin PM, Meijers KA, Brand R, et al. Analysis of the synovial cell infiltrate in early rheumatoid synovial tissue in relation to local disease activity. Arthritis Rheum. 1997;40:217–25.

26. Koch A. Angiogenesis as a target in rheumatoid arthritis. Ann Rheum Dis. 2003;62:ii60–7.

27. Firestein GS. Starving the synovium: angiogenesis and inflammation in rheumatoid arthritis. J Clin Invest. 1999;103:3–4.

28. Karmakar S, Kay J, Gravallese EM. Bone damage in rheumatoid arthritis – mechanistic insights and approaches to prevention. Rheum Dis Clin North Am. 2010;36:385–404.

29. Shiozawa S, Shiozawa K, Fujita T. Morphologic observations in the early phase of the cartilage-pannus junction. Light and electron microscopic studies of active cellular pannus. Arthritis Rheum. 1983;26:472–8.

30. Bromley M, Woolley DE. Histopathology of the rheumatoid lesion. Identification of cell types at sites of cartilage erosion. Arthritis Rheum. 1984;27:857–63.

31. Pitzalis C, Kelly S, Humby F. New learnings on the pathophysiology of RA from synovial biopsies. Curr Opin Rheumatol. 2013;25:334–44.

32. Farahat MN, Yanni G, Poston R, Panayi GS. Cytokine expression in synovial membranes of patients with rheumatoid arthritis and osteoarthritis. Ann Rheum Dis. 1993;52:870–5.

33. Takemura S, Braun A, Crowson C, Kurtin PJ, Cofield RH, O'Fallon WM, et al. Lymphoid neogenesis in rheumatoid synovitis. J Immunol Baltim Md 1950. 2001;167:1072–80.

34. Kraan MC, Reece RJ, Smeets TJM, Veale DJ, Emery P, Tak PP. Comparison of synovial tissues from the knee joints and the small joints of rheumatoid

arthritis patients: Implications for pathogenesis and evaluation of treatment. Arthritis Rheum. 2002;46:2034–8.

35. Kraan MC, Haringman JJ, Post WJ, Versendaal J, Breedveld FC, Tak PP. Immunohistological analysis of synovial tissue for differential diagnosis in early arthritis. Rheumatol Oxf Engl. 1999;38:1074–80.

36. Tak PP, van der Lubbe PA, Cauli A, Daha MR, Smeets TJ, Kluin PM, et al. Reduction of synovial inflammation after anti-CD4 monoclonal antibody treatment in early rheumatoid arthritis. Arthritis Rheum. 1995;38:1457–65.

37. van de Sande MGH, de Hair MJH, Schuller Y, van de Sande GPM, Wijbrandts CA, Dinant HJ, et al. The features of the synovium in early rheumatoid arthritis according to the 2010 ACR/EULAR classification criteria. PLoS One. 2012;7:e36668.

38. Edwards JC. Fibroblast biology. Development and differentiation of synovial fibroblasts in arthritis. Arthritis Res. 2000;2:344–7.

Concurrent validity of different functional and neuroproteomic pain assessment methods in the rat osteoarthritis monosodium iodoacetate (MIA) model

Colombe Otis[1,2], Julie Gervais[1], Martin Guillot[1,2], Julie-Anne Gervais[1], Dominique Gauvin[1,2], Catherine Péthel[1,3], Simon Authier[4], Marc-André Dansereau[3], Philippe Sarret[3], Johanne Martel-Pelletier[2], Jean-Pierre Pelletier[2], Francis Beaudry[1,2] and Eric Troncy[1,2*] (iD)

Abstract

Background: Lack of validity in osteoarthritis pain models and assessment methods is suspected. Our goal was to 1) assess the repeatability and reproducibility of measurement and the influence of environment, and acclimatization, to different pain assessment outcomes in normal rats, and 2) test the concurrent validity of the most reliable methods in relation to the expression of different spinal neuropeptides in a chemical model of osteoarthritic pain.

Methods: Repeatability and inter-rater reliability of reflexive nociceptive mechanical thresholds, spontaneous static weight-bearing, treadmill, rotarod, and operant place escape/avoidance paradigm (PEAP) were assessed by the intraclass correlation coefficient (ICC). The most reliable acclimatization protocol was determined by comparing coefficients of variation. In a pilot comparative study, the sensitivity and responsiveness to treatment of the most reliable methods were tested in the monosodium iodoacetate (MIA) model over 21 days. Two MIA (2 mg) groups (including one lidocaine treatment group) and one sham group (0.9 % saline) received an intra-articular (50 μL) injection.

Results: No effect of environment (observer, inverted circadian cycle, or exercise) was observed; all tested methods except mechanical sensitivity (ICC <0.3), offered good repeatability (ICC ≥0.7). The most reliable acclimatization protocol included five assessments over two weeks. MIA-related osteoarthritic change in pain was demonstrated with static weight-bearing, punctate tactile allodynia evaluation, treadmill exercise and operant PEAP, the latter being the most responsive to analgesic intra-articular lidocaine. Substance P and calcitonin gene-related peptide were higher in MIA groups compared to naïve (adjusted P (adj-P) = 0.016) or sham-treated (adj-P = 0.029) rats. Repeated post-MIA lidocaine injection resulted in 34 times lower downregulation for spinal substance P compared to MIA alone (adj-P = 0.029), with a concomitant increase of 17 % in time spent on the PEAP dark side (indicative of increased comfort).

(Continued on next page)

* Correspondence: eric.troncy@umontreal.ca
Colombe Otis and Julie Gervais are first co-authors.
[1]Groupe de Recherche en Pharmacologie Animale du Québec (GREPAQ),
Department of Biomedical Sciences, Faculty of veterinary medicine,
Université de Montréal, 1500 des Vétérinaires Street, P.O. Box 5000,
St-Hyacinthe, Quebec J2S 7C6, Canada
[2]Osteoarthritis Research Unit, Research Center Hospital of Montreal University
(CRCHUM), Montreal, Quebec, Canada
Full list of author information is available at the end of the article

(Continued from previous page)

Conclusion: This study of normal rats and rats with pain established the most reliable and sensitive pain assessment methods and an optimized acclimatization protocol. Operant PEAP testing was more responsive to lidocaine analgesia than other tests used, while neuropeptide spinal concentration is an objective quantification method attractive to support and validate different centralized pain functional assessment methods.

Keywords: Animal preclinical model, Osteoarthritis, Monosodium iodoacetate, Methods, Validation, Acclimatization, Pain metrology, Neuropeptide

Background

Osteoarthritis (OA), the most common of all arthropathies in our aging population, is a leading cause of disability and represents a large (and growing) worldwide socio-economic cost [1]. It affects approximately 30 million adults in the USA [2], and this number is expected to double by 2020 [3], with longer life expectancy and the increasing incidence of obesity, two major risk factors for the disease. Despite critical importance in drug development, translation of OA therapies focusing either on structure (disease-modifying OA drugs) or pain (symptom-modifying OA drugs) from the bench to bedside has slowed [1, 4, 5]. Differences between preclinical OA models and the disease evaluated in clinical trials contribute to this failure. Rising criticism is noted over the classic translational research, which has failed to predict the efficacy of chronic pain treatments [6–9]. Most critics have targeted the poor validity and clinical relevance of experimental pain models using laboratory animals [10, 11]. It has also been hypothesized that current animal models are too reliant on evoked (reflexive) withdrawal responses and that development of meaningful assessment tools allowing, for instance, the measurement of continuous spontaneous pain, might help to translate experimental data to clinical practice [6, 12].

Naturally occurring OA models are recognized to present pathophysiological changes closest to clinical OA, particularly in large animals [13], but also entail experimental disadvantages (long period to onset, and variability of disease development). In contrast, chemical models cause the most rapidly progressing OA, requiring less invasive procedures and enabling standardization (with increased sample homogeneity). The monosodium iodoacetate (MIA) chemical OA model as described 25 years ago induces cartilage degeneration by disruption of chondrocyte metabolism (i.e., breaking down the cellular aerobic glycolysis). In rats, the MIA model is well-established and resembles the histological and pain-related characteristics of human degenerative OA [14–29]. Owing to the extensive description of the pain response in rats, the MIA OA model was proposed as a standard OA model for pain assessment [23, 30].

The quality of pain assessment methodologies is a cornerstone of preclinical studies targeting new analgesics

[7, 10–12, 16, 31, 32]. Three different categories of pain expression can be evaluated in rats: reflexive measures, spontaneous measures, and operant responses [8, 31]. First, reflexive measures using stimulus-evoked responses are commonly used in rats to assess potential hyperalgesia and allodynia, recognized as a clinical expression of the neuropathic pain (nociceptive sensitization) component [8, 33–35]. These measures are generated by exposure to thermal, mechanical, or electrical stimulus, involving mainly spinal-level pain processing, and are also increasingly present in human quantitative sensory testing characterization of pain [36–38]. Second, spontaneous measures can be useful to quantify pain and/or wellbeing [8]. For example, kinetic (static or dynamic weight distribution) [14] or kinematic [39] (ambulation evaluation or characterization) measurement, and spontaneous activity [24] can indirectly assess quality of life in OA models. Pain-induced behaviors (scratching/licking/biting, hypophagia, vocalization, etc.) should also be considered in this category [37]. Finally, operant responses have been more recently introduced to characterize pain in animal models [8, 34, 40–44]. Operant testing is opposite to reflexive response testing as it allows the quantification of behavioral responses at higher levels of the brain, reproducing multiple dimensions of pain, including affective and cognitive changes and not only sensory-discriminative perception [42, 43, 45, 46]. This type of measure allows the observer to evaluate the aversive component of pain as operant tests give the animal an opportunity to avoid the painful condition [33, 40–43, 47–49].

In patients OA of the knee joint, pain is a combination of inflammatory, immune and neurogenic components participating in the hypersensitivity syndrome. Central sensitization mechanisms [50] include various biochemical processes such as increased spinal release of neurotransmitters and neuromodulators, and increased excitability of postsynaptic neurons. In an OA [51] and arthritis [52] rat model, higher levels of neuropeptides, such as substance P (SP) and calcitonin gene-related peptide (CGRP) have been found in the spinal cord. Thus, nervous system modulation seems to play a critical role in the development of the disease [53]. The contribution of these spinal neuromediators to neurogenic inflammation-mediated chronic pain in OA, and concomitant changes in functional pain assessment methods has not been fully established.

With such a variety of methods for pain and analgesic response assessment, it is difficult to opt for the method(s) most adapted to specific conditions. The current study undertook to establish, the reliability of a panel of pain assessment methods (including reflexive, spontaneous, and operant testing) in normal rats, and the influence of environmental conditions, including acclimatization and experimental conditions of manipulation (observer, inverted circadian cycle, and exercise). The most reliable methods were then used to characterize OA pain in the well-established chemical MIA model in rats, while conducting concurrent validation of pain assessment methods in relation to the expression of different spinal neuropeptides and their responsiveness to treatment with intra-articular lidocaine.

Methods

Ethics statement

During the study, care and use of animals were subject to and approved by the Comité d'Éthique de l'Utilisation des Animaux of Université de Montréal (#Rech-1495) and conducted in accordance with principles outlined in the current Guide to the Care and Use of Experimental Animals published by the Canadian Council on Animal Care and the Guide for the Care and Use of Laboratory Animals published by the US National Institutes of Health.

Animals

The present study was conducted on female (n = 63; excluding spares) Sprague-Dawley rats (Charles River Laboratories, Saint-Constant, QC, Canada) ranging from 225–300 g in weight at the beginning of experiment. The animals were housed under regular laboratory conditions and maintained under a light-dark cycle with food and water provided *ad libitum*. Body weight was obtained weekly. At the end of each experiment, the animals were returned to their housing colony.

Phase 1: reliability of pain assessment methods in normal rats

Experimental design

Phase 1 included a total of 39 normal rats distributed into 8 groups. First, the repeatability of measurements was tested for the influence of environment, including observer, inverted circadian cycle (activity during the day), and exercise (two groups of five animals in crossover). Additionally, repeatability over an extended period was tested again for static weight-bearing (SWB; one group of four animals also tested for exercise effect), and for tactile sensitivity and place escape/avoidance paradigm (PEAP) operant test (one group of five animals).

Second, using the most reliable methods only, the influence of four acclimatization protocols (four groups of five animals) was tested to determine the most effective approach to obtain predictable data with low variability. Different pain assessment methods were selected to include reflexive, spontaneous behavior and operant measures.

Influence of environment

First, rats (n = 10) were randomly distributed into two groups of five. Animals were acclimated to the test apparatus on two occasions at day -3 and -1 before starting the experimentation. In a crossover design, the animals were subsequently assessed for three repeated days during light (1000–1400 h) and dark (2000–2400 h) cycles to test the influence of inverted circadian cycles. Both cycles were separated by a 3-day washout period without assessment. Dark cycle evaluations were performed under low-intensity red light. Animals were tested on each of six assessment days by two observers, with the following methods in this order of evaluation: mechanical and tactile sensitivity, SWB, treadmill exercise, mechanical and tactile sensitivity, SWB, PEAP operant test (without nociceptive stimulation) and rotarod acceptance. The mechanical and tactile nociceptive thresholds and SWB evaluation were performed before and after the treadmill exercise to verify the influence of exercise on these three pain assessment methods. Finally, PEAP and rotarod were performed at the end of the evaluation schedule to ensure respectively, that the length of the test, and possible falling from the test device would not impair the other outcomes. To test inter-rater reliability, two female observers were selected for their different levels of experience in laboratory animals (one intermediate, one with advanced expertise).

Second, in complementary studies about test repeatability (after acclimatization on two occasions, at day -3 and -1), SWB was specifically retested over 15 days with two SWB assessments separated by a treadmill session (then testing again the potential effect of exercise on SWB) in a group of four rats. This evaluation was done daily, from days 1 to 5, then on days 8 and 15.

Finally, the repeatability of measurements of tactile sensitivity and PEAP (with nociceptive stimulation) was tested in a group of five rats over 25 days. These evaluations were done daily, from days 1 to 15, and repeated on days 18 and 25.

Influence of acclimatization protocols

In order to determine the most efficient acclimatization protocol associated with the most repeatable data (previously obtained), the next experiment was conducted in a total of 20 animals (four groups of 5 animals). Briefly, over 2 weeks, different acclimatization protocols were tested and included 8 (days -14, -13, -12, -11, -10, -8, -6, and -1), 6 (days -14, -8, -7, -6, -5, and -1), 5 (days -14, -7, -5, -3, and -1) or 4 (days -14, -8, -6, and -1) days of evaluation. The order of assessment was SWB, tactile and mechanical sensitivity, PEAP with nociceptive stimulation, and treadmill. The schedule of pain evaluation methods was determined to obtain nociceptive threshold values before placing the animal on the operant testing device where many paw stimulations were elicited (see subsequent description).

Pain assessment methods

Mechanical sensitivity Mechanical sensitivity was assessed by measuring the paw withdrawal threshold (PWT) to an increasing pressure stimulus placed on the dorsal surface of the hind paw using an algorimeter (Randall Selitto test Paw Pressure Meter®, IITC Life Science Inc., Woodland Hills, CA, USA), employing a wedge-shaped probe (1.75 mm² of surface) and a cutoff value set at 250 g. The animals were placed in a sling apparatus (Lomir Biomedical Inc., Notre-Dame-de-l'Île-Perrot, QC, Canada). The probe was applied once on the dorsal surface at a steadily increasing pressure. The PWT was determined when the animal removed the paw from the apparatus, and the required pressure was recorded. Withdrawal thresholds were measured on the right and left hind paws. The data were expressed as PWT in grams.

Tactile sensitivity First, the animal was placed inside an elevated metal grid cage to allow just enough space for the rat to move while being restricted. After the rat exploration session during the first 2 minutes, tactile sensitivity was assessed using an Electronic von Frey Anesthesiometer® (IITC Life Science Inc., Woodland Hills, CA, USA) applied to the plantar surface of the hind paws and by measuring the PWT to von Frey ascending mechanical stimuli. Gradually increasing pressure was applied with a mechanical von Frey polypropylene probe (0.7 mm², Rigid Tip®, IITC Life Science Inc., Woodland Hills, CA, USA) fitted to a handheld force transducer. The rigid tip was placed perpendicularly into the mid-plantar surface of the paw. The stimulus was continued until the hind paw was withdrawn or elevated such that the force leveled off. Actions such as vocalization, agitation, jumping, and avoidance were considered indicative of the PWT. Voluntary movements associated with locomotion were not considered to be a withdrawal response. The peak of force in grams was recorded with a cutoff value at 100 g. For each animal, triplicates of each hind paw were taken with a 60-s interval between each stimulus.

Static weight bearing The weight distribution through the right and left knee was assessed using an Incapacitance Meter® (IITC Life Science Inc., Woodland Hills, CA, USA) to measure SWB distribution in the two hind limbs. The force exerted by each hind limb was measured and analyzed in grams, but reported in percentage of total body weight (%BW) to normalize the data. Rats were allowed to acclimate to the testing apparatus and when stationary, readings were taken over a 3-s period. Triplicates were taken simultaneously for each limb at each time point.

Treadmill exercise All rats underwent forced training over a 20-minute period at constant treadmill speed (11 m/minute) (IITC Life Science Inc., Woodland Hills, CA, USA). To force the animal to exercise on the treadmill belt, each lane was equipped with an independent shocker grid. The intensity of the shocker grid was kept at the minimum required to keep the animal on the exercise belt. The treadmill number of total crossings (TNTC) was recorded over the whole period, but also reported in blocks of 5 minutes, to potentially detect a within-time change in activity. A total crossing was considered completed when the animal crossed the entire length of the lane. The TNTC was used as an indicator of exercise and/or performance. When the rats were running continuously on the belt, they were exposed to maximal intensity exercise, as they were not pausing, causing them to cross the entire length of the motorized lane.

Operant testing The PEAP was used as operant testing apparatus [33, 40, 49]. Rats were placed into test cage apparatus that was painted half white and half black. Neither side was illuminated with additional light. With the cage on an elevated metal grid, the observer, located below, determined the preferential location of the rat. The 20-minute observation period began after 2 minutes of acclimatization/exploration to the test environment on each occasion.

Operant testing without nociceptive stimulation The percentage of time spent on the black or white side of the test apparatus was calculated from observation of the preferential location every 15 s.

Operant testing with nociceptive stimulation If the rat was on the black side of the test apparatus, the plantar surface of the right (ipsilateral to possible MIA intra-articular injection) hind paw (RHP) was stimulated with a thin wire (60 g) every 15 s, to prompt withdrawal of the limb. When the rat was on the white side of the cage, a similar mechanical stimulation was applied, but to the plantar surface of the left (contralateral) hind paw (LHP). The percentage of time in the black and white side of the test apparatus was calculated from observation of the preferential location every 15 s. The calculations were sequenced by successive blocks (n = 4) of 5-minute periods. Moreover, the total number of crossings from the white to the dark side was noted to detect any decrease in activity. If a rat remained in the crossing tunnel, it would be stimulated to advance and complete its crossing.

Rotarod Using a Rotamex 4/8® (Columbus Instruments Inc., Columbus, OH, USA) with a previously published protocol [29], the rats were exposed to an acceleration speed of 5 to 16 rpm, over 60 s, before being maintained at this speed, while the time before falling was monitored with a cutoff time of 3 minutes.

Phase 2: concurrent validity with the MIA model
Experimental design
In the second phase, a pilot study (n = 24 rats) was conducted to test the concurrent validity of different functional and neuropeptide pain assessment methods in the MIA rat OA model. A single intra-articular injection of MIA was performed in the right knee of 16 animals distributed among two groups (n = 8 each). An additional sham group (n = 8) received a single intra-articular injection (50 μL) of 0.9 % NaCl. For the purpose of the study, one of the two MIA groups also received a punctual lidocaine (L) injection (MIA-L group) in the right knee on days 7, 14 and 21. At the end of the 21 days of the experimentation, all animals were euthanized with an overdose of isoflurane and a sacrifice by transection of the cervical spine before spinal cord collection.

Acclimatization period and baseline assessment
The study began with an acclimatization period for the selected optimal outcomes (SWB, tactile sensitivity, PEAP, rotarod, and treadmill), according to the optimal acclimatization protocol of five occurrences (days -14, -7, -5, -3, and -1) obtained in phase 1. Because of pain induction in phase 2, tactile sensitivity could be considered as punctate tactile allodynia evaluation (PTAE). Baseline values were acquired at day -1 in this order of evaluation, following the above-described testing procedures: SWB, PTAE, and PEAP with nociceptive stimulation, rotarod and treadmill, with intra-articular injection of MIA at day 0 in the right knee.

Intra-articular injection
On day 0, fasted (3–6 h) rats from all groups were premedicated with buprenorphine hydrochloride (0.02 mg/ kg IM; Buprenex® injectable, Reckitt Benckiser Inc., Mississauga, ON, Canada) and mask-anesthetized with a 2 % isoflurane–O_2 mixture. After surgical preparation, a single intra-articular injection of 2 mg MIA (monosodium iodoacetate, BioUltra®, ≥98 %, Sigma-Aldrich Canada Co., no. I9148-5G, Oakville, ON, Canada)

dissolved in isotonic saline, or saline 0.9 % (both 50 μL volume) was administered through the infrapatellar ligament of the right knee, using a 26-gauge, 0.5-inch needle mounted on a 0.5-mL syringe. On days 7, 14, and 21 post-MIA injection, 25 minutes before functional assessment, rats from the MIA-L group were again similarly anesthetized with a single intra-articular injection of lidocaine through the infrapatellar ligament of the right knee. Lidocaine Neat® (2 %, Zoetis Canada, Kirkland, QC, Canada) was injected at a volume of 50 μL using a 26-gauge, 0.5-inch needle mounted on a 0.5-mL syringe.

Post-injection evaluation
The assessments were performed according to the specific schedules of the different groups on days 3, 7, 14, and 21 post injection, and conducted as described for phase 1. For the MIA-L group on days 7, 14, and 21, the evaluation started 25 minutes after the animals recovered from anesthesia. The evaluation sequence was as follows: SWB (%BW), PTAE (grams), PEAP (percentage of time spent on the dark side), rotarod (seconds) and treadmill (TNTC). The schedule of evaluation was designed to obtain the SWB at rest and the PTAE data before the operant testing evaluation, as this test elicits many PWT stimulations.

Proteomic analysis
Reagents and solutions Acetic anhydride 99.5 % (Ac_2O) and ammonium bicarbonate (NH_4HCO_3) were obtained from Sigma-Aldrich Inc. (St Louis, MO, USA). SP and CGRP were purchased from Phoenix Pharmaceuticals Inc. (Belmont, CA, USA). Acetonitrile was purchased from Thermo Fisher Scientific Inc. (NJ, USA), and trifluoroacetic acid, formic acid and ammonium hydroxide 28.0–30.0 % (NH4OH) were purchased from J.T. Baker® (Phillipsburg, NJ, USA). Standard solutions were prepared as previously performed [54].

Instrumentation The tandem mass spectrometry coupled to high-performance liquid chromatography (HPLC-MS/MS) system comprises a Thermo Surveyor autosampler, a Thermo Surveyor MS pump and a Thermo LCQ Advantage Ion Trap Mass Spectrometer (Thermo Fisher Scientific Inc., San Jose, CA, USA). Data were acquired and analyzed with Xcalibur™ 1.4 (Thermo Fisher Scientific Inc., San Jose, CA, USA), and regression analysis were performed with PRISM® (version 5.0d) (GraphPad software Inc., La Jolla, CA, USA) using the nonlinear curve fitting module with an estimation of the goodness of fit. The calibration lines were constructed from the peak-area ratios of targeted neuropeptides (SP or CGRP) and the acetylated SP analog internal standard.

Bioanalytical methods Acetylated SP was used as the internal standard. The reaction was performed as previously described [54] and the analytical method used was also based on a previously published method [55]. The internal standard solution was tested by HPLC-MS/MS in multiple reactions monitoring (MRM) mode and no residual SP were detected.

Spinal cord sample preparation At the end of the 21 days of experimentation, the entire spinal cord tissue of rats (n = 24) was rapidly collected by a flush of saline within the lumbar spinal canal following deep anesthesia with isoflurane and sacrifice by transection of the cervical spine. Samples were snap-frozen in liquid nitrogen and stored at −80 °C pending analysis. Each spinal cord was weighed accurately and homogenized using a tissue tear or following the addition of phosphate-buffered saline solution (PBS) 0.01 M at a ratio of 1:5 (v/v) and protease inhibitor cocktail (Sigma-Aldrich Inc., Oakville, ON, Canada, number PP8340) at the same ratio. The samples were sonicated and the homogenate was mixed with acetonitrile at a ratio of 1:1 (v/v) to remove larger proteins. The samples were vortexed and centrifuged for 10 minutes (×12,000 g) and the supernatant was transferred into an injection vial then spiked with the internal standard solution at a ratio of 1:1 (v/v). The spinal cords from a naive group (n = 5) in phase 1 were also collected to obtain a baseline value from normal rats to normalize values obtained from the MIA, MIA-L, and sham groups.

Statistical analysis

All statistical analyses were performed two-sided with an alpha value set at 0.05 (phase 1) or 0.10 (phase 2) using a statistical software program (SAS system for Windows, version 9.2, Cary, NC, USA). The alpha value for phase 2 was set at 0.1 because this phase was an exploratory study. In a pilot study, it is acceptable to set a higher alpha value when the study has the hopes of finding an effect that could lead to a promising scientific discovery [56] in order to increase the power (consequently decreasing the risk of type II error), but increasing the chances of type I error (i.e., saying there is a difference when there is not). To be consistent with the statistical rules of correction for multiple comparisons, phase 2 results were presented as adjusted p values (adj-P) because the values obtained in the statistical report need to be multiplied by the total number of comparisons. The normality of the outcomes was verified using the Shapiro-Wilk test and the homogeneity of variance was assessed using the absolute values of the residuals of the mixed model, when appropriate.

Phase 1: reliability of pain assessment methods in normal rats

For mechanical nociceptive thresholds and SWB, the effect of the circadian cycle was assessed using the paired t test adapted for a crossover design. Moreover, the effect of covariates of interest, namely observer, exercise, limb (when both left and right limbs were tested), or trials (when replicates were conducted), was assessed using a general linear model. Generalized linear mixed model analyses for repeated measures were conducted to test the effect of groups on TNTC and rotarod (lognormal distribution), and PEAP (Poisson distribution). Models accounted for baseline measurements using the baseline as covariates. This enabled assessment of the effect of the procedure over time using each subject as its own control. For each model, the best structure of the covariance model was assessed using information criteria that measure the relative fit of competing covariance models. When comparing the 5-minute periods, the Bonferroni adjustment was applied (initial alpha value divided by 4).

Outcome repeatability (test-retest reliability) was assessed by computing the intraclass correlation coefficient (ICC). The ICC is a measure of the proportion of variance that is attributable to objects of measurement. Quantifying the test-retest reliability, the closer the ICC is to 1.0, the higher the reliability and the lower the error variance [57]. A ratio of 0.3–0.4 indicates fair agreement, 0.5–0.6 moderate agreement, 0.7–0.8 strong agreement, and >0.8 almost perfect agreement. Moreover, the coefficient of variation (CV), as a normalized measure of dispersion of the distribution, was used to test the effect of the proposed acclimatization protocols. The CV for each variable was calculated at day -14 (initial assessment), and the variation in CV was assessed at the end of each acclimatization protocol as the CV ratio of day -1 (final assessment) to day -14. At the initial assessment (day -14), the CV interpretation was as follows: <10 % indicated almost perfect dispersion, 11–25 % light dispersion, and 26–40 % fair dispersion. The day -1/day -14 CV ratio indicated improvement (decrease in variability) related to the acclimatization protocol if it was <1, and deterioration (increase in variability) if >1.

Phase 2: concurrent validity with the MIA model

The SWB and PTAE data were expressed as the average obtained from the three trials on the RHP. Data were then analyzed using linear mixed models (SWB and PTAE) or generalized linear mixed models for repeated measures. Treatment groups and day were considered as fixed effects and animals in groups as random effects. Models accounted for baseline measurement using the baseline as a covariate. For each model, the best structure of the covariance model was assessed using a graphical method (plots of covariance versus lag in time between pairs of observations compared to different covariance models), and using information criteria that measure the relative fit of competing covariance models. When multiple comparisons were carried out, the Tukey-Kramer adjustment was used to obtain adj-P values. Neuropeptide data were analyzed using the unpaired exact Wilcoxon test with an alpha value set at 0.10 following non-parametric Kruskal-Wallis one-way analysis of variance.

Results

Phase 1: reliability of pain assessment methods in normal rats

Data variability and influence of environment

The repeatability of measurements made with different assessment methods was tested in normal rats, and the influence of environment, including observer, inverted circadian cycle (activity during the day), exercise, limb, and trial, was assessed on testing.

Mechanical sensitivity We did not find any effect of observer, circadian cycle, exercise, or limb in the PWT measured with the Randall Selitto test Paw Pressure Meter®. However, the data obtained with this test were highly variable among individuals and not repeatable (ICC <0.3).

Tactile sensitivity The PWT measured with the Electronic von Frey Anesthesiometer® in normal rats gave average values of 40–80 g in both hind limbs. The observer, the circadian cycle, and exercise did not produce any effect on tactile sensitivity. No significant difference between the right and left hind limbs, or trial effect (in the triplicates) was observed. However, the data were markedly variable over the whole period (6 days in total) with an ICC for both hind limbs <0.5. Following repetition of the experiment in five rats over 25 days, the ICC improved after excluding the first 2 weeks of daily evaluation. More precisely, the ICC for days 15, 18, and 25 was >0.8 for both hind limbs (Table 1).

Static weight bearing In normal animals, the Incapacitance Meter® apparatus measured average values of weight distributed over each hind limb between 35 and 38 % BW. The observer, the circadian cycle, and exercise did not produce any effect on SWB. No significant difference between the right and left hind limbs, or trial effect (in the triplicates) was observed. When analyzing the last two days of assessment (in comparison to the whole period of 6 days), the ICC improved (Table 2), and this was particularly evident for the SWB ICC after exercise (ICC >0.7 in both hind limbs for the last 2 days of assessment). This suggests that the treadmill exercise slightly decreased the inter-individual variability in SWB measurement. Finally, following repetition of evaluation over 15 days with in four rats, the ICC improved after excluding the first week of daily evaluation (days 1 to 5), with a value ≥0.66 for days 8 and 15 in both hind limbs (Table 2).

Treadmill The treadmill exercise sessions were generally well accepted by female Sprague-Dawley rats (84 % acceptability). Neither the observer, nor the circadian cycle produced any effect on the TNTC. The TNTC was extremely repeatable with an ICC of 0.84. A period effect was demonstrated ($P = 0.003$) in the 15-day study in four rats (Fig. 1). Post hoc analysis showed that the initial and final 5-minute periods were different for TNTC ($P = 0.0002$), whereas both intermediate 5-minute periods (numbers 2 and 3) were highly repeatable with an ICC of 0.73 and 0.92, respectively.

Place escape/avoidance paradigm The first experiment with operant testing was done without nociceptive stimulus. Neither the observer, nor the circadian cycle produced any effect on the preferential localization. The localization was highly repeatable among animals, with an ICC of 0.90, where the rats spent 91 % of their time on the black side. A period effect was demonstrated ($P < 0.0001$) in the 25-day study of five rats (Fig. 2). The PEAP assessment with nociceptive stimulation once again demonstrated robust repeatability, with an ICC of 0.83, and rats spent 81 % of their time on the black side. The post hoc analysis showed that the intermediate 5-minute periods (numbers 2 and 3) were similar in the percentage of time, and were highly repeatable

Table 1 Test-retest reliability of the tactile sensitivity evaluation

	LHP	RHP
ICC over the whole period	0.78	0.26
ICC for days 7, 15, 18, and 25	0.79	0.27
ICC for days 15, 18, and 25	0.84	0.81

A group of normal rats (n = 5) was tested with the Electronic von Frey Anesthesiometer® daily from days 1 to 15 and then on days 18 and 25. The intraclass correlation coefficients (ICCs) for values calculated for the entire evaluation period were compared to values calculated after exclusion of the first week and the first two weeks of assessment. *LHP* left hind paw, *RHP* right hind paw

Table 2 Test-retest reliability of the static weight bearing

	Before exercise		After exercise	
	LHP	RHP	LHP	RHP
ICC over the whole period	0.00	0.00	0.00	0.23
ICC for days 8 and 15	0.67	0.66	0.66	0.76

A group of normal rats (n = 4) was tested for static weight bearing before and after treadmill exercise daily from days 1 to 5 and then on days 8 and 15. The intraclass correlation coefficients (ICCs) calculated for the entire evaluation period were compared to ICCs calculated after exclusion of the first week of assessment. *LHP* left hind paw, *RHP* right hind paw

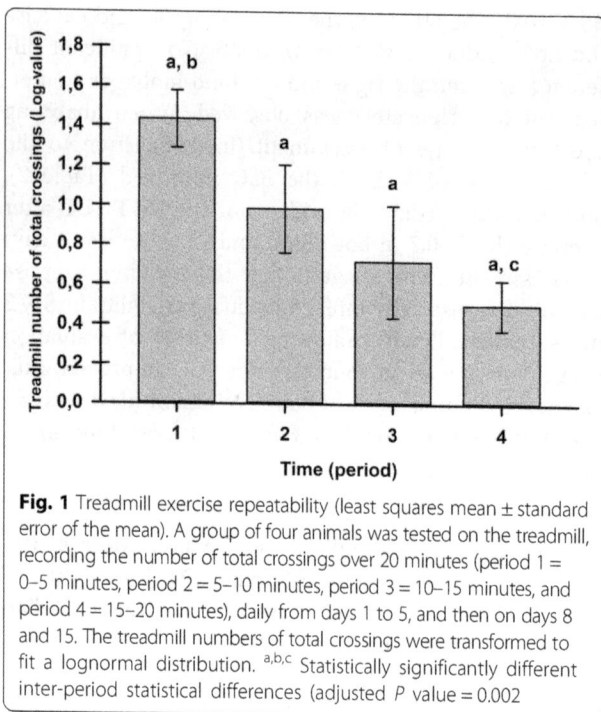

Fig. 1 Treadmill exercise repeatability (least squares mean ± standard error of the mean). A group of four animals was tested on the treadmill, recording the number of total crossings over 20 minutes (period 1 = 0–5 minutes, period 2 = 5–10 minutes, period 3 = 10–15 minutes, and period 4 = 15–20 minutes), daily from days 1 to 5, and then on days 8 and 15. The treadmill numbers of total crossings were transformed to fit a lognormal distribution. [a,b,c] Statistically significantly different inter-period statistical differences (adjusted P value = 0.002

and different ($P \leq 0.0216$) from the initial and final 5-minute periods.

Rotarod Neither the observer, nor the circadian cycle produced any effect on the performance time in the rotarod, and this performance time was highly repeatable with an ICC of 0.92.

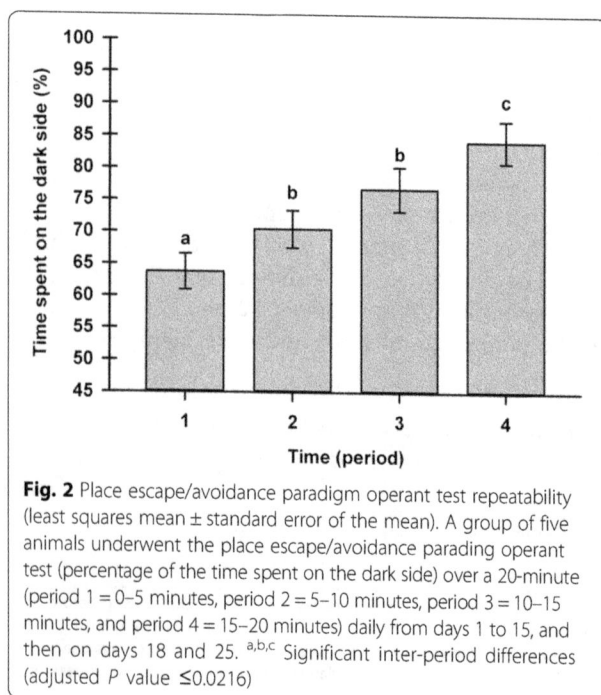

Fig. 2 Place escape/avoidance paradigm operant test repeatability (least squares mean ± standard error of the mean). A group of five animals underwent the place escape/avoidance parading operant test (percentage of the time spent on the dark side) over a 20-minute (period 1 = 0–5 minutes, period 2 = 5–10 minutes, period 3 = 10–15 minutes, and period 4 = 15–20 minutes) daily from days 1 to 15, and then on days 18 and 25. [a,b,c] Significant inter-period differences (adjusted P value ≤0.0216)

Influence of acclimatization protocols and comparison of assessment method variability

When looking at the different assessment methods for the initial day of acclimatization (day -14), inter-individual variability (CV) appeared lower for the SWB, followed by PEAP, tactile sensitivity, and treadmill (TNTC) evaluation, with mechanical sensitivity last (Table 3). The variation in CV at day -1, normalized to day -14, as tested by the day -1/day -14 CV ratio, was compared between acclimatization protocols for the different pain assessment methods (Table 3). The most intensive protocol with the highest number of acclimatization procedures (n = 8) presented the lowest variability between days -1 and -14, similar to the protocol with 6 or 5 days of acclimatization. The protocol with only 4 days of acclimatization yielded the highest variations in CV. The acclimatization protocol using five occurrences of exposition to different assessment methods appeared the most appropriate to limit variability in assessment.

Phase 2: concurrent validity with the MIA model

The MIA injection successfully induced pain-related changes as assessed by SWB, PTAE, PEAP, and TNTC. However, the rotarod was not sensitive to MIA-induced pain, as all groups had similar (maximal) time of acceptance. In consequence, no further analysis was conducted with this testing modality. The sham injection was not totally neutral when compared to baseline values: while no effect was present for SWB or TNTC, the sham group had a transient decrease in PTAE (days 7 and 14) and PEAP (days 3 and 7). The response to lidocaine injection varied by assessment method: a clear analgesic effect was noted with PTAE (on days 7 and 14), and PEAP (on days 7, 14 and 21); a trend toward better performance was observed with TNTC, but no difference was observed with MIA for SWB. Neuropeptide spinal quantification permitted validation of the lidocaine treatment effect and the pain generated by MIA injection.

Static weight bearing

Analysis of SWB data demonstrated a group effect ($P = 0.0005$), a time effect ($P < 0.0001$) and a time x group effect ($P = 0.005$). In the MIA group, the nadir of weight force was observed on day 3 and was different from values recorded on days 7 (adj-$P = 0.005$), 14 (adj-$P = 0.01$) and 21 (adj-$P = 0.001$) (Fig. 3). No significant difference within time was observed for the sham group, whereas in the MIA-L group, day 3 RHP SWB (without lidocaine injection) was lower than on day 14 (adj-$P = 0.001$). Compared to the sham group, the RHP SWB decreased on day 3 in the MIA (adj-$P = 0.002$) and the MIA-L (adj-$P = 0.001$) groups. Subsequently, the RHP SWB in the MIA group returned to levels similar to

Table 3 Coefficient of variation (CV) for each outcome and variation in CV between four protocols of acclimatization

Functional evaluation[a]	8 Days		6 Days		5 Days		4 Days	
	CV (D-14)	CV* ratio	CV (D-14)	CV* ratio	CV (D-14)	CV* ratio	CV (D-14)	CV* ratio
SWB	17.3	*0.72*	31.2	*0.30*	11.7	*0.62*	12.2	*0.67*
PEAP	23.8	1.01	24.1	1.07	21.3	0.97	22.8	1.11
TS	42.9	*0.85*	22.9	1.24	20.4	1.01	27.4	1.80
TNTC	36.9	1.10	106.5	*0.54*	31.2	0.91	38.0	1.92
MS	63.3	*0.74*	71.8	1.07	72.2	*0.71*	75.3	*0.53*

[a]The functional evaluation includes the values recorded for the right hind limb, when available (static weight bearing (SWB), tactile sensitivity (TS), mechanical sensitivity (MS)), or the response of the animal (place escape/avoidance paradigm (PEAP) and treadmill number of total crossings (TNTC)). *The CV values calculated on day -1 were normalized to the CV values on day -14 (D-14) to test the influence of the acclimatization protocol on the outcome measures. A day -1/day -14 CV ratio value <1 was indicative of improvement in variability and is presented in bold italics

those in the sham group, and at no time point of evaluation did the lidocaine injection provide any benefit.

Punctate tactile allodynia evaluation

Descriptive statistics for the RHP PTAE over the evaluation days are provided in Table 4. The PWT was lower after the MIA injection on days 3, 7, 14, and 21. This was also the case for the sham group on days 7 and 14. In the MIA-L group, the nadir in PWT was observed on day 3, whereas a significant increase was observed on days 7 and 14. There was a difference between MIA and MIA-L on days 7 (adj-P = 0.07) and 14 (adj-P = 0.08) (Fig. 4).

Place escape/avoidance paradigm

Between-group analysis confirmed a significant treatment effect of lidocaine, in which MIA-L was different

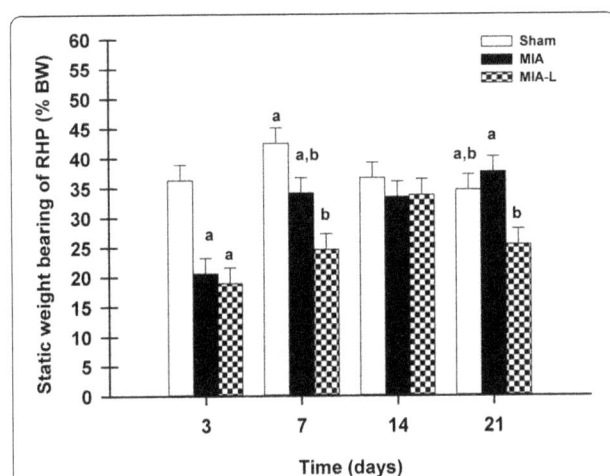

Fig. 3 Static weight-bearing (SWB) evolution after induction of osteoarthritis (least squares mean ± standard error of the mean). On day 3, the monosodium iodoacetate (*MIA*) intra-articular injection in the right knee induced asymmetrical weight distribution in the rats injected with MIA (adjusted P value (adj-P) = 0.0024) and rats injected with MIA and punctual lidocaine (*MIA-L*) (adj-P = 0.0011) compared to rats injected with 0.9 % saline (sham). Subsequently, a statistically significant difference in right hind paw SWB was only observed between the sham and MIA-L groups at days 7 and 21. *%BW* percentage of body weight. [a,b]Significant inter-group statistical differences

from MIA (P = 0.07) and different from sham (P = 0.01) (Fig. 5). The group difference was particularly present for the two intermediate periods 2 and 3 of PEAP assessment previously observed as the most repeatable ones (see "Phase 1").

Treadmill

There was close similarity in the type of performance on the treadmill in the MIA-L and sham groups, in which their TNTC remained comparable to baseline values. Inversely, the TNTC in the MIA group decreased from day 7 onward. However, the observed between-group difference was not significant (P = 0.14).

Neuropeptides

The mean relative ratio (RR) of neuropeptide concentrations of SP and CGRP 21 days after induction of OA are shown in Fig. 6. The absolute values of the concentration of neuropeptides have all been normalized to the function of the naive group values and are shown as the RR. Compared to the naive group (Table 5 and Fig. 6) with a RR of 1, the SP concentrations were significantly increased in the MIA model (adj-P = 0.016) with 2 mg of MIA (RR 1.77 ± 0.16) as in the lidocaine treatment group (MIA-L) (RR 1.43 ± 0.09). The level of this peptide was statistically higher in the MIA group (adj-P = 0.029) compared to the sham group injected with saline 0.9 % (RR 1.26 ± 0.14). However, both the sham and MIA-L groups have significantly lower SP concentrations when compared to the MIA group (adj-P = 0.029). The concentration of CGRP was significantly increased in both MIA models (RR 2.29 ± 0.39 and 2.09 ± 0.29 for MIA and MIA-L, respectively). The sham group (RR 1.22 ± 0.07) had an increase too, in comparison with the naive group (adj-P = 0.016). On the other hand, both MIA groups had a statistically significantly higher level of CGRP than the sham group (adj-P = 0.029). When compared to the MIA group, the MIA-L group had a statistically similar level of CGRP neuropeptide (adj-P = 0.200).

Table 4 Mean and standard deviation of the punctate tactile allodynia evaluation by experimental group over time

Experimental group	Days									
	-1		3		7		14		21	
	Mean	SD	Mean	SD	Mean	SD	Mean	SD	Mean	SD
MIA	53.8	11.2	39.2	13.1	43.1	13.7	40.0	10.0	39.8	8.5
MIA-L	70.4	16.8	35.0	13.8	52.6	12.7	47.8	14.3	36.2	17.8
Sham	56.3	16.9	49.0	14.8	39.2	16.6	37.0	17.6	45.6	17.0

Descriptive statistics of the punctate tactile allodynia evaluation (PTAE) of the right hind paw. The measure was obtained for the three groups (eight animals per group) in grams on days 3, 7, 14, and 21 following the intra-articular injection of monosodium iodoacetate (MIA). Intra-articular injection was performed on day 0 (2 mg of MIA for the MIA and rats injected with monosodium iodoacetate and punctual lidocaine (MIA-L) groups and 0.9 % NaCl for the sham group). The MIA-L group also received an intra-articular injection of lidocaine in the right knee on days 7, 14, and 21, at 25 minutes before the PTAE. *SD* standard deviation

Discussion

Rat models are common in OA research as they are easy to customize and are cost-effective [58]. The MIA model in particular can be standardized and is associated with rapidly developing well-characterized lesions [23, 30]. In an effort to improve the translation of preclinical OA research to the clinical field, we conducted a two-phase study, first, to determine the most reliable pain assessment method protocol, and second, to validate this protocol in the most common chemical model of OA in rats with concomitant changes in spinal neuropeptide concentrations.

Initially, the effect of the environment (inverted circadian cycle, activity level (treadmill exercise), and observer) was tested using well-known pain assessment tools. Prior studies have demonstrated an effect of the inverted circadian cycle on pain research protocols with rodents [59–61]. Our results did not suggest any impact of conducting the evaluation during daytime (more convenient for the investigator). Our group reported a significant

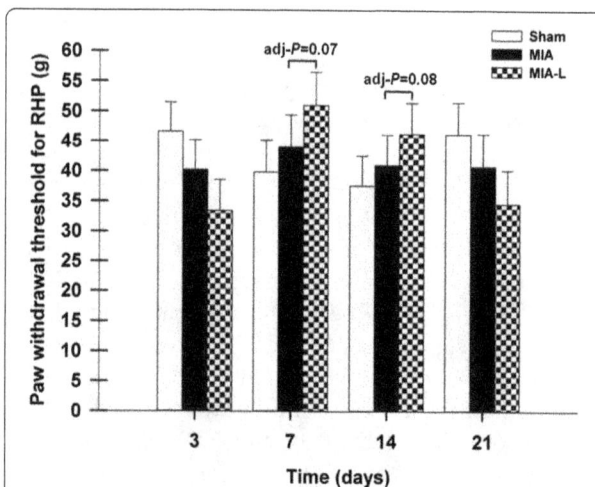

Fig. 4 Right hind paw (*RHP*) withdrawal threshold evolution after induction of osteoarthritis (least squares mean ± standard error of the mean). On days 7 (adjusted *P* value (adj-*P*) = 0.07) and 14 (adj-*P* = 0.08), the RHP paw withdrawal threshold was increased for the rats injected with monosodium iodoacetate and punctual lidocaine (*MIA-L*) when compared with rats injected with MIA

reduction in variability of kinetics measures after exercise in cats [62] and dogs [63] with OA. The current study confirmed beneficial effects of exercise to reduce SWB (or other outcome) variability in the MIA rat model of OA. This study also qualified TNTC as a quantitative pain measure using spontaneous behavior. Importantly, the study tested reliability and validity of TNTC, and the potential impact on results obtained with other pain assessment methods, which may be used concurrently. Our results confirmed that a broad range of methods can be combined for pain assessment in the same animals while maintaining reliability and scientific validity.

Finally, as different observers can introduce some degree of bias in pain assessment outcomes, inter-rater reliability was tested by observers with different levels of expertise (one intermediate and one advanced). The methodology included in the current study was accessible to an observer with intermediate experience, as no significant difference was identified during analysis based on the level of experience. As a limitation, the number of observers was minimal, as both observers were women, and only objective assessment methods were selected for this study (limiting any bias related to subjective observation). Therefore, such a hypothesis (the potential influence of experience, and/or gender) would need to be tested further before making inferences from the results. This is particularly important, as recent work has established the influence of the observer's gender in inducing stress-related analgesia in rodents [64]. Similarly, for limiting the influence of interferential factors in studying the effect of environment, only female rats were used. A possible gender effect would need to be tested in future experiments. Indeed, male rodents are recognized as more sensitive to olfactory exposure to males, including men, causing stress and related analgesia [64]. Moreover, sexual dimorphism [65] and hormonal influence [66, 67] have been observed in endogenous pain modulation mechanisms. Finally, women are more represented in the field of chronic pain [68]; however, many reasons have been explored to investigate this finding [69]. Also, for decades, males have been overrepresented

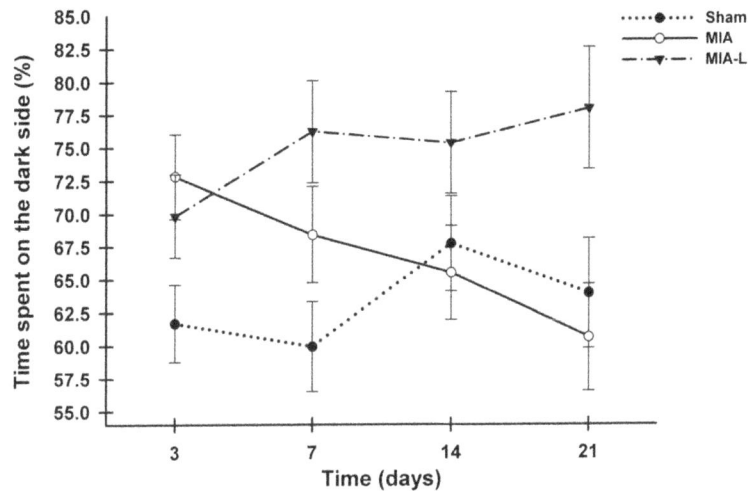

Fig. 5 Place escape/avoidance paradigm (PEAP) evolution after osteoarthritis induction (least squares mean ± standard error of the mean). The percentage of time spent on the PEAP dark side was statistically higher in the lidocaine-treated rats with monosodium iodoacetate (*MIA-L*) when compared to the rats injected with monosodium iodoacetate (*MIA*) (*P* = 0.07) and the sham group (*P* = 0.01) group. Data presented here were collected for the whole period of assessment (20 minutes) at each day, but the observed between-group differences were the most obvious during the intermediate periods 2 (5–10 minutes) and 3 (10–15 minutes)

in preclinical research. This situation can definitely lead to a certain bias [70]. All these previous studies justify our decision to use female rats.

As a recognized indicator of test-retest reliability [57], the ICC demonstrated that assessment of mechanical sensitivity using the Randall Selitto test presents poor repeatability, and this outcome cannot be recommended for a valid reflexive measure of pain. The phase 1 experiments demonstrated that SWB and tactile sensitivity can produce more repeatable data when animals (and the observer) are allowed to acclimate to the test device for at least one week. Similarly, there was a slight reduction in the variability of SWB when measured after treadmill exercise. However, the beneficial effects of exercise were not as significant in the chemically induced OA rat model as those observed in cats with naturally

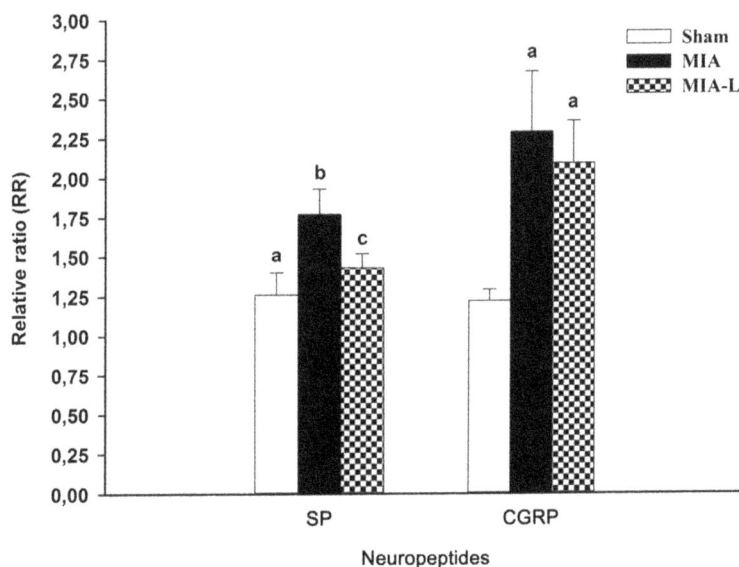

Fig. 6 Spinal substance P (*SP*) and calcitonin gene-related peptide (*CGRP*) concentrations 21 days after monosodium iodoacetate (*MIA*) injection (relative ratio (*RR*) mean and SD). Mean RR spinal cord concentration was normalized to the naive group. An RR of 1 indicated the concentration of normal rats from the naive group. The RR for SP and CGRP were increased in all groups (including the sham group) but had a higher peak after MIA injection. Lidocaine treatment (*L*) induced a lesser liberation of SP and CGRP (albeit not statistically significant for the latter) in the spinal cord of the MIA-L group. [a,b,c]Significant inter-group statistical differences (adjusted *P* value <0.10)

Table 5 Neuropeptides inter-group comparisons in the monosodium iodoacetate osteoarthritis rat model

Inter-group comparisons	SP	CGRP
Three groups vs. naive rats	0.016*	0.016*
MIA vs. sham	0.029*	0.029*
MIA-L vs. sham	0.057*	0.029*
MIA-L vs. MIA	0.029*	0.200

MIA monosodium iodoacetate, *MIA-L* rats injected with monosodium iodoacetate and treated with punctual lidocaine injection, *SP* substance P, *CGRP* calcitonin gene related-peptide. *Inter-group statistically significant difference (adjusted *P* value)

occurring OA [62, 71]. The PEAP, rotarod, and treadmill activity measured as TNTC appeared to be highly repeatable without requiring prolonged acclimatization. It must be noted that in both treadmill and PEAP, the intermediate periods 2 and 3 (i.e., 5–10 minutes, and 10–15 minutes, respectively) demonstrated the highest repeatability. These results also suggest that the treadmill and PEAP sessions are a little too long, so for future experimentation the session could be reduced in both cases to 15 minutes instead of 20 minutes. To our knowledge, this study is the first to evaluate the test-retest (repeatability) and inter-rater (reproducibility) reliability of a complete set of pain assessment methods in normal rodents.

As a measure of distribution dispersion that does not require similar units and therefore allows comparison of different variables, the CV of each pain assessment method was verified. At the first evaluation, we again observed the poor metrological property of mechanical sensitivity, presenting the highest inter-individual variability (around 70 % CV). Moreover, the different acclimatization protocols did not help to decrease this variability as the variation in CV from the last to the first evaluation was between 0.53 and 1.07. On the other side, our results support the importance of choosing the optimal acclimatization protocol for pain assessment in the rat model. To our knowledge, this study represents the first systematic evaluation of the effect on data variability of different acclimatization protocols, including four to eight assessments over a 2-week period, with a series of tests near or far from the others. The most reliable acclimatization protocol included five assessments with exposure to the testing methods every other day for the last week (days -14, -7, -5, -3, and -1), with baseline values acquired at day -1.

The second exploratory phase of our project evaluated the validity of the most promising pain assessment methods as determined during phase 1, when applied to the MIA model of OA in rats. Briefly, SWB, PTAE, PEAP, and TNTC detected pain-related changes following OA induction with an intra-articular MIA injection and were validated by increased release of spinal neuropeptides such as SP and CGRP. However, the rotarod assessment, as used in our experimental conditions, was not sensitive to induction of OA pain. Moreover, the PTAE and PEAP methods demonstrated that the sham injection of 0.9 % NaCl was not totally neutral, which was confirmed by the augmentation of spinal liberation of SP (26 times higher) and CGRP (22 times higher) in the sham group. Interestingly, PTAE and PEAP also confirmed the analgesic effect of intra-articular lidocaine injection by the downregulation of spinal neuropeptides, whereas TNTC and SWB did not detect the expected analgesic effect. These results suggest that SWB detects more biomechanical alterations of the joint than ongoing pain and consequently, could be a sensitive method to detect knee joint dysfunction. Of the four pain assessment methods evaluated for concurrent validity, only PEAP detected a treatment effect of lidocaine with a significant difference between the MIA-L group and both the sham and MIA groups. Interestingly, body weight was not affected, either by possible manipulation-related stress in phase 1, or by MIA induction of pain in phase 2. This confirms the possible lack of sensitivity of different endpoints used in research, such as feeding, drinking, etc., for determining quality of life.

The enhanced escape/avoidance behavior and lower PWT were previously demonstrated in both neuropathic and inflammatory pain models [33, 41, 47, 72, 73]. The higher sensitivity of PEAP compared to PTAE in detecting the efficacy of pain relief was also demonstrated in other studies [33].

It would be logical to consider that animals would allocate roughly a similar amount of time in both environments if they do not show natural preference or aversion to one of the two environments in the PEAP testing. This study clearly establishes a strong preference of the rat, a nocturnal animal, to the dark side of the test apparatus. The acclimatization of rats to the test apparatus is fast, the establishment of a baseline is preferable, and both intermediate periods 2 and 3 are highly repeatable. Moreover, PEAP assessment includes both classical (Pavlovian) and operant conditioning in the process of training [42]. When compared with PEAP, PTAE required a longer acclimatization period for both the animal and the observer (at least one week as demonstrated in this study). However, assessing the escape/avoidance behavior using the PEAP required a much longer evaluation time (with 20 to 30 minutes required for each animal), being too labor-intensive to the experimenters, while no automated apparatus is commercially available for this test.

Interestingly, the intra-articular lidocaine injection affected both PTAE and PEAP, and to a lesser degree TNTC, but did not alter changes in weight bearing on the RHP. The lack of effect of lidocaine on SWB could be related to reduced pain in the absence of movement in this model. In a recent study [25], intra-articular lidocaine (200 μL) was efficient to reduce the shift in weight bearing at day 14 post-MIA injection, but only for the highest dose of MIA (4.8 mg). The lower MIA dose and volume in our study (2 mg and 50 μL) combined with the lower sensitivity of SWB may be responsible for the lack of effect with this method, while PEAP and PTAE accurately captured the expected pharmacological effects of lidocaine. Intra-articular lidocaine was chosen for the analgesic test in this study, because of the apparently controversial results obtained in conditioning procedures with non-steroidal anti-inflammatory and opioid drugs (for review, see [42]).

These findings may be useful when designing studies of the efficacy of analgesia using the MIA-induced OA rat model. Moreover, there is also some evidence that the combination of the quick-acting effect of lidocaine (reaching a peak effect at 10 minutes after the intra-articular injection on a CatWalk) [74] and the necessary time to induce a change in the distribution of gait in supraspinal locomotor areas in patients with OA [75], seems to explain the lack of detection of lidocaine analgesia by SWB. Previous studies combined with our results, provide evidence for future use of a continuous infusion of lidocaine to obtain a more sustained analgesic effect, attaining higher lidocaine synovial levels for a prolonged time period.

The intra-articular injection of saline (sham group) generated some hyperalgesia or allodynia, as assessed by PTAE and reflected by the observed change in the operant testing. This is supported by the recent finding of some increased NF-kB activity on days 3 and 7 measured by in vivo luminescent imaging in a transgenic mouse model receiving an intra-articular injection of saline [76]. Moreover, in the MIA mouse model tested in the same study, temporal kinetics of NF-kB activity were strongly correlated with mechanical allodynia (PTAE) and serum interleukin (IL)-6 levels in the inflammatory phase (day 3) of this model, while serum IL-1β was strongly correlated with pain sensitivity in the chronic pain phase (up to day 28) [76]. An increase in the intra-articular pressure and possible injection-related inflammation are proposed to explain this finding. Based on these results, a neutral control group (without intra-articular injection) may be valuable in future experiments.

The MIA model is recognized as valuable in OA research for its ability to detect analgesic effects of different drugs and compounds. The initial inflammatory phase of this model allows the evaluation of various non-steroidal anti-inflammatory drugs and cyclo-oxygenase inhibitors [14, 24, 27, 77]. Moreover, the efficacy of morphine, gabapentin, pregabalin, and the transient receptor potential

vanilloid receptor antagonist was successfully demonstrated in this model [15–17, 24, 77]. Moreover, some studies showed that MIA-induced OA leads to an increase in the neuron firing rate and a reduced activation threshold of the afferent nerve fibers [78], which consequently leads to sensitization of spinal neurons in the dorsal horn [79]. In this study, spinal cord neuropeptide quantification suggests and supports development of central sensitization in this model. Indeed, our study confirms an increase in spinal biomarkers of SP and CGRP, as previously observed in the MIA model [51].

The upregulation of spinal neuropeptides observed in this study suggests activation of the peptidergic afferent C-fibers, resulting in central sensitization. It has been well-demonstrated [80], by relative increasing expression of target gene mRNA like pro-inflammatory cytokines (IL-1 and tumor necrosis factor) and pain mediators (CGRP, SP, neuropeptide Y, and galanin), that MIA-induced joint degeneration in rats generates an animal model suitable for mechanistic and pharmacologic studies on nociceptive pain pathways caused by OA. Altogether, this provides further key in vivo evidence that OA pain could be caused by central sensitization through communication between peripheral OA nociceptors and the central sensory system [81, 82]. Despite the fact that SWB did not detect lidocaine treatment on day 21, or asymmetry of weight distribution, our study clearly demonstrated that lidocaine analgesic effects noted by PEAP were translated by concomitant significant downregulation of spinal SP, which was 34 times lower, and of CGRP, which was 20 times lower on day 21.

These results mimic similar therapeutic effects on behavior and SP and CGRP spinal cord expression of intra-articular resiniferatoxin [83] and proteasome inhibitor MG132 [84] in the MIA OA pain model in rats. Unfortunately, we observed that the MIA model caused temporary changes of short duration (return to baseline values at day 21 post injection) and relies on a disease mechanism (chemical inhibition of glyceraldehyde-3-phosphate dehydrogenase activity in chondrocytes, resulting in cell death following the disruption of its cellular glycolysis process [15, 16, 18]) that differs from human natural OA, which could limit the predictability of the therapeutic effect of analgesic and disease-modifying agents. Finally, higher levels of spinal neuropeptides at sacrifice clearly confirms that our model caused some long-term pain or OA damage.

Conclusion

Pain assessment methods used with the MIA model should be selected and scheduled appropriately. In this study only mechanical sensitivity had poor metrological properties, but SWB, the operant PEAP testing, tactile sensitivity, rotarod, and treadmill (TNTC) were repeatable under different environmental conditions. The rotarod test did not achieve sufficient sensitivity to detect OA pain induced by MIA injection in rats and may not be included in future studies. For detecting the analgesic effect of local administration of lidocaine, the pain assessment method that demonstrated the best results was the operant testing, which had the greatest sensitivity, followed by PTAE, whereas SWB had some limitation in sensitivity. Spinal neuropeptide quantification at the end of the experiment has allowed us to validate the effect of positive lidocaine treatment in a more objective manner, as MIA can induce pain. However, the main limitation of this study was the small sample size. Furthermore, it was possible to increase the validity and reliability of pain assessment methods with an optimal acclimatization protocol (five assessments over 2 weeks). In addition, the sham intra-articular saline injection was not totally neutral, particularly with more sensitive methods such as PEAP, PTAE, and this was confirmed by the release of spinal neuropeptides. We therefore recommend the addition of a naive control group (without intra-articular injection). Moreover, increased neuropeptide levels obviously support the central sensitization observed in the MIA rat model. The present results highlight potential for these neuro-mediators as pharmacological biomarkers for analgesic testing in association with sensitive functional assessment methods.

Abbreviations
Adj-P, adjusted *p* value; BW, body weight; CGRP, calcitonin gene-related peptide; CV, coefficient of variation; D, day; HPLC-MS/MS, tandem mass spectrometry coupled to high-performance liquid chromatography; ICC, intraclass correlation coefficient; IL, interleukin; L, lidocaine; LHP, left hind paw; LS-Mean, least square means; MIA, monosodium iodoacetate; MRM, multiple reactions monitoring; MS, mechanical sensitivity; n, number of animals; OA, osteoarthritis; P, probability; PEAP, place escape/avoidance paradigm; PTAE, punctate tactile allodynia evaluation; PWT, paw withdrawal threshold; RHP, right hind paw; RPM, revolutions per minute; RR, relative ratio; SD, standard deviation; SEM, standard error of the mean; SP, substance P; SWB, static weight bearing; TNTC, treadmill number of total crossings; TS, tactile sensitivity; V/V, volume/volume.

Acknowledgements
The authors would like to address special thanks to Mrs Virgina Wallis for editing the manuscript. The authors would like to thank ArthroLab Inc. and CiToxLAB North-America Inc. personnel for their contributions to this work.

Funding
This study was partly supported by a Discovery grant (#327158-2008; #441651-2013; Eric Troncy) and a Collaborative Research and Development grant ((#418399-2011 with ArthroLab Inc.; Eric Troncy) from the Natural Sciences and Engineering Research Council of Canada (NSERC), supporting pain bio-analyses, by an ongoing New Opportunities Fund grant (#9483) and a Leader Opportunity Fund grant (#24601; Eric Troncy) from the Canada Foundation for Innovation, supporting pain equipment, and ArthroLab, Inc. and CiToxLAB North America, Inc. for their collaboration, access to animals, personnel and related facilities. This study was funded by a Pfizer Neuropathic Pain Research award (#WS386180; Eric Troncy) from Pfizer Canada, Inc.

Authors' contributions
Each co-author has taken an active part in this project from the conception and design of the content (CO, JG, SA, JMP, JPP, and ET), to the technical manipulations (CO, JG, JAG, DG, CP, SA, MAD, PS, FB, and ET), analysis, and interpretation of published data (CO, JG, MG, FB, and ET), and drafting and revising of the article (all co-authors) with the final approval of the submitted version. Each of them completely agrees with the presented data, and believes that the manuscript represents honest work.

Authors' information
This manuscript is part of the PhD thesis of CO. Several authors are recognized experts in the field of animal pain assessment (ET and FB), laboratory animal pain assessment (ET, PS, and SA), rheumatology (JMP, JPP, and ET) and others are their graduate students (CO, JG, MG, JAG, DG, CP, and MAD).

Competing interests
The authors declare that they have no competing interests.

Author details
[1]Groupe de Recherche en Pharmacologie Animale du Québec (GREPAQ), Department of Biomedical Sciences, Faculty of veterinary medicine, Université de Montréal, 1500 des Vétérinaires Street, P.O. Box 5000, St-Hyacinthe, Quebec J2S 7C6, Canada. [2]Osteoarthritis Research Unit, Research Center Hospital of Montreal University (CRCHUM), Montreal, Quebec, Canada. [3]Department of Physiology and Biophysics, Faculty of Medicine and Health Sciences, Université de Sherbrooke, Sherbrooke, Quebec, Canada. [4]CiToxLAB North America Inc., Laval, Quebec, Canada.

References
1. Little CB, Hunter DJ. Post-traumatic osteoarthritis: from mouse models to clinical trials. Nat Rev Rheumatol. 2013;9:485–97.
2. Lawrence RC, Felson DT, Helmick CG, Arnold LM, Choi H, Deyo RA, et al. Estimates of the prevalence of arthritis and other rheumatic conditions in the United States. Part II. Arthritis Rheum. 2008;58:26–35.
3. Hootman JM, Helmick CG. Projections of US prevalence of arthritis and associated activity limitations. Arthritis Rheum. 2006;54:226–9.
4. Kissin I. The development of new analgesics over the past 50 years: a lack of real breakthrough drugs. Anesth Analg. 2010;110:780–9.
5. Palmer AM, Sundstrom L. Translational medicines research. Drug Discov Today. 2013;18:503–5.
6. Dolgin E. Animalgesic effects. Nat Med. 2010;16:1237–40.
7. Mao J. Translational pain research: achievements and challenges. J Pain. 2009;10:1001–11.
8. Mogil JS. Animal models of pain: progress and challenges. Nat Rev Neurosci. 2009;10:283–94.
9. Yezierski RP, Vierck CJ. Should the hot-plate test be reincarnated? J Pain. 2011;12:936–7. author reply 938-939.
10. Blackburn-Munro G. Pain-like behaviours in animals - how human are they? Trends Pharmacol Sci. 2004;25:299–305.
11. Vierck CJ, Hansson PT, Yezierski RP. Clinical and pre-clinical pain assessment: are we measuring the same thing? Pain. 2008;135:7–10.
12. Mogil JS, Crager SE. What should we be measuring in behavioral studies of chronic pain in animals? Pain. 2004;112:12–5.
13. Moreau M, Pelletier JP, Lussier B, d'Anjou MA, Blond L, Pelletier JM, et al. *A posteriori* comparison of natural and surgical destabilization models of canine osteoarthritis. Biomed Res Int. 2013;2013:180453.
14. Bove SE, Calcaterra SL, Brooker RM, Huber CM, Guzman RE, Juneau PL, et al. Weight bearing as a measure of disease progression and efficacy of anti-inflammatory compounds in a model of monosodium iodoacetate-induced osteoarthritis. Osteoarthritis Cartilage. 2003;11:821–30.

15. Combe R, Bramwell S, Field MJ. The monosodium iodoacetate model of osteoarthritis: a model of chronic nociceptive pain in rats? Neurosci Lett. 2004;370:236–40.

16. Fernihough J, Gentry C, Malcangio M, Fox A, Rediske J, Pellas T, et al. Pain related behaviour in two models of osteoarthritis in the rat knee. Pain. 2004; 112:83–93.

17. Ferreira-Gomes J, Adaes S, Sousa RM, Mendonca M, Castro-Lopes JM. Dose-dependent expression of neuronal injury markers during experimental osteoarthritis induced by monoiodoacetate in the rat. Mol Pain. 2012;8:50.

18. Guingamp C, Gegout-Pottie P, Philippe L, Terlain B, Netter P, Gillet P. Mono-iodoacetate-induced experimental osteoarthritis: a dose-response study of loss of mobility, morphology, and biochemistry. Arthritis Rheum. 1997;40: 1670–9.

19. Guzman RE, Evans MG, Bove S, Morenko B, Kilgore K. Mono-iodoacetate-induced histologic changes in subchondral bone and articular cartilage of rat femorotibial joints: an animal model of osteoarthritis. Toxicol Pathol. 2003;31:619–24.

20. Kelly S, Dunham JP, Murray F, Read S, Donaldson LF, Lawson SN. Spontaneous firing in C-fibers and increased mechanical sensitivity in A-fibers of knee joint-associated mechanoreceptive primary afferent neurones during MIA-induced osteoarthritis in the rat. Osteoarthritis Cartilage. 2012;20:305–13.

21. Kobayashi K, Imaizumi R, Sumichika H, Tanaka H, Goda M, Fukunari A, et al. Sodium iodoacetate-induced experimental osteoarthritis and associated pain model in rats. J Vet Med Sci. 2003;65:1195–9.

22. Liu P, Okun A, Ren J, Guo RC, Ossipov MH, Xie J, et al. Ongoing pain in the MIA model of osteoarthritis. Neurosci Lett. 2011;493:72–5.

23. Marker CL, Pomonis JD. The monosodium iodoacetate model of osteoarthritis pain in the rat. Methods Mol Biol. 2012;851:239–48.

24. Nagase H, Kumakura S, Shimada K. Establishment of a novel objective and quantitative method to assess pain-related behavior in monosodium iodoacetate-induced osteoarthritis in rat knee. J Pharmacol Toxicol Methods. 2012;65:29–36.

25. Okun A, Liu P, Davis P, Ren J, Remeniuk B, Brion T, et al. Afferent drive elicits ongoing pain in a model of advanced osteoarthritis. Pain. 2012;153: 924–33.

26. Orita S, Ishikawa T, Miyagi M, Ochiai N, Inoue G, Eguchi Y, et al. Pain-related sensory innervation in monoiodoacetate-induced osteoarthritis in rat knees that gradually develops neuronal injury in addition to inflammatory pain. BMC Musculoskelet Disord. 2011;12:134.

27. Pomonis JD, Boulet JM, Gottshall SL, Phillips S, Sellers R, Bunton T, et al. Development and pharmacological characterization of a rat model of osteoarthritis pain. Pain. 2005;114:339–46.

28. Thakur M, Rahman W, Hobbs C, Dickenson AH, Bennett DL. Characterisation of a peripheral neuropathic component of the rat monoiodoacetate model of osteoarthritis. PLoS One. 2012;7, e33730.

29. Vonsy JL, Ghandehari J, Dickenson AH. Differential analgesic effects of morphine and gabapentin on behavioural measures of pain and disability in a model of osteoarthritis pain in rats. Eur J Pain. 2009;13:786–93.

30. Lampropoulou-Adamidou K, Lelovas P, Karadimas EV, Liakou C, Triantafillopoulos IK, Dontas I, et al. Useful animal models for the research of osteoarthritis. Eur J Orthop Surg Traumatol. 2014;24:263–71.

31. Barrot M. Tests and models of nociception and pain in rodents. Neuroscience. 2012;211:39–50.

32. Edwards RR, Sarlani E, Wesselmann U, Fillingim RB. Quantitative assessment of experimental pain perception: multiple domains of clinical relevance. Pain. 2005;114:315–9.

33. Boyce-Rustay JM, Zhong C, Kohnken R, Baker SJ, Simler GH, Wensink EJ, et al. Comparison of mechanical allodynia and the affective component of inflammatory pain in rats. Neuropharmacology. 2010;58:537–43.

34. Vierck CJ Jr, Kline R 4th, Wiley RG. Comparison of operant escape and innate reflex responses to nociceptive skin temperatures produced by heat and cold stimulation of rats. Behav Neurosci. 2004;118:627–35.

35. Yalcin I, Charlet A, Freund-Mercier MJ, Barrot M, Poisbeau P. Differentiating thermal allodynia and hyperalgesia using dynamic hot and cold plate in rodents. J Pain. 2009;10:767–73.

36. Cruz-Almeida Y, Fillingim RB. Can quantitative sensory testing move us closer to mechanism-based pain management? Pain Med. 2014;15:61–72.

37. Negus SS, Vanderah TW, Brandt MR, Bilsky EJ, Becerra L, Borsook D. Preclinical assessment of candidate analgesic drugs: recent advances and future challenges. J Pharmacol Exp Ther. 2006;319:507–14.

38. Suokas AK, Walsh DA, McWilliams DF, Condon L, Moreton B, Wylde V, et al. Quantitative sensory testing in painful osteoarthritis: a systematic review and meta-analysis. Osteoarthritis Cartilage. 2012;20:1075–85.

39. Allen KD, Mata BA, Gabr MA, Huebner JL, Adams Jr SB, Kraus VB, et al. Kinematic and dynamic gait compensations resulting from knee instability in a rat model of osteoarthritis. Arthritis Res Ther. 2012;14:R78.

40. Fuchs PN, McNabb CT. The place escape/avoidance paradigm: a novel method to assess nociceptive processing. J Integr Neurosci. 2012;11:61–72.

41. LaBuda CJ, Fuchs PN. A behavioral test paradigm to measure the aversive quality of inflammatory and neuropathic pain in rats. Exp Neurol. 2000;163: 490–4.

42. Li JX. The application of conditioning paradigms in the measurement of pain. Eur J Pharmacol. 2013;716:158–68.

43. Navratilova E, Xie JY, King T, Porreca F. Evaluation of reward from pain relief. Ann NY Acad Sci. 2013;1282:1–11.

44. Vierck CJ Jr, Kline RH, Wiley RG. Intrathecal substance p-saporin attenuates operant escape from nociceptive thermal stimuli. Neuroscience. 2003;119: 223–32.

45. King CD, Devine DP, Vierck CJ, Rodgers J, Yezierski RP. Differential effects of stress on escape and reflex responses to nociceptive thermal stimuli in the rat. Brain Res. 2003;987:214–22.

46. Mauderli AP, Acosta-Rua A, Vierck CJ. An operant assay of thermal pain in conscious, unrestrained rats. J Neurosci Methods. 2000;97:19–29.

47. Pedersen LH, Blackburn-Munro G. Pharmacological characterisation of place escape/avoidance behaviour in the rat chronic constriction injury model of neuropathic pain. Psychopharmacology (Berl). 2006;185:208–17.

48. Vierck CJ, Acosta-Rua A, Nelligan R, Tester N, Mauderli A. Low dose systemic morphine attenuates operant escape but facilitates innate reflex responses to thermal stimulation. J Pain. 2002;3:309–19.

49. Zhang XJ, Zhang TW, Hu SJ, Xu H. Behavioral assessments of the aversive quality of pain in animals. Neurosci Bull. 2011;27:61–7.

50. Woolf CJ. Windup and central sensitization are not equivalent. Pain. 1996;66: 105–8.

51. Ferland CE, Pailleux F, Vachon P, Beaudry F. Determination of specific neuropeptides modulation time course in a rat model of osteoarthritis pain by liquid chromatography ion trap mass spectrometry. Neuropeptides. 2011;45:423–9.

52. Calza L, Pozza M, Zanni M, Manzini CU, Manzini E, Hokfelt T. Peptide plasticity in primary sensory neurons and spinal cord during adjuvant-induced arthritis in the rat: an immunocytochemical and in situ hybridization study. Neuroscience. 1998;82:575–89.

53. Levine JD, Collier DH, Basbaum AI, Moskowitz MA, Helms CA. Hypothesis: the nervous system may contribute to the pathophysiology of rheumatoid arthritis. J Rheumatol. 1985;12:406–11.

54. Beaudry F, Ferland CE, Vachon P. Identification, characterization and quantification of specific neuropeptides in rat spinal cord by liquid chromatography electrospray quadrupole ion trap mass spectrometry. Biomed Chromatogr. 2009;23:940–50.

55. Che FY, Fricker LD. Quantitation of neuropeptides in Cpe(fat)/Cpe(fat) mice using differential isotopic tags and mass spectrometry. Anal Chem. 2002;74: 3190–8.

56. Curran-Everett D, Benos DJ. Guidelines for reporting statistics in journals published by the American Physiological Society. Am J Physiol Regul Integr Comp Physiol. 2004;287:R247–249.

57. Weir JP. Quantifying test-retest reliability using the intraclass correlation coefficient and the SEM. J Strength Cond Res. 2005;19:231–40.

58. Gregory MH, Capito N, Kuroki K, Stoker AM, Cook JL, Sherman SL. A review of translational animal models for knee osteoarthritis. Arthritis. 2012;2012: 764621.

59. Jansen van't Land C, Hendriksen CF. Change in locomotor activity pattern in mice: a model for recognition of distress? Lab Anim. 1995;29:286–93.

60. John TM, Brown MC, Wideman L, Brown GM. Melatonin replacement nullifies the effect of light-induced functional pinealectomy on nociceptive rhythm in the rat. Physiol Behav. 1994;55:735–9.

61. Perissin L, Facchin P, Porro CA. Diurnal variations in tonic pain reactions in mice. Life Sci. 2000;67:1477–88.

62. Moreau M, Guillot M, Pelletier JP, Martel-Pelletier J, Troncy E. Kinetic peak vertical force measurement in cats afflicted by coxarthritis: data management and acquisition protocols. Res Vet Sci. 2013;95:219–24.

63. Beraud R, Moreau M, Lussier B. Effect of exercise on kinetic gait analysis of dogs afflicted by osteoarthritis. Vet Comp Orthop Traumatol. 2010;23:87–92.

64. Sorge RE, Martin LJ, Isbester KA, Sotocinal SG, Rosen S, Tuttle AH, et al. Olfactory exposure to males, including men, causes stress and related analgesia in rodents. Nat Methods. 2014;11:629–32.

65. Gaumond I, Spooner MF, Marchand S. Sex differences in opioid-mediated pain inhibitory mechanisms during the interphase in the formalin test. Neuroscience. 2007;146:366–74.

66. Coulombe MA, Spooner MF, Gaumond I, Carrier JC, Marchand S. Estrogen receptors beta and alpha have specific pro- and anti-nociceptive actions. Neuroscience. 2011;184:172–82.

67. Liu X, Li W, Dai L, Zhang T, Xia W, Liu H, et al. Early repeated administration of progesterone improves the recovery of neuropathic pain and modulates spinal 18 kDa-translocator protein (TSPO) expression. J Steroid Biochem Mol Biol. 2014;143:130–40.

68. Fillingim RB, King CD, Ribeiro-Dasilva MC, Rahim-Williams B, Riley 3rd JL. Sex, gender, and pain: a review of recent clinical and experimental findings. J Pain. 2009;10:447–85.

69. Mogil JS. Sex differences in pain and pain inhibition: multiple explanations of a controversial phenomenon. Nat Rev Neurosci. 2012;13:859–66.

70. Mogil JS, Chanda ML. The case for the inclusion of female subjects in basic science studies of pain. Pain. 2005;117:1–5.

71. Guillot M, Moreau M, Heit M, Martel-Pelletier J, Pelletier JP, Troncy E. Characterization of osteoarthritis in cats and meloxicam efficacy using objective chronic pain evaluation tools. Vet J. 2013;196:360–7.

72. Baastrup C, Jensen TS, Finnerup NB. Pregabalin attenuates place escape/ avoidance behavior in a rat model of spinal cord injury. Brain Res. 2011; 1370:129–35.

73. LaGraize SC, Labuda CJ, Rutledge MA, Jackson RL, Fuchs PN. Differential effect of anterior cingulate cortex lesion on mechanical hypersensitivity and escape/avoidance behavior in an animal model of neuropathic pain. Exp Neurol. 2004;188:139–48.

74. Ferreira-Gomes J, Adaes S, Mendonca M, Castro-Lopes JM. Analgesic effects of lidocaine, morphine and diclofenac on movement-induced nociception, as assessed by the Knee-Bend and CatWalk tests in a rat model of osteoarthritis. Pharmacol Biochem Behav. 2012;101:617–24.

75. Jahn K, Deutschlander A, Stephan T, Kalla R, Hufner K, Wagner J, et al. Supraspinal locomotor control in quadrupeds and humans. Prog Brain Res. 2008;171:353–62.

76. Bowles RD, Mata BA, Bell RD, Mwangi TK, Huebner JL, Kraus VB, et al. In Vivo luminescent imaging of NF-kappaB activity and serum cytokine levels predict pain sensitivities in a rodent model of osteoarthritis. Arthritis Rheum. 2014;66:637–46.

77. Ivanavicius SP, Ball AD, Heapy CG, Westwood FR, Murray F, Read SJ. Structural pathology in a rodent model of osteoarthritis is associated with neuropathic pain: increased expression of ATF-3 and pharmacological characterisation. Pain. 2007;128:272–82.

78. Schuelert N, McDougall JJ. Electrophysiological evidence that the vasoactive intestinal peptide receptor antagonist VIP6-28 reduces nociception in an animal model of osteoarthritis. Osteoarthritis Cartilage. 2006;14:1155–62.

79. Harvey VL, Dickenson AH. Behavioural and electrophysiological characterisation of experimentally induced osteoarthritis and neuropathy in C57Bl/6 mice. Mol Pain. 2009;5:18.

80. Im HJ, Kim JS, Li X, Kotwal N, Sumner DR, van Wijnen AJ, et al. Alteration of sensory neurons and spinal response to an experimental osteoarthritis pain model. Arthritis Rheum. 2010;62:2995–3005.

81. Zhang RX, Ren K, Dubner R. Osteoarthritis pain mechanisms: basic studies in animal models. Osteoarthritis Cartilage. 2013;21:1308–15.

82. Abaei M, Sagar DR, Stockley EG, Spicer CH, Prior M, Chapman V, et al. Neural correlates of hyperalgesia in the monosodium iodoacetate model of osteoarthritis pain. Mol Pain. 2016;12:1–12.

83. Kim Y, Kim EH, Lee KS, Lee K, Park SH, Na SH, et al. The effects of intra-articular resiniferatoxin on monosodium iodoacetate-induced osteoarthritic pain in rats. Korean J Physiol Pharmacol. 2016;20:129–36.

84. Ahmed AS, Li J, Erlandsson-Harris H, Stark A, Bakalkin G, Ahmed M. Suppression of pain and joint destruction by inhibition of the proteasome system in experimental osteoarthritis. Pain. 2012;153:18–26.

Integrating genome-wide DNA methylation and mRNA expression profiles identified different molecular features between Kashin-Beck disease and primary osteoarthritis

Yan Wen[1], Ping Li[1], Jingcan Hao[1,2], Chen Duan[1], Jing Han[1], Awen He[1], Yanan Du[1], Li Liu[1], Xiao Liang[1], Feng Zhang[1*] and Xiong Guo[1*]

Abstract

Background: Kashin-Beck disease (KBD) is an endemic osteochondropathy of unknown etiology. Osteoarthritis (OA) is a form of degenerative joint disease sharing similar clinical manifestations and pathological changes to articular cartilage with KBD.

Methods: A genome-wide DNA methylation profile of articular cartilage from five KBD patients and five OA patients was first performed using the Illumina Infinium HumanMethylation450 BeadChip. Together with a previous gene expression profiling dataset comparing KBD cartilage with OA cartilage, an integrative pathway enrichment analysis of the genome-wide DNA methylation and the mRNA expression profiles conducted in articular cartilage was performed by InCroMAP software.

Results: We identified 241 common genes altered in both the DNA methylation profile and the mRNA expression profile of articular cartilage of KBD versus OA, including CHST13 (NM_152889, fold-change = 0.5979, P_{methy} = 0.0430), TGFBR1 (NM_004612, fold-change = 2.077, P_{methy} = 0.0430), TGFBR2 (NM_001024847, fold-change = 1.543, P_{methy} = 0.037), TGFBR3 (NM_001276, fold-change = 0.4515, P_{methy} = 6.04 × 10^{-4}), and ADAM12 (NM_021641, fold-change = 1.9768, P_{methy} = 0.0178). Integrative pathway enrichment analysis identified 19 significant KEGG pathways, including mTOR signaling (P = 0.0301), glycosaminoglycan biosynthesis-chondroitin sulfate/dermatan sulfate (P = 0.0391), glycosaminoglycan biosynthesis-keratan sulfate (P = 0.0278), and PI3K-Akt signaling (P = 0.0243).

Conclusion: This study identified different molecular features between Kashin-Beck disease and primary osteoarthritis and provided novel clues for clarifying the pathogenetic differences between KBD and OA.

Keywords: Kashin-Beck disease, Osteoarthritis, Methylation, Gene expression

* Correspondence: fzhxjtu@mail.xjtu.edu.cn; guox@mail.xjtu.edu.cn
[1]Key Laboratory of Trace Elements and Endemic Diseases of National Health and Family Planning Commission, School of Public Health, Xi'an Jiaotong University, Health Science Center, No.76 Yan Ta West Road, Xi'an 710061, People's Republic of China
Full list of author information is available at the end of the article

Background

Kashin-Beck disease (KBD) is an endemic and chronic osteochondropathy in China. According to the China Health Statistic Yearbook in 2013, there are still 645,000 people suffering from KBD. The original pathological changes of KBD appear in the deep zone of the growth plate cartilage and articular cartilage [1], which will result in premature closure of the epiphyseal plate and impaired endochondral ossification. Some genetic factors, such as ITPR2, HLA-DRB1, and ABI3BP, are thought to be causes of KBD and lead to a difference between individuals in the incidence of KBD [2–4].

Primary osteoarthritis (OA) is a form of degenerative joint disease. It is highly prevalent worldwide and affects about 10% of men and 18% of women over 60 years of age [5]. The biological and pathological alterations of OA mainly happen in the cartilage, subchondral bone, and synovium. Recently, systemic inflammation has also been found to be associated with OA [6]. Generally, the etiology of OA is complex and multifactorial, with genetic, biological, and biomechanical components involved.

KBD and OA share common characteristics regarding the manifestation and pathological changes in the articular cartilage. For example, necrosis and apoptosis of chondrocytes can both appear in the articular cartilage of KBD and OA. Additionally, the narrowed joint space, movement disorder of joints, painful joints, and osteophytes can be seen both in KBD and OA cartilage. However, KBD is an endemic disease causing by environmental risk factors. The etiology and molecular mechanism of KBD are different from OA [7], and clarifying the differences between KBD and OA would be helpful for pathogenetic and therapeutic studies of both KBD and OA. Previously, we compared the genome-wide expression profiles of KBD and OA [7]. Recent studies have demonstrated the important role of DNA methylation in the development of OA [8]. Therefore, integrative analysis of genome-wide DNA methylation and mRNA expression profiles may provide novel clues for understanding the pathogenesis of both KBD and OA.

DNA methylation, as an epigenetic control mechanism, plays an important role in the regulation of gene expression and, therefore, various biological processes and diseases. It is tissue-specific, dynamic, and sequence context-dependent [9]; thus, it has great significance in deciphering the complex methylation patterns needed for answering biological questions. Recent studies have demonstrated an association between the epigenetic changes and the progression of OA [8, 10–13]. Shi et al. also found that there is a difference in the methylation status of KBD blood compared to normal blood [14].

Facilitated by recent technological advances, it has become easier and quicker to obtain high-throughput data at one time point regarding the genomic, epigenomic,

transcriptomic, and proteomic scales. It is thought that there will be an exciting potential for answering more biological questions by integrating these together [15]; to take DNA methylation as an example, to show that the epigenetic feature can regulate transcriptional results, it will be helpful to correlate the epigenomic data and transcriptomic data. Gao et al. matched DNA methylation data to the RNA-seq data of breast cancer and regarded the epigenetic silencing of WNT signaling antagonists and bone morphogenetic proteins as key events underlying breast cancer [16]. Therefore, it is necessary to conduct an integrative analysis between DNA methylation and gene expression data rather than studying them individually.

In this study, a genome-wide methylation study was conducted on the articular cartilage of KBD and comparing this to OA. Furthermore, by utilizing previously published gene expression profiling study data comparing the articular cartilage of KBD with OA, an integrative analysis was conducted in these two datasets using InCroMAP software. Our results illustrated different molecular features and biological networks underlying KBD compared to OA.

Methods

Sample collection

Cartilage specimens were collected from the femoral condyles of knee joints of KBD and OA patients undergoing total knee joint arthroplasty. DNA samples were extracted from the cartilage specimens using QIAamp DNA Mini Kit (QIAGEN, Germany). All study subjects were Chinese Han. KBD donors came from the KBD prevalent area of Yongshou county, Xi'an city of the Shaanxi province, while OA donors were from Xi'an city of the Shaanxi province. Written informed consent was obtained from all subjects. KBD patients were diagnosed strictly according to national diagnostic criteria of Kashin-Beck disease in China (WS/T 207-2010). OA patients were diagnosed strictly according to the Western Ontario and McMaster Universities Osteoarthritis Index (WOMAC). Any subjects who had a history of other bone or joint diseases were excluded from this study.

Finally, five KBD patients (three males and two females) and five OA patients (three males and two females) were collected and divided into five pairs matched according to their age and sex for the DNA methylation study. The average ages of KBD patients and OA patients were 57.4 ± 7.12 and 64.6 ± 5.01 years, respectively.

Genome-wide DNA methylation study

In this study, the Illumina Infinium HumanMethylation450 BeadChip (Illumina, Inc., USA) was used to carry out the genome-wide DNA methylation study. Genomic DNA was extracted from articular cartilage. A total of 500 ng DNA was used for bisulfite conversion according to the standard protocol for the EZ DNA Methylation Kit (Zymo Research, USA). The DNA solution was mixed with NaOH and then melted into a single-stranded molecular sample. Then, the whole-genome amplification was conducted and the prepared sample was incubated at 37 °C overnight. After hybridization to the HumanMethylation450 array, the array was washed and stained followed the protocol of the Infinium HD Assay Methylation. The fluorescence signal was scanned by the IScan SQ scanner (iScan System, Illumina, USA), and the obtained raw image intensity data were processed using GenomeStudio software (Illumina, USA).

For the genome-wide DNA methylation study, the β value was defined as the expression of the average percentage of methylated cytosine at a given CpG site, which varied from 0 (completely unmethylated) to 1 (completely methylated). Differentially methylated CpG sites were identified using the empirical Bayes moderated t test, which was described by the Illumina Methylation Analyzer package. For each CpG site, the false discovery rate (FDR)-adjusted P value was calculated using the Benjiamini-Hochberg method. The definition of significant CpG was: 1) FDR-adjusted P value ≤ 0.05; and 2) β-value difference ($\Delta\beta$) ≥ 0.2. For quality control, the samples with more than 90% missing values or detection P value > 0.05 in more than 90% of cartilage specimens were eliminated.

Gene expression profiling study

The dataset of gene expression profiling for KBD and OA from our previous study was used here [7]. Briefly, KBD donors came from the KBD prevalent areas of Yongshou county and Linyou county of Xi'an city of the Shaanxi province, while OA donors were collected from Xi'an city of the Shaanxi province. Cartilage specimens were collected from the femoral condyles of knee joints of four KBD patients (three males and one female) and four OA patients (three males and one female) undergoing total knee joint arthroplasty. The average ages of KBD patients and OA patients were 59 ± 1.63 and 62 ± 2.94 years, respectively. Total RNA was isolated from the patient's articular cartilage using the Agilent Total RNA Isolation Mini kit (Agilent Technologies, Santa Clara, CA, USA). The integrity and concentration of RNA samples were detected by agarose gel electrophoresis and spectrophotometer. The RNA was reverse-transcribed into cDNA and then the cDNA was transcribed into cRNA in the presence of Cy3- or Cy5-CTP. The labeled cRNA of KBD and OA was purified separately and mixed with hybridization buffer. The hybridization solution was prepared using the In Situ Hybridization Plus Kit (Agilent Technologies). Then, the hybridization was carried out using the Agilent 4 × 44 k Whole Human Genome microarrays

(G4112F; Agilent Technologies). The hybridization experiment was completed in in the Agilent G2545A hybridization oven.

Hybridization signals were recorded by an Agilent G52565BA scanner and analyzed using Feature Extraction 9.3 (Agilent Technologies) and Spotfire 8.0 (Spotfire Inc., Cambridge, MA, USA) software. Spots that failed to pass the quality control procedures were flagged and excluded from further analysis. A possible dye-related bias in the microarray results was eliminated using an algorithm that involved application of normalization factors. The generated data were imported into spreadsheets (Excel; Microsoft, Redmond, WA, USA) for downstream data analysis and statistical evaluation. To identify differentially expressed genes, fold-change was calculated for each gene through dividing the fluorescent value of the KBD patient by that of the OA subject. Genes with fold-change ≥ 1.5 and $P < 0.05$ were regarded as differently expressed in KBD patients compared with OA patients. To further validate the microarray results, four upregulated genes (EPHA3, TRPC6, DOK5, and BIRC5) and four downregulated genes (BBC3, SMAD9, SLC25A37, and RASD1) were selected for quantitative reverse-transcription polymerase chain reaction (qRT-PCR) in our previous study [7]. The results of qRT-PCR experiment of the eight genes were entirely consistent with those of the microarray study, confirming the accuracy of the microarray experiment [7].

Statistical analysis

In this study, InCroMAP software was applied for single-platform and cross-platform integrative pathway enrichment analysis [17]. The dataset sheet was formatted as required by InCroMAP . After importing the data into InCroMAP, data pairing was firstly performed to match the two datasets according to each probe's identifier, and the genes which were commonly differentially expressed and methylated between KBD and OA were identified. Integrated gene set enrichment analysis was then conducted in InCroMAP by applying the threshold of $P_{methy} < 0.05$ and fold-change ≥ 1.5 [17].

Results
The main commonly differentially expressed and methylated genes

Six hundred and ninety-four genes were identified to be differently methylated between KBD and OA, including 285 hypermethylated CpG sites and 951 hypomethylated CpG sites, corresponding to 189 hypermethylated genes and 505 hypomethylated genes.

By performing the "pair-data" command in InCroMAP, 241 genes were identified to be commonly differentially expressed and methylated between KBD and OA. The family members of transforming growth factor (TGF) beta receptor, including

TGFBR1 (NM_004612, fold-change = 2.077, P_{methy} = 0.0430), TGFBR2 (NM_001024847, fold-change = 1.543, P_{methy} = 0.037), and TGFBR3 (NM_001276, fold-change = 0.4515, P_{methy} = 6.04 × 10^{-4}), were found to have different expression and methylation levels in KBD relative to OA. Additionally, CHST13 and ADAM12 were also identified to be commonly differentially expressed and methylated in KBD compared to OA (CHST13: NM_152889, fold-change = 0.5979, P_{methy} = 0.0430; ADAM12: NM_021641, fold-change = 1.9768, P_{methy} = 0.0178). Among these, TGFBR2 and ADAM12 showed increased mRNA expression levels and decreased DNA methylation levels in KBD cartilage compared with OA cartilage. TGFBR3 and CHST13 presented reduced mRNA expression and DNA methylation levels, while TGFBR1 showed increased mRNA expression and DNA methylation levels in KBD cartilage compared with OA cartilage. The main commonly differentially expressed and methylated genes can be seen in (Additional file 1: Table S1).

Pathway enrichment analysis of DNA methylation data
Thirteen pathways were identified to be significantly enriched in the differentially methylated genes between KBD and OA cartilage (Additional file 2: Table S2), such as other types of O-glycan biosynthesis (path:hsa00514, P = 2.44 × 10^{-3}), ABC transporters (path:hsa02010, P = 7.54 × 10^{-3}), insulin secretion (path:hsa04911, P = 0.0132), mammalian target of rapamycin (mTOR) signaling pathway (path:hsa04150, P = 0.0144), and glycosaminoglycan (GAG) degradation (path:hsa00531, P = 0.0168).

Integrative pathway enrichment analysis
Nineteen pathways were identified to be significantly altered regarding both expression and methylation levels (Table 1). The top five significant pathways included adherens junction (path:hsa04520, P = 5.34 × 10^{-3}), insulin secretion (path:hsa04911, P = 7.32 × 10^{-3}), other types of O-glycan biosynthesis (path:hsa00514, P = 0.0101), pathways in cancer (path:hsa05200, P = 0.0148), and pancreatic cancer (path:hsa05212, P = 0.0156).

The pathways related to glycosaminoglycan biosynthesis (path:hsa00532 and path:hsa00533) and the pathway related to osteoclast differentiation (path:hsa04380) were found to be altered significantly in KBD compared with OA (path:hsa00532, P = 0.0391; path:hsa00533, P = 0.0278; and path:hsa04380, P = 0.0325), and the mTOR signaling pathway (path:hsa04150) was also one of the significantly altered pathways (P = 0.0301; Fig. 1).

Table 1 Integrative pathway enrichment analysis results of DNA methylation and mRNA expression profiles between KBD and OA cartilage

Pathway name	KEGG ID	P value	No. of significantly different genes*	No. of genes in KEGG pathway
Adherens junction	path:hsa04520	5.34 × 10^{-3}	5	60
Insulin secretion	path:hsa04911	7.32 × 10^{-3}	5	65
Other types of O-glycan biosynthesis	path:hsa00514	0.010	3	24
Pathways in cancer	path:hsa05200	0.015	10	247
Pancreatic cancer	path:hsa05212	0.016	4	52
Chronic myeloid leukemia	path:hsa05220	0.017	4	53
Valine, leucine and isoleucine biosynthesis	path:hsa00290	0.020	1	4
Type II diabetes mellitus	path:hsa04930	0.021	3	32
PI3K-Akt signaling pathway	path:hsa04151	0.024	9	233
Glycosaminoglycan biosynthesis—keratan sulfate	path:hsa00533	0.028	2	14
mTOR signaling pathway	path:hsa04150	0.030	3	37
Nicotinate and nicotinamide metabolism	path:hsa00760	0.031	2	15
Osteoclast differentiation	path:hsa04380	0.033	5	99
Glycosaminoglycan biosynthesis—chondroitin sulfate/dermatan sulfate	path:hsa00532	0.039	2	17
Transcriptional misregulation in cancer	path:hsa05202	0.041	6	143
Acute myeloid leukemia	path:hsa05221	0.047	3	45
Vascular smooth muscle contraction	path:hsa04270	0.048	4	77
Chagas disease (American trypanosomiasis)	path:hsa05142	0.048	4	77
Insulin signaling pathway	path:hsa04910	0.049	4	78

KEGG Kyoto Encyclopedia of Genes and Genomes, *mTOR* mammalian target of rapamycin, *PI3K* phosphatidylinositol 3′-kinase
* Number of genes differently expressed and methylated in Kashin-Beck disease (KBD) compared with osteoarthritis (OA) within the given pathway

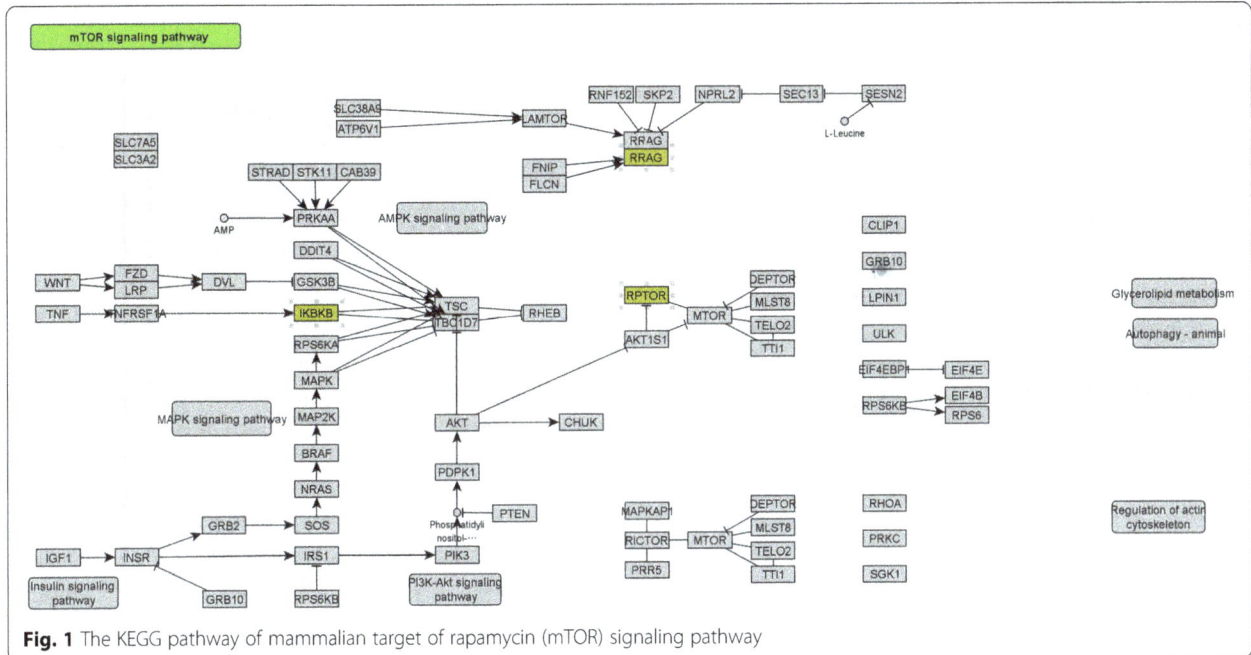

Fig. 1 The KEGG pathway of mammalian target of rapamycin (mTOR) signaling pathway

Discussion

In this study, an integrative analysis of global DNA methylation and mRNA expression profiles was performed using InCroMAP; 241 genes were identified to be commonly differentially expressed and methylated between KBD and OA, and 19 pathways were found to be altered in KBD relative to OA.

The family of TGF-beta receptors was found to be commonly differentially expressed and methylated in KBD compared with OA, including TGFBR1, TGFBR2, TGFBR3 (Additional file 1: Table S1). TGF-beta can encode a secreted ligand of the TGF-beta superfamily of proteins and regulate cell differentiation and growth by binding to various TGF-beta receptors. TGFBR1 can form a heteromeric complex with TGFBR2 when bound to TGF-beta, transducing the TGF-beta signal from the cell surface to the cytoplasm. TGFBR3 is a membrane proteoglycan that often functions as a co-receptor with other TGF-beta receptor superfamily members. The TGF-beta superfamily consists of the TGF-beta subfamily and the bone morphogenetic protein subfamily. The balance between the two subfamilies is essential for the development of growth plate. In a previous study, TGF-beta was also found to have an enhanced expression level in the articular cartilage of KBD compared with that of normal cartilage [18]. Another study observed that after treatment with T-2 toxin, an important environmental risk for KBD, the chondrocytes had an elevated mRNA expression level of TGFB3 [19]. Therefore, based on others and our previous study results, we might infer that the disturbance of the TGF-beta superfamily induced by T-2 toxin led to the impaired development of the growth plate in KBD, but

further biological studies were needed to confirm our finding. Additionally, TGF-beta has also played an important role in the development of OA by reducing collagen cleavage and chondrocyte differentiation [20]. However, the difference in the roles played by the TGF-beta superfamily in KBD and OA was still unclear.

We also found that ADAM12 showed increased mRNA expression levels and hypomethylated DNA levels in KBD cartilage compared to OA cartilage. ADAM12 belongs to the family of ADAMs (a disintegrin and metalloproteases). ADAM12 has been implicated in a variety of biological processes, involving cell-cell and cell-matrix interactions [21]. ADAM12-S transgenic mice were found to exhibit a pronounced increase in longitudinal bone growth and an increased number of proliferating chondrocytes [22]. In a previous genome-wide association study involving 2471 study subjects, ADAM12 polymorphism was identified to be significantly associated with joint destruction and growth retardation phenotypes of KBD and showed a decreased protein expression level in KBD cartilage compared to healthy control cartilage [23]. Given the impaired bone development in KBD children, ADAM12 might be involved in the skeletal growth retardation of KBD, but further biological studies were needed to reveal the roles of the identified genes in the development of KBD and OA.

Additionally, we observed that hypermethylated/hypomethylated genes did not always have lower/higher mRNA expression levels, such as TGFBR3 and CHST13. A similar phenomenon has been reported by previous studies [10, 24]. These results might be partly explained by the complicated transcriptional regulation of DNA methylation [25, 26].

The mTOR signaling pathway was one of the pathways which were found to be altered on the gene expression and DNA methylation scales in KBD relative to OA. mTOR is a highly conversed serine/threonine protein kinase that can integrate stimuli, such as nutrients and growth factors, to regulate several biological processes, including metabolism, autophagy, protein synthesis, and ribosome biogenesis. mTOR can be inhibited by rapamycin and induce the autophagy process [27]. Recently, the important role of mTOR signaling in the progression of OA was shown in several studies [28, 29]. Intra-articular injection of rapamycin could attenuate the articular cartilage degradation caused by OA through reducing the expression of mTOR [29]. The cartilage-specific ablation of mTOR in a mouse model could result in increased autophagy signaling and a significant protection from medial meniscus-induced OA [28]. Additionally, mTOR signaling was also thought to be related to skeletal growth in mammals. Genetic deletion of mTOR1 or mTOR2, the two distinct complexes of mTOR, could diminish embryonic skeletal growth due to severe delays in chondrocyte hypertrophy and impaired bone formation [30, 31].

However, little was previously known about mTOR signaling in KBD chondrocytes. For the first time, we found the mTOR signaling pathway to be altered in KBD chondrocytes compared with OA in this study. A previous study identified that defective autophagy could be seen in KBD chondrocytes with reduced Beclin1 and LC3, and several autophagy-related genes were found to be differentially expressed in KBD chondrocytes compared with the normal control [32]. Due to the significant effects of mTOR signaling on the autophagy process and skeletal growth, it was considered worthy to further study mTOR in KBD chondrocytes.

The pathways related to the glycosaminoglycan (GAG) biosynthesis, including chondroitin sulfate (CS)/dermatan sulfate (DS) and keratan sulfate (KS), were also found to be altered on the gene expression and DNA methylation scales in KBD chondrocytes relative to OA. GAGs, a heterogeneous family of unbranched polysaccharides, exist either as a free state or attached to proteins to form proteoglycans (PGs) and can be found both on the cell surface and in the extracellular matrix (ECM) [33]. PGs and GAGs are the ECM components of articular cartilage, whose functions are critical for the articular cartilage [34]. There are three classes of GAGs in cartilage, including hyaluronan (HA), CS, and KS. Since DS is a modified form of CS, DS was included into the CS class here. CS can account for 80% of GAGs and KS can account for 5–20% of GAGs in articular cartilage [35]. They together provide cartilage resistance to the physical stress and load [35].

Previous studies have shown that CS and KS dramatically decrease in the articular cartilage of KBD children compared with normal controls [36]. Urine hydroxyproline, a marker of catabolism levels of PGs in vivo, was also higher in children from the KBD endemic areas [37]. Moreover, a series of enzymes involved in CS metabolism were identified to be abnormally expressed in KBD cartilage—for example, the anabolic enzymes including PAPSS2, PAPST1, and CHST15 were significantly lower in KBD samples than those found in the controls; in contrast, the catabolic enzymes including ARSB and GALNS were significantly higher than in the control samples [38]. This evidence suggests a global disruption of glycosaminoglycan biosynthesis in KBD cartilage. In this study, CHST13, another kind of sulfotransferase responsible for the anabolism of CS, was also found to be lower in KBD chondrocytes relative to OA. Additionally, an abnormal DNA methylation level of other genes related to glycosaminoglycan biosynthesis, such as UST, was also identified in this study. Because of the lack of DNA methylation studies in KBD chondrocytes, how DNA methylation regulates the expression of GAG-related genes remains unknown, and further efforts should be made to study this field.

Interestingly, the pathway for osteoclast differentiation was also found to be altered in the cartilage in this study. The pathway for osteoclast differentiation can regulate the genesis of osteoclasts, a kind of multinucleate cell originating from the hematopoietic monocyte-macrophage lineage and responsible for bone resorption. The dynamic balance of bone-forming osteoblasts and bone-resorbing osteoclasts is essential for the homeostasis of the bony skeleton. Impaired osteoclasts can result in osteoporosis (OP) [39]. KBD, but not OA, is characteristic of OP [40]. In addition, KBD and OP phenotypes were found to have pleiotropic effects and share common risk genes in a previous study [40]. However, this study was conducted in cartilage chondrocytes but not in osteoclasts, and it lacked further evidence to conclude what role these osteoclast differentiation-related genes played in chondrocytes and what the situation was regarding KBD osteoclasts.

The phosphatidylinositol 3'-kinase (PI3K)-Akt signaling pathway was another altered pathway identified in this study. The PI3K-Akt signaling pathway can regulate fundamental cellular functions such as cell growth, survival, and movement. If this pathway is inhibited in chondrocytes, the cells show a reduced level of survival and proteoglycan synthesis [41]. This pathway was additionally thought to be a potential target for the treatment of OA [42–44]. In a previous study conducted in KBD chondrocytes compared with normal controls, the PI3K-Akt signaling pathway was identified to be significantly differentially expressed, and it was concluded that an environmental risk factor for KBD, selenium deficiency, might induce chondrocyte apoptosis and cell death through the PI3K-Akt signaling pathway [45]. Moreover, in this study, the PI3K-Akt signaling pathway showed different levels of gene expression and DNA methylation in KBD cartilage relative to OA. Based on previous studies and our study results, we suggest that the PI3K-Akt pathway exerts its effect in different ways in KBD compared with OA. However, the interaction of genes within the PI3K-Akt pathway is complicated and needs further study.

There were some limitations to this study. Firstly, articular cartilage specimens were collected from severe KBD and OA patients undergoing total joint arthroplasty. Currently, there are limited numbers of severe KBD patients who need surgical treatment [46]. Due to articular cartilage degradation, the amount of DNA and mRNA samples extracted from collected cartilage specimens is generally not enough for both genome-wide DNA methylation and mRNA expression profiling experiments. Therefore, a relative small sample of five KBD and five OA patients was used for DNA methylation profiling and another independent sample of four KBD patients and four OA patients was used for mRNA expression profiling. A similar sampling design has been used by previous studies [47, 48]. Secondly, because it was impossible to collect articular cartilage specimens from early-stage patients all the study subjects were at the end-stage of KBD or OA. Therefore, our study results trend to reflect the alterations in end-stage disease. Third, utilizing the pathway enrichment analysis approach of InCroMAP software, we identified multiple pathways that were significantly enriched in the differentially expressed and differentially methylated gene sets between KBD and OA. However, according to the pathway enrichment analysis results of InCro-MAP, we could not determine whether the identified pathways were activated or inhibited. Further biological studies are warranted to reveal the mechanisms of the identified pathways implicated in the development of KBD and OA.

In summary, this was the first integrative study in KBD combining gene expression profiling and DNA methylation profiling datasets. By performing integrative enrichment analysis with two datasets, 19 pathways were identified to be altered in KBD cartilage relative to OA. For the first time, the autophagy and ECM metabolism-related pathways (mTOR signaling pathway, glycosaminoglycan biosynthesis) were especially found to be differentially methylated and expressed in KBD relative to OA.

Conclusion

This study suggests a different molecular feature in the pathology of KBD and OA and provides new clues for the study of KBD and OA.

Abbreviations

CS: Chondroitin sulfate; DS: Dermatan sulfate; ECM: Extracellular matrix; FDR: False discovery rate; GAG: Glycosaminoglycan; HA: Hyaluronan; KBD: Kashin-Beck disease; KS: Keratan sulfate; mTOR: Mammalian target of rapamycin; OA: Osteoarthritis; OP: Osteoporosis; PG: Proteoglycan; PI3K: Phosphatidylinositol 3′-kinase; qRT-PCR: Quantitative reverse-transcription polymerase chain reaction; TGF: Transforming growth factor

Acknowledgements
Not applicable.

Funding
This study is supported by the National Natural Science Foundation of China (No. 81472925, 81673112 and 81302392), the Technology Research and Development Program of Shaanxi Province of China (2013KJXX-51), the National Key R&D Program of China (2016YFE0119100), and the Fundamental Research Funds for the Central Universities.

Authors' contributions
FZ designed the study, performed the methylation study, and analyzed the data. XG designed the study and conducted the disease diagnosis. YW analyzed and processed the data and wrote the manuscript. JH and PL conducted the experiments in this study. CD conducted the gene expression profile study and supplied the data. JH, AH, YD, LL, and XL participated in the sample collection. All authors read and approved the final manuscript.

Consent for publication
All authors have read the final manuscript and approved the manuscript for publication.

Competing interests
The authors declare that they have no competing interests.

Author details
[1]Key Laboratory of Trace Elements and Endemic Diseases of National Health and Family Planning Commission, School of Public Health, Xi'an Jiaotong University, Health Science Center, No.76 Yan Ta West Road, Xi'an 710061, People's Republic of China. [2]The First Affiliated Hospital of Xi'an Jiaotong University, Xi'an 710061, People's Republic of China.

References
1. Wang SJ, Guo X, Zuo H, Zhang YG, Xu P, Ping ZG, Zhang Z, Geng D. Chondrocyte apoptosis and expression of Bcl-2, Bax, Fas, and iNOS in articular cartilage in patients with Kashin-Beck disease. J Rheumatol. 2006;33(3):615–9.
2. Zhang F, Wen Y, Guo X, Zhang Y, Wang X, Yang T, Shen H, Chen X, Tian Q, Deng HW. Genome-wide association study identifies ITPR2 as a susceptibility gene for Kashin-Beck disease in Han Chinese. Arthritis Rheumatol. 2015;67(1):176–81.
3. Zhang F, Guo X, Zhang Y, Wen Y, Wang W, Wang S, Yang T, Shen H, Chen X, Tian Q. Genome-wide copy number variation study and gene expression analysis identify ABI3BP as a susceptibility gene for Kashin-Beck disease. Hum Genet. 2014;133(6):793–9.
4. Lu AL, Guo X, Aisha MM, Shi XW, Zhang Y, Zhang YY. Kashin-Beck disease and Sayiwak disease in China: prevalence and a comparison of the clinical manifestations, familial aggregation, and heritability. Bone. 2011;48(2):347–53.
5. Woolf AD, Pfleger B. Burden of major musculoskeletal conditions. Bull World Health Organ. 2003;81(9):646–56.
6. Glyn-Jones S, Palmer AJR, Agricola R, Price AJ, Vincent TL, Weinans H, Carr AJ. Osteoarthritis. Lancet. 2015;386(9991):376–87.

7. Duan C, Guo X, Zhang XD, Yu HJ, Yan H, Gao Y, Ma WJ, Gao ZQ, Xu P, Lammi M. Comparative analysis of gene expression profiles between primary knee osteoarthritis and an osteoarthritis endemic to Northwestern China, Kashin-Beck disease. Arthritis Rheum. 2010;62(3):771–80.

8. Fernandez-Tajes J, Soto-Hermida A, Vazquez-Mosquera ME, Cortes-Pereira E, Mosquera A, Fernandez-Moreno M, Oreiro N, Fernandez-Lopez C, Fernandez JL, Rego-Perez I, et al. Genome-wide DNA methylation analysis of articular chondrocytes reveals a cluster of osteoarthritic patients. Ann Rheum Dis. 2014;73(4):668–77.

9. Yong WS, Hsu FM, Chen PY. Profiling genome-wide DNA methylation. Epigenetics Chromatin. 2016;9:26.

10. Jeffries MA, Donica M, Baker LW, Stevenson ME, Annan AC, Humphrey MB, James JA, Sawalha AH. Genome-wide DNA methylation study identifies significant epigenomic changes in osteoarthritic cartilage. Arthritis Rheumatol. 2014;66(10):2804–15.

11. Rushton MD, Reynard LN, Barter MJ, Refaie R, Rankin KS, Young DA, Loughlin J. Characterization of the cartilage DNA methylome in knee and hip osteoarthritis. Arthritis Rheumatol. 2014;66(9):2450–60.

12. Zhang Y, Fukui N, Yahata M, Katsuragawa Y, Tashiro T, Ikegawa S, Lee MT. Genome-wide DNA methylation profile implicates potential cartilage regeneration at the late stage of knee osteoarthritis. Osteoarthr Cartil. 2016; 24(5):835–43.

13. Roach HI, Yamada N, Cheung KS, Tilley S, Clarke NM, Oreffo RO, Kokubun S, Bronner F. Association between the abnormal expression of matrix-degrading enzymes by human osteoarthritic chondrocytes and demethylation of specific CpG sites in the promoter regions. Arthritis Rheum. 2005;52(10):3110–24.

14. Shi XW, Shi BH, Lyu AL, Zhang F, Zhou TT, Guo X. Exploring genome-wide DNA methylation profiles altered in Kashin-Beck Disease Using Infinium Human Methylation 450 Bead Chips. Biomed Environ Sci. 2016;29(7):539–43.

15. Hawkins RD, Hon GC, Ren B. Next-generation genomics: an integrative approach. Nat Rev Genet. 2010;11(7):476.

16. Gao Y, Jones A, Fasching PA, Ruebner M, Beckmann MW, Widschwendter M, Teschendorff AE. The integrative epigenomic-transcriptomic landscape of ER positive breast cancer. Clin Epigenetics. 2015;7:16.

17. Wrzodek C, Eichner J, Buchel F, Zell A. InCroMAP: integrated analysis of cross-platform microarray and pathway data. Bioinformatics. 2013;29(4):506–8.

18. Guo X, Zuo H, Cao CX, Zhang Y, Geng D, Zhang ZT, Zhang YG, Von der Mark K, von de Mark H. Abnormal expression of Col X, PTHrP, TGF-beta, bFGF, and VEGF in cartilage with Kashin-Beck disease. J Bone Miner Metab. 2006;24(4):319–28.

19. Yang L, Zhang J, Zhao G, Wu C, Ning Y, Guo X, Wang X, Lammi MJ. Gene expression profiles and molecular mechanism of cultured human chondrocytes' exposure to T-2 toxin and deoxynivalenol. Toxicon. 2017;140:38–44.

20. Tchetina EV, Antoniou J, Tanzer M, Zukor DJ, Poole AR. Transforming growth factor-β2 suppresses collagen cleavage in cultured human osteoarthritic cartilage, reduces expression of genes associated with chondrocyte hypertrophy and degradation, and increases prostaglandin E 2 production. Am J Pathol. 2006;168(1):131–40.

21. Kveiborg M, Albrechtsen R, Couchman JR, Wewer UM. Cellular roles of ADAM12 in health and disease. Int J Biochem Cell Biol. 2008;40(9):1685–702.

22. Kveiborg M, Albrechtsen R, Rudkjaer L, Wen G, Damgaard-Pedersen K, Wewer UM. ADAM12-S stimulates bone growth in transgenic mice by modulating chondrocyte proliferation and maturation. J Bone Miner Res. 2006;21(8):1288.

23. Hao J, Wang W, Yan W, Xiao X, He A, Xiong G, Yang T, Liu X, Hui S, Chen X. A bivariate genome-wide association study identifies ADAM12 as a novel susceptibility gene for Kashin-Beck disease. Sci Rep. 2016;6:31792.

24. Delgado-Calle J, Fernández AF, Sainz J, Zarrabeitia MT, Sañudo C, García-Renedo R, Pérez-Núñez MI, García-Ibarbia C, Fraga MF, Riancho JA. Genome-wide profiling of bone reveals differentially methylated regions in osteoporosis and osteoarthritis. Arthritis Rheumatol. 2013;65(1):197.

25. Zhang X, Yazaki J, Sundaresan A, Cokus S, Chan SW, Chen H, Henderson IR, Shinn P, Pellegrini M, Jacobsen SE, et al. Genome-wide high-resolution mapping and functional analysis of DNA methylation in arabidopsis. Cell. 2006;126(6):1189–201.

26. Schubeler D. Function and information content of DNA methylation. Nature. 2015;517(7534):321–6.

27. Shimobayashi M, Hall MN. Making new contacts: the mTOR network in metabolism and signalling crosstalk. Nat Rev Mol Cell Biol. 2014;15(3):155.

28. Zhang Y, Vasheghani F, Li YH, Blati M, Simeone K, Fahmi H, Lussier B, Roughley P, Lagares D, Pelletier JP, et al. Cartilage-specific deletion of mTOR upregulates autophagy and protects mice from osteoarthritis. Ann Rheum Dis. 2015;74(7):1432–40.

29. Takayama K, Kawakami Y, Kobayashi M, Greco N, Cummins JH, Matsushita T, Kuroda R, Kurosaka M, Fu FH, Huard J. Local intra-articular injection of rapamycin delays articular cartilage degeneration in a murine model of osteoarthritis. Arthritis Res Ther. 2014;16(6):10.

30. Chen JQ, Holguin N, Shi Y, Silva MJ, Long FX. mTORC2 signaling promotes skeletal growth and bone formation in mice. J Bone Miner Res. 2015;30(2):369–78.

31. Chen JQ, Long FX. mTORC1 signaling controls mammalian skeletal growth through stimulation of protein synthesis. Development. 2014;141(14):2848–54.

32. Wu C, Zheng J, Yao X, Shan H, Li Y, Xu P, Guo X. Defective autophagy in chondrocytes with Kashin-Beck disease but higher than osteoarthritis. Osteoarthr Cartil. 2014;22(11):1936–46.

33. Ghiselli G. Drug-mediated regulation of glycosaminoglycan biosynthesis. Med Res Rev. 2017;37(5):1051.

34. Hardingham TE, Fosang AJ. Proteoglycans: many forms and many functions. FASEB J. 1992;6(3):861.

35. Kuiper NJ, Sharma A. A detailed quantitative outcome measure of glycosaminoglycans in human articular cartilage for cell therapy and tissue engineering strategies. Osteoarthr Cartil. 2015;23(12):2233–41.

36. Guiqin Z, Jinxian L, Yuxia S, Xie X, Liu Y. The obeservation of components of articular cartilage proteoglycan in Kashin-Beck disease children. Chinese J Control Endem Dis. 1990;04:200–2.

37. Mengyu T. Study on cartilage metabolism of Kashin-Beck Disease—a comparative analysis of urine hydroxyproline and acid aminopolysaccharides. J Xi'an Jiaotong Univ. 1979;03:41–7.

38. Luo M, Chen J, Li S, Sun H, Zhang Z, Fu Q, Li J, Wang J, Hughes CE, Caterson B, et al. Changes in the metabolism of chondroitin sulfate glycosaminoglycans in articular cartilage from patients with Kashin-Beck disease. Osteoarthr Cartil. 2014;22(7):986–95.

39. Teitelbaum SL, Ross FP. Genetic regulation of osteoclast development and function. Nat Rev Genet. 2003;4(8):638.

40. Wen Y, Guo X, Hao J, Xiao X, Wang W, Wu C, Wang S, Yang T, Shen H, Chen X. Integrative analysis of genome-wide association studies and gene expression profiles identified candidate genes for osteoporosis in Kashin-Beck disease patients. Osteoporos Int. 2016;27(3):1041–6.

41. Cravero JD, Carlson CS, Im HJ, Yammani RR, Long D, Loeser RF. Increased expression of the Akt/PKB inhibitor TRB3 in osteoarthritic chondrocytes inhibits insulin-like growth factor 1-mediated cell survival and proteoglycan synthesis. Arthritis Rheum. 2009;60(2):492.

42. Chen JZ, Crawford R, Xiao Y. Vertical inhibition of the PI3K/Akt/mTOR pathway for the treatment of osteoarthritis. J Cell Biochem. 2013;114(2):245–9.

43. Lee HH, Chang CC, Shieh MJ, Wang JP, Chen YT, Young TH, Hung SC. Hypoxia enhances chondrogenesis and prevents terminal differentiation through PI3K/Akt/FoxO dependent anti-apoptotic effect. Sci Rep. 2013;3:12.

44. Jia GH, Xia C, Xin PZ, Yi TT, Xiao YW, Gang S, Bing Z. 17β-Estradiol promotes cell proliferation in rat osteoarthritis model chondrocytes via PI3K/Akt pathway. Cell Mol Biol Lett. 2011;16(4):564–75.

45. Yu FF, Zhang YX, Zhang LH, Li WR, Guo X, Lammi MJ. Identified molecular mechanism of interaction between environmental risk factors and differential expression genes in cartilage of Kashin-Beck disease. Medicine. 2016;95(52):e5669.

46. Guo X, Ma WJ, Zhang F, Ren FL, Qu CJ, Lammi MJ. Recent advances in the research of an endemic osteochondropathy in China: Kashin-Beck disease. Osteoarthritis Cartil. 2014;22(11):1774–83.

47. Rani L, Mathur N, Gupta R. Genome-wide DNA methylation profiling integrated with gene expression profiling identifies PAX9 as a novel prognostic marker in chronic lymphocytic leukemia. Clin Epigenetics. 2017;9:57.

48. Zhang L, Ma S, Wang H, Su H, Su K, Li L. Identification of pathogenic genes related to rheumatoid arthritis through integrated analysis of DNA methylation and gene expression profiling. Gene. 2017;634:62–7.

Association between general joint hypermobility and knee, hip, and lumbar spine osteoarthritis by race

Portia P. E. Flowers[1], Rebecca J. Cleveland[1,2], Todd A. Schwartz[1,3,4], Amanda E. Nelson[1,2], Virginia B. Kraus[5], Howard J. Hillstrom[6], Adam P. Goode[7], Marian T. Hannan[8], Jordan B. Renner[1,9], Joanne M. Jordan[1,2,10] and Yvonne M. Golightly[1,10,11*]

Abstract

Background: Osteoarthritis (OA) prevalence differs by race. General joint hypermobility (GJH) may be associated with OA, but differences by race are not known. This community-based study examined the frequency of GJH and its relationship with knee, hip, and lumbar spine OA by race (African American vs. Caucasian).

Methods: Data were from the Johnston County OA project, collected 2003–2010. GJH was defined as Beighton score ≥ 4. OA symptoms were defined as the presence of pain, aching, or stiffness on most days separately at the knee, hip, and lower back. Radiographic OA (rOA) of the knee or hip was defined as Kellgren-Lawrence grade 2–4. Lumbar spine rOA was disc space narrowing grade ≥ 1 and osteophyte grade ≥ 2 in ≥ 1 at the same lumbar level. Lumbar spine facet rOA was present in ≥ 1 lumbar levels. Separate logistic regression models stratified by race were used to examine the association between hypermobility and rOA or OA symptoms at each joint site, adjusting for age, sex, previous joint injury, and body mass index (BMI).

Results: Of 1987 participants, 1/3 were African-American and 2/3 were women (mean age 65 years, mean BMI 31 kg/m^2). Nearly 8% of Caucasians were hypermobile vs. 5% of African-Americans ($p = 0.03$). Hypermobility was associated with lower back symptoms in Caucasians (adjusted odds ratio (aOR) 1.54, 95% confidence interval (CI) 1.00, 2.39), but not in African-Americans (aOR 0.77, 95% CI 0.34, 1.72). Associations between hypermobility and other knee, hip, or lumbar spine/facet OA variables were not statistically significant.

Conclusions: General joint hypermobility was more common in Caucasians than African-Americans. Although there were no associations between hypermobility and rOA, the association between hypermobility and lower back symptoms may differ by race.

Keywords: Osteoarthritis, General joint hypermobility, Cohort, Race, Pain

* Correspondence: golight@email.unc.edu
[1]Thurston Arthritis Research Center, University of North Carolina, 3300 Doc J. Thurston Bldg, CB#7280, Chapel Hill 27599-7280, NC, USA
[10]Department of Epidemiology, Gillings School of Global Public Health, University of North Carolina, Chapel Hill 27599, NC, USA
Full list of author information is available at the end of the article

Background

Osteoarthritis (OA) is a painful and debilitating joint disease and is a leading cause of disability. Although OA is common in all adults, the prevalence and severity of OA in some joints is greater among African-Americans than Caucasians. For example, compared to Caucasians, African-Americans experience a higher rate of progression [1] and higher prevalence of knee OA [2, 3] and have more severe superior hip joint space narrowing and more hip osteophytes than Caucasians [4]. At the lumbar spine, African-Americans also have a higher prevalence of disc space narrowing, vertebral osteophytes, and facet joint OA compared to Caucasians [5]. These observed differences in OA by race may in part be related to underlying biomechanical factors that alter joint mechanics or increase joint stresses, such as obesity or repetitive occupational activities.

General joint hypermobility (GJH), a condition involving abnormally large range of motion in the joints [6], is a biomechanical factor that may contribute to OA and joint pain [7–11]. Prior studies show variation in the relationship of hypermobility and OA or symptoms by joint site [12–14] and across populations [15–17]. For example, in a study of women 50+ years of age in the United Kingdom, hypermobility was associated with knee OA but had an inverse association with hand OA [12]. Hypermobility is more commonly associated with younger populations and women [15], but few studies have examined whether it varies by race. In a study of 81 Caucasian and 45 African-American women, Wood [18] reported that Caucasians were more likely to have hypermobility of the elbow (18% vs. 6%), the proximal interphalangeal (PIP) joints II–IV (90% vs. 74%), and PIP V (46% vs. 36%) when compared to African-Americans. Conversely, African-Americans exhibited hypermobility of the distal interphalangeal joints II–IV (79% v. 88%) and hyperextension of the thumb interphalangeal joints (52% vs. 66%) more frequently than Caucasians. In a study of US military personnel (male and female), Scher and colleagues [19] observed a higher adjusted incidence rate of a GJH syndrome diagnosis code in Caucasians compared to African-Americans (adjusted incidence rate ratio 1.44, 95% confidence interval 1.19, 1.75). Differences between Caucasians and African-Americans in the occurrence of hypermobility, particularly when including lower body joints, have not been examined in a large, community-based older adult population. Furthermore, it is not known whether the relationship between GJH and OA varies by race.

Considering the potential link between hypermobility and OA along with their independent variation by race, the purpose of this cross-sectional study of a large community-based sample was to (1) describe the frequency of GJH by race and (2) examine the relationship between GJH and radiographic OA (rOA) and symptoms consistent with OA at the knee, hip, and lumbar spine by race. We hypothesized that (1) Caucasians would be more likely to have GJH than African-Americans and (2) the relationship between GJH and rOA or OA symptoms would differ between Caucasians and African-Americans.

Methods
Study design

Participants were from the Johnston County OA Project, a community-based cohort study of individuals with and without OA [2]. Non-institutionalized Caucasian and African-American residents aged 45 years or older were recruited from six communities within Johnston County, North Carolina. Because the parent study was designed to examine racial differences in OA development and progression longitudinally, African-Americans were oversampled to allow for such comparisons. This study was approved by the Institutional Review Boards of the University of North Carolina School of Medicine and the Centers for Disease Control and Prevention (UNC 14–3219). All participants provided written informed consent prior to data collection.

Hypermobility

GJH data were collected during 2003–2010 and were assessed using the Beighton score [20]. For analyses, the first available Beighton score was used. When the Beighton measure was added to the parent project, only eight participants from the original cohort (enrolled 1991–1997) who attended their first follow up clinic visit completed this measure; most original cohort participants who returned for their second follow up visit (2006–2010) completed the Beighton measure ($N = 1115$, Fig. 1). Nearly all of the participants in the enrichment cohort (enrolled in 2003–2004) completed the Beighton measure as part of their baseline clinic visit; 22 enrichment cohort participants completed their first Beighton measure during their first follow up clinic visit (2006–2010, Fig. 1).

For the Beighton criteria, participants were evaluated on their ability to complete nine tasks involving joint range of motion: forward trunk flexion with palms on floor and knees extended, right and left knee hyperextension $\geq 10°$, right and left elbow hyperextension $\geq 10°$, right and left passive dorsiflexion of the 5th finger $\geq 90°$, and right and left passive apposition of thumb to forearm. One point was given for the completion of each maneuver, with scores ranging from 0 (unable to complete any maneuver) to 9 (able to complete all maneuvers). Based on previous literature, general joint hypermobility was defined as a Beighton score ≥ 4 [6]. Two examiners were trained by the Principal Investigator of the parent study to conduct musculoskeletal assessments and were re-trained prior to follow up data collection of the original cohort and the enrollment or follow up of the enhancement cohort. Inter-rater reliability was high ($\kappa > 0.80$) between the two

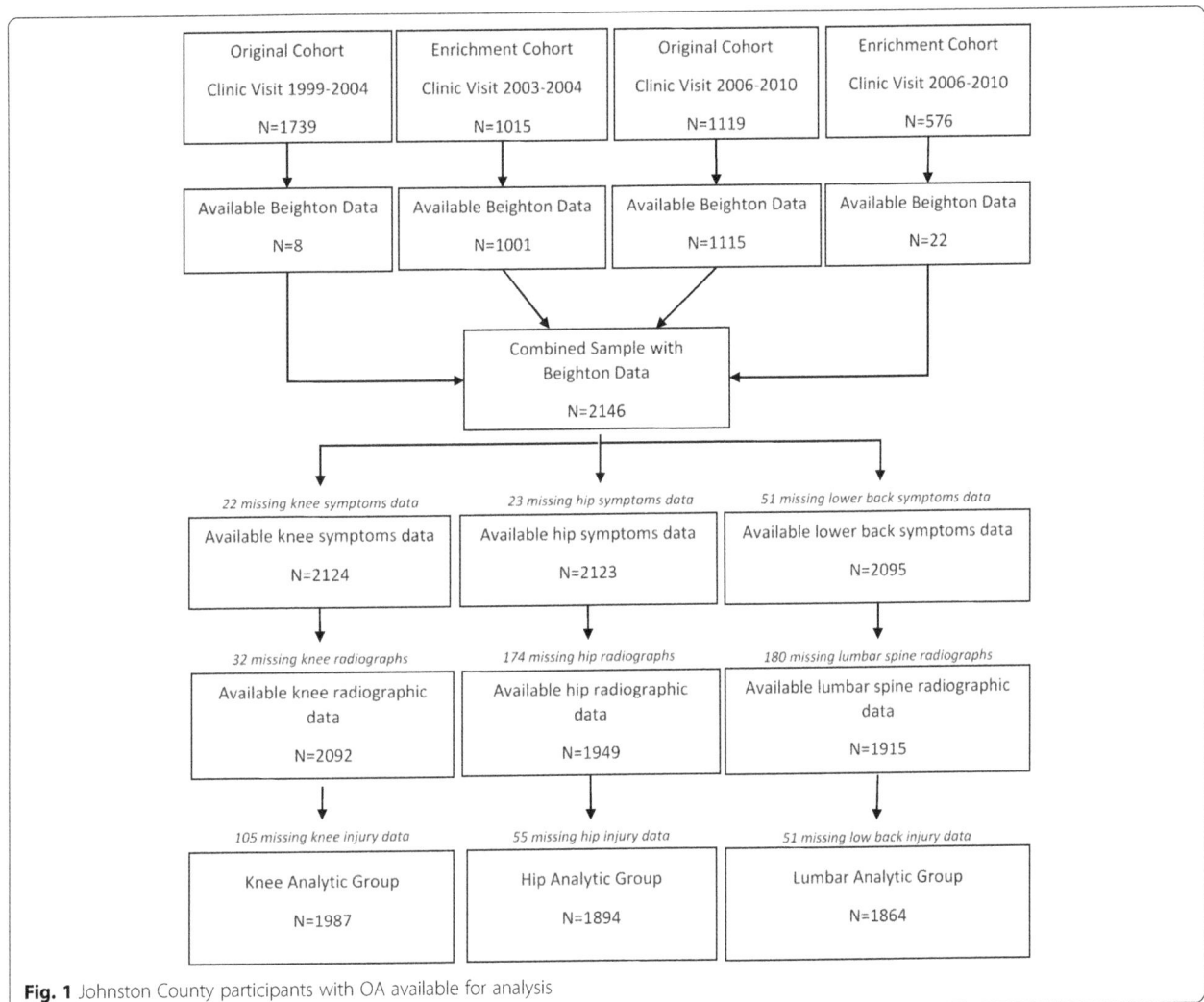

Fig. 1 Johnston County participants with OA available for analysis

examiners for each of the Beighton maneuvers (see Additional file 1: Table S1).

Osteoarthritis and symptoms

Knee and hip rOA was defined as a Kellgren Lawrence (KL) grade ≥2. Lumbar spine rOA was defined as disc space narrowing (DSN) grade ≥1 and presence of osteophytes (OST) grade ≥2 at the same lumbar level in at least one lumbar spine level. Lumbar spine facet joint rOA was defined as the presence or absence of OA features (e.g., osseous overgrowth, sclerosis) in at least one lumbar level. Radiographs at each site were evaluated by a single expert radiologist (JBR) who previously conducted intra-rater reliability analysis in a random sample of participants (intra-rater reliability for evaluation of hip/knee [21], κ = 0.89; of DSN [22], κ = 0.89; of OST [22], κ = 0.90; and of facet joints [22], κ = 0.73). Information on the presence of symptoms consistent with OA was obtained via questionnaire with the following question: "On most days, do you have pain, aching, or stiffness in your [right/left] hip/[right/left]

knee/lower back?" An affirmative answer determined the presence of symptoms at each particular joint. No time period for the duration of symptoms was specified.

Covariates

Race, age, and sex were collected via self-report, with race (African-American/Caucasian) and sex (men/women) treated as dichotomous variables. Age and body mass index (BMI; kg/m^2) were considered as continuous variables. History of joint injury was obtained via questionnaire consisting of two questions: "Has a doctor ever told you that you broke or fractured your [right/left] hip/[right/left] knee/lower back?" and "Other than a fracture, have you injured your [right/left] hip/[right/left] knee/lower back enough to require a cane, cast, or crutch for two weeks or longer?" Injury was defined as a "yes" response to at least one of the questions for a given joint site. BMI was calculated as Weight (kg) / (Height (m))^2 [2]. Height was measured using a calibrated stadiometer, and weight was measured using a balance-beam scale. Both measures were taken without shoes.

Statistical analysis

Means and standard deviations for continuous variables, and frequencies and percentages for categorical variables, were calculated for demographic and clinical characteristics at each joint site (knee, hip, and lumbar spine). Differences in percentages of hypermobility, symptoms, and rOA by racial group were assessed using chi-square statistics with a significance level of $p = 0.05$; no adjustments were made to p values for multiple comparisons. Separate logistic regression analyses, stratified by race (Caucasian vs. African-American), were carried out to examine the association between hypermobility and symptoms or rOA at the knee, hip, lumbar spine, and lumbar facet joints. Because the occurrence of GJH and OA are known to substantially differ by age, one set of models was adjusted for age only, and another set was adjusted for known OA risk factors including age [23], sex [24], history of joint injury [25, 26], and BMI [27]. All statistical analyses were completed using SAS System Software 9.4 (SAS Institute, Inc., Cary, NC, USA).

Results

A total of 2146 participants in the Johnston County OA parent study had available Beighton data (1123 participants from the original cohort, and 1023 participants from the enrichment cohort; Fig. 1). For the knee analytic group, 1987 participants were considered for analysis (Fig. 1; Table 1). For the hip analytic group, 1894 participants had available data, and 1864 participants were included in the lumbar spine analytic group (Fig. 1; Table 1). Participant characteristics were generally similar across the three analytic groups; all groups had a mean age of approximately 65 years and mean BMI of 31 kg/m^2. Nearly two thirds of participants were women, and one third was African-American. In the knee

analytic group, 16% of participants had a history of knee injury. Few participants in the hip and lumbar spine analytic groups reported a history of hip (5.0%) and back injury (2.4%). Patient characteristics for all three analytic groups were also similar to the total available participants ($N = 2146$).

Frequency of GJH, joint symptoms, and rOA by race

GJH was more common in Caucasians than in African-Americans (7.8% vs. 5.2%, $p = 0.03$; Table 2). Compared to Caucasians, symptoms at the knee occurred more frequently in African-Americans (49.0% vs. 42.6%, $p < 0.01$); a similar but non-significant difference was observed for knee rOA (41.2% vs. 37.2%, $p = 0.08$). Although not statistically significant, hip symptoms and hip rOA were slightly more common in Caucasians than African-Americans (34.3% vs. 30.6%, $p = 0.11$; 34.5% vs. 30.3%, $p = 0.07$, respectively). There was no difference by race in the occurrence of lower back symptoms (40.2% vs. 40.5%), but lumbar spine rOA and lumbar spine facet joint rOA were more common in Caucasians than in African-Americans (61.9% vs. 52.8%, $p < 0.01$; 73.7% vs. 60.5%, $p < 0.01$, respectively).

Association between GJH and symptoms or rOA by race

As shown in Table 3, there was a positive association between GJH and OA symptoms at the lumbar spine among Caucasians (adjusted odds ratio (aOR) 1.54, 95% confidence interval (CI) 1.00, 2.39), but a non-significant inverse relationship among African-Americans (aOR 0.77, 95% CI 0.34, 1.72). There were no statistically significant associations between hypermobility and knee, hip, lumbar spine rOA, or facet joint rOA for either race group. However, parameter estimates suggested an inverse association of GJH and rOA of the knee, hip, lower back symptoms or lumbar spine rOA and facet joint rOA among African-Americans, while estimates for Caucasians either appeared to be attenuated toward the null (knee rOA, lumbar spine rOA) or suggested a positive association (hip rOA, lumbar spine facet joint rOA).

Discussion

To our knowledge, this is the first study to examine GJH and its relationship to OA and OA symptoms among African-Americans and Caucasians in a large community-based sample of middle-to-older-aged adults. Results of this study suggest that the frequency of GJH may be lower in African-Americans than Caucasians and that the link between hypermobility and lower back symptoms may vary by race.

The frequency of GJH in the total sample was modest (around 7%), but Caucasians were somewhat more likely to have GJH than African-Americans, corresponding with previous studies reporting higher frequencies of general hypermobility and hypermobility at the elbow

Table 1 Distribution of GJH and patient characteristics (total sample and by joint site)

	Total sample and analytic groups			
	Total (N = 2146)	Knee (N = 1987)	Hip (N = 1894)	Lumbar spine (N = 1864)
Age (years), mean ± SD	65 ± 11	65 ± 11	66 ± 10	66 ± 10
Women, n (%)	1432 (66.7%)	1322 (66.5%)	1237 (65.3%)	1210 (64.9%)
African-American, n (%)	735 (34.3%)	670 (33.7%)	624 (33.0%)	615 (33.0%)
Body mass index (kg/m^2), mean ± SD	31 ± 7	31 ± 7	31 ± 7	31 ± 7
Prior joint injury, n (%)	461 (21.5%)	323 (16.3%)	94 (5.0%)	44 (2.4%)

GJH general joint hypermobility, *SD* standard deviation

Table 2 Distribution of GJH, joint symptoms and radiographic OA by race, Johnston County OA Project, 2003–2010

	Race		
	Caucasian (N = 1317)	African-American (N = 670)	p value
GJH, n/N (%)	103/1317 (7.8%)	35/670 (5.2%)	0.03
Knee symptoms, n/N (%)	561/1317 (42.6%)	328/670 (49.0%)	<0.01
Knee rOA, n/N (%)	490/1317 (37.2%)	276/670 (41.2%)	0.08
Hip symptoms, n/N (%)	435/1270 (34.3%)	191/624 (30.6%)	0.11
Hip rOA, n/N (%)	438/1270 (34.5%)	189/624 (30.3%)	0.07
Lower back symptoms, n/N (%)	502/1249 (40.2%)	249/615 (40.5%)	0.90
Lumbar spine rOA, n/N (%)	773/1249 (61.9%)	325/615 (52.8%)	<0.01
Lumbar spine facet joint rOA, n/N (%)	937/1272 (73.7%)	370/612 (60.5%)	<0.01

GJH general joint hypermobility, *OA* osteoarthritis, *rOA* radiographic osteoarthritis

and PIP joints for Caucasians compared to African-Americans [18, 19]. Considering previous reports of African Americans having more severe OA than Caucasians, it is possible that these results may be a reflection of disease severity with subsequent decreases in hypermobility. However, because we do not know the severity of symptoms or radiographic evidence of OA, we are unable to make this determination. In addition, African-Americans had a higher frequency of knee symptoms compared to Caucasians, corresponding with previous literature [2, 28, 29]. However, more Caucasians had rOA in the lumbar region compared to African-Americans; these results agree with a previous study of the Johnston County population, which reported a higher prevalence of lumbar spine disc space narrowing, vertebral osteophytes, and facet joint rOA in Caucasians compared to African-Americans [5].

The present study showed that hypermobility was positively associated with lower back symptoms in Caucasians. Though racial make-up was not reported by Larsson et al. [16] in a study of musicians, a positive association between GJH and lower back symptoms was also reported; specifically, 23% of musicians with hypermobility in the spine (i.e., positive Beighton trunk maneuver) had back symptoms (e.g.

Table 3 Race-specific multivariable logistic regression models for joint symptoms and radiographic OA with GJH

	Beighton ≥4	Beighton <4	Age-adjusted[a] OR (95% CI)	Multivariably adjusted[b] OR (95% CI)
Knee symptoms				
Caucasian	42/103 (40.8%)	519/1214 (42.8%)	0.92 (0.61–1.39)	1.00 (0.65–1.56)
African-American	14/35 (40.0%)	314/635 (49.4%)	0.67 (0.33–1.35)	0.70 (0.34–1.47)
Knee rOA				
Caucasian	29/103 (28.2%)	461/1214 (38.0%)	0.77 (0.49–1.23)	0.90 (0.55–1.47)
African-American	9/35 (25.7%)	267/635 (42.0%)	0.45 (0.20–1.02)	0.45 (0.19–1.09)
Hip symptoms				
Caucasian	33/90 (36.7%)	402/1180 (34.1%)	1.13 (0.73–1.77)	1.19 (0.75–1.87)
African-American	9/29 (31.0%)	182/595 (30.6%)	1.02 (0.46–2.29)	0.99 (0.43–2.27)
Hip rOA				
Caucasian	33/90 (36.7%)	405/1180 (34.3%)	1.26 (0.79–1.99)	1.30 (0.82–2.07)
African-American	8/29 (27.6%)	181/595 (30.4%)	0.84 (0.35–2.00)	0.79 (0.33–1.89)
Lower back symptoms				
Caucasian	45/91 (49.5%)	457/1158 (39.5%)	1.50 (0.98–2.30)	**1.54 (1.00–2.39)**
African-American	10/29 (34.5%)	239/586 (40.8%)	0.76 (0.35–1.67)	0.77 (0.34–1.72)
Lumbar Spine rOA				
Caucasian	51/91 (56.0%)	722/1158 (62.3%)	0.77 (0.51–1.18)	0.91 (0.58–1.43)
African-American	12/29 (41.4%)	313/586 (53.4%)	0.62 (0.29–1.31)	0.57 (0.25–1.28)
Lumbar facet rOA				
Caucasian	69/93 (74.2%)	868/1179 (73.6%)	1.03 (0.64–1.67)	1.31 (0.78–2.19)
African-American	16/28 (57.1%)	354/584 (60.6%)	0.87 (0.40–1.86)	0.74 (0.31–1.76)

OA osteoarthritis, *GJH* general joint hypermobility, *rOA* radiographic osteoarthritis
[a]Adjusted for age only
[b]Adjusted for age, gender, prior joint injury, and body mass index. Statistically significant odds ratios are represented in bold

, pain, weakness, stiffness) compared to 11% without hypermobility ($p < 0.001$). Interestingly, however, when assessing trunk hypermobility in the present study, we found inverse relationships between trunk hypermobility and lower back symptoms in both Caucasians (aOR = 0.37 (0.20–0.68)) and African Americans (aOR = 0.44 (0.20–0.99)) and 22% of individuals with trunk hypermobility had lower back symptoms compared to 41% without trunk hypermobility. With an average age of 65 ± 11 years in the present study compared to 25 ± 9 years in the study by Larsson et al. [16], this discrepancy may be a reflection of joint stiffening with age corresponding to decreasing hypermobility and increasing joint symptoms common to the presence of OA. Though no racial differences are apparent, future studies should further investigate the influence of age on changes in joint mobility and joint symptoms. In our study hypermobility was inversely associated with knee rOA in African-Americans, though it was not statistically significant (aOR = 0.45 (0.19–1.09)) . Again, this may be a reflection of more progressive joint disease and in African Americans compared to Caucasians, making the relationship between hypermobility and OA less apparent. Though it remains unclear why African-Americans with GJH were less likely to have knee rOA than those without hypermobility, this inverse relationship is not unprecedented as shown in previous studies reporting reduced risk of knee rOA in mostly Caucasian postmenopausal women with GJH [14] and inverse associations between hypermobility and knee rOA in a family-based prospective study of participants of mixed African-American and native American ancestry [13].

The present study benefits from the large community-based sample, the inclusion of African-American and Caucasian participants, the presence of participants who were 45 years of age and older to allow examination of OA, and the detailed data on GJH, rOA, and joint symptoms. However, there were several limitations of this study. These analyses were cross-sectional, and consequently, the contribution of GJH to rOA and progression of joint symptoms is not known. The Beighton criteria provide a general assessment of overall hypermobility, and results may differ if one examines hypermobility and rOA or symptoms at a single joint site (e.g., trunk hypermobility and lower back symptoms). In addition, this study assessed current hypermobility (i.e., at the time of the study visit) in our older adult sample. GJH is a condition found more commonly in younger individuals, potentially contributing to challenges with identifying relationships between hypermobility (waning with age as joints tend to stiffen over time [30, 31]) and OA (increasing with age). Thus, the lack of statistically significant associations between hypermobility and joint symptoms and rOA in our study may reflect the older age of our population. Studies that assess hypermobility in youth and subsequent rOA or joint symptom development and/or progression would clarify this association. The injury variables used as

covariates in these analyses were based on self-report, and there may be recall bias in which those with rOA or joint symptoms were more likely to recall a prior injury than those who were asymptomatic or free of joint disease. However, the use of medical records to assess history of injury may not be reliable either, since not all joint injuries are reported to health professionals (particularly if the individual considers the injury to be minor or recurrent), and retrospective retrieval would be difficult for those who had sustained an injury several decades prior to study assessments. The benefit of self-report over medical records is that it may capture more occurrences of injury.

Conclusions

In conclusion, Caucasians had a somewhat higher prevalence of GJH than African-Americans, although it was not a common condition in either group in this older adult population. Although our study results should be interpreted with caution, patterns suggest that associations of GJH and lower body OA symptoms may differ by race. Caucasians with hypermobility were more likely to have lumbar symptoms than those without hypermobility, but similar associations were not observed in African-Americans. Longitudinal studies of the changing relationship between hypermobility and rOA or OA symptom progression can further advance our understanding of the roles of hypermobility and race in OA.

Abbreviations

aOR: Adjusted odds ratio; BMI: Body mass index; DSN: Disc space narrowing; GJH: General joint hypermobility; KL: Kellgren Lawrence; OA: Osteoarthritis; OST: Osteophytes; PIP: Proximal interphalangeal; rOA: Radiographic OA

Acknowledgments

We are very thankful to the participants and staff in the Johnston County Osteoarthritis Project. This work would not be possible without their diligence and their dedication to this project.

Funding

This study was supported by National Institute of Arthritis and Musculoskeletal and Skin Diseases (NIAMS) (R01AR067743, R01AR067743-02S1, R01AR071440-01A1), NIH/NIAMS Multipurpose Arthritis and Musculoskeletal Diseases Center (P60AR30701), NIH/NIAMS Multidisciplinary Clinical Research Center (P60AR064166), Centers for Disease and Prevention Control (CDC)/Association of Schools of Public Health (S043, S3486), and Centers for Disease and Prevention Control (U01DP006266).

Authors' contributions

All authors were involved with the conception and design of the present study. JBR and JMJ were responsible for the design of and data acquisition for the parent study (Johnston County OA Project). All authors analyzed and interpreted data, drafted or revised the manuscript critically for important intellectual content, and approved the final version of the manuscript.

Consent for publication
Not applicable.

Competing interests
The authors declare that they have no competing interests.

Author details
[1]Thurston Arthritis Research Center, University of North Carolina, 3300 Doc J. Thurston Bldg, CB#7280, Chapel Hill 27599-7280, NC, USA. [2]School of Medicine, University of North Carolina, Chapel Hill 27599, NC, USA. [3]Department of Biostatistics, Gillings School of Global Public Health, University of North Carolina, Chapel Hill 27599, NC, USA. [4]School of Nursing, University of North Carolina, Chapel Hill 27599, NC, USA. [5]Department of Medicine, Duke Molecular Physiology Institute, School of Medicine, Duke University, Durham 27701, NC, USA. [6]Motion Analysis Laboratory, Hospital for Special Surgery, New York 10021, NY, USA. [7]Department of Orthopedic Surgery, Duke Clinical Research Institute, School of Medicine, Duke University, Durham 27708, NC, USA. [8]Institute for Aging Research, Hebrew SeniorLife, Boston 02131, MA, USA. [9]Department of Radiology, University of North Carolina, Chapel Hill 27599, NC, USA. [10]Department of Epidemiology, Gillings School of Global Public Health, University of North Carolina, Chapel Hill 27599, NC, USA. [11]Injury Prevention Research Center, University of North Carolina, Chapel Hill 27599, NC, USA.

References
1. Kopec JA, Sayre EC, Schwartz TA, Renner JB, Helmick CG, Badley EM, et al. Occurrence of radiographic osteoarthritis of the knee and hip among African Americans and whites: a population-based prospective cohort study. Arthritis Care Res (Hoboken). 2013;65:928–35.
2. Jordan JM, Helmick CG, Renner JB, Luta G, Dragomir AD, Woodard J, et al. Prevalence of knee symptoms and radiographic and symptomatic knee osteoarthritis in African Americans and Caucasians: the Johnston County Osteoarthritis Project. J Rheumatol. 2007;34:172–80.
3. Nelson AE, Renner JB, Schwartz TA, Kraus VB, Helmick CG, Jordan JM. Differences in multijoint radiographic osteoarthritis phenotypes among African Americans and Caucasians: the Johnston County Osteoarthritis Project. Arthritis Rheumatol. 2011;63:3843–52.
4. Nelson AE, Braga L, Renner JB, Atashili J, Woodard J, Hochberg MC, et al. Characterization of individual radiographic features of hip osteoarthritis in African American and white women and men: the Johnston County Osteoarthritis Project. Arthritis Care Res (Hoboken). 2010;62:190–7.
5. Goode AP, Marshall SW, Renner JB, Carey TS, Kraus VB, Irwin DE, et al. Lumbar spine radiographic features and demographic, clinical, and radiographic knee, hip, and hand osteoarthritis. Arthritis Care Res (Hoboken). 2012;64:1536–44.
6. Wolf JM, Cameron KL, Owens BD. Impact of joint laxity and hypermobility on the musculoskeletal system. J Am Acad Orthop Surg. 2011;19:463–71.
7. Golightly YM, Nelson AE, Hannan MT, Hillstrom HJ, Kraus VB, Cleveland RJ, et al. SAT0614 joint hypermobility and ankle osteoarthritis in a community-based cohort. Ann Rheum Dis. 2016;75:892.
8. Golightly YM, Goode AP, Cleveland RJ, Nelson AE, Hannan MT, Hillstrom HJ, et al. FRI0598 Relationship of joint hypermobility with low back pain and lumbar spine osteoarthritis: a cohort study. Ann Rheum Dis. 2016;75:659.
9. Grahame R. How often, when and how does joint hypermobility lead to osteoarthritis? Rheumatology (Oxford). 1989;28:320.
10. Golightly YM, Nelson AE, Kraus VB, Renner JB, Jordan JM. General joint hypermobility and hip osteoarthritis: the Johnston County osteoarthritis project [abstract]. Osteoarthr Cartil. 2012;20:S182.
11. Golightly YM, Hannan MT, Nelson A, Cleveland RJ, Kraus V, Schwartz TA,

Hillstrom HJ, Goode AP, Renner JB, Jordan JM. Is Joint Hypermobility Related to Foot Osteoarthritis and Symptoms? [abstract]. Arthritis Rheumatol. 2016;68(suppl 10):2852–4. http://acrabstracts.org/abstract/is-joint-hypermobility-related-to-foot-osteoarthritis-and-symptoms/. Accessed 1 Aug 2017.
12. Scott D, Bird H, Wright V. Joint laxity leading to osteoarthrosis. Rheumatol Rehabil. 1979;18:167–9.
13. Chen H-C, Shah SH, Li Y-J, Stabler TV, Jordan JM, Kraus VB. Inverse association of general joint hypermobility with hand and knee osteoarthritis and serum cartilage oligomeric matrix protein levels. Arthritis Rheumatol. 2008;58:3854–64.
14. Dolan AL, Hart DJ, Doyle DV, Grahame R, Spector TD. The relationship of joint hypermobility, bone mineral density, and osteoarthritis in the general population: the Chingford Study. J Rheumatol. 2003;30:799–803.
15. Remvig L, Jensen DV, Ward RC. Epidemiology of general joint hypermobility and basis for the proposed criteria for benign joint hypermobility syndrome: review of the literature. J Rheumatol. 2007;34:804–9.
16. Larsson L-G, Baum J, Mudholkar GS, Kollia GD. Benefits and disadvantages of joint hypermobility among musicians. N Engl J Med. 1993;329:1079–82.
17. Decoster LC, Bernier JN, Lindsay RH, Vailas JC. Generalized joint hypermobility and its relationship to injury patterns among NCAA lacrosse players. J Athl Train. 1999;34:99–105.
18. Wood PH. Is hypermobility a discrete entity? Proc R Soc Med. 1971;64:690–2.
19. Scher DL, Owens BD, Sturdivant RX, Wolf JM. Incidence of joint hypermobility syndrome in a military population: impact of gender and race. Clin Orthop Relat Res. 2010;468:1790–5.
20. Beighton P, Solomon L, Soskolne CL. Articular mobility in an African population. Ann Rheum Dis. 1973;32:413–8.
21. Jordan JM, Linder GF, Renner JB, Fryer JG. The impact of arthritis in rural populations. Arthritis Rheum. 1995;8:242–50.
22. Goode AP, Nelson AE, Kraus VB, Renner JB, Jordan JM. Biomarkers reflect differences in osteoarthritis phenotypes of the lumbar spine: the Johnston County Osteoarthritis Project. Osteoarthr Cartil. 2017;25:1672–9.
23. Oliveria SA, Felson DT, Reed JI, Cirillo PA, Walker AM. Incidence of symptomatic hand, hip, and knee osteoarthritis among patients in a health maintenance organization. Arthritis Rheumatol. 1995;38:1134–41.
24. Srikanth VK, Fryer JL, Zhai G, Winzenberg TM, Hosmer D, Jones G. A meta-analysis of sex differences prevalence, incidence and severity of osteoarthritis. Osteoarthr Cartil. 2005;13:769–81.
25. Moss AS, Murphy LB, Helmick CG, Schwartz TA, Barbour KE, Renner JB, et al. Annual incidence rates of hip symptoms and three hip OA outcomes from a U.S. population-based cohort study: the Johnston County Osteoarthritis Project. Osteoarthr Cartil. 2016;24:1518–27.
26. Gelber AC, Hochberg MC, Mead LA, Wang N-Y, Wigley FM, Klag MJ. joint injury in young adults and risk for subsequent knee and hip osteoarthritis. Ann Intern Med. 2000;133:321–8.
27. Cooper C, Snow S, McAlindon TE, Kellingray S, Stuart B, Coggon D, et al. Risk factors for the incidence and progression of radiographic knee osteoarthritis. Arthritis Rheumatol. 2000;43:995–1000.
28. Dillon CF, Rasch EK, Gu Q, Hirsch R. Prevalence of knee osteoarthritis in the United States: arthritis data from the Third National Health and Nutrition Examination Survey 1991-94. J Rheumatol. 2006;33:2271–9.
29. Sowers M, Lachance L, Hochberg M, Jamadar D. Radiographically defined osteoarthritis of the hand and knee in young and middle-aged African American and Caucasian women. Osteoarthr Cartil. 2000;8:69–77.
30. Chapman EA, de Vries HA, Swezey R. Joint stiffness: effects of exercise on young and old men. J Gerontol. 1972;27:218–21.
31. Such CH, Unsworth A, Wright V, Dowson D. Quantitative study of stiffness in the knee joint. Ann Rheum Dis. 1975;34:286–91.

From osteoarthritic synovium to synovial-derived cells characterization: synovial macrophages are key effector cells

Cristina Manferdini[1,2], Francesca Paolella[1], Elena Gabusi[2], Ylenia Silvestri[1], Laura Gambari[1], Luca Cattini[1], Giuseppe Filardo[3], Sandrine Fleury-Cappellesso[4] and Gina Lisignoli[1,2]*

Abstract

Background: The aim of the study was to characterize synovial cells from OA synovium with low-grade and moderate-grade synovitis and to define the role of synovial macrophages in cell culture.

Methods: Synovial tissue explants were analyzed for the expression of typical markers of synovial fibroblasts (SF), synovial macrophages (SM) and endothelial cells. Synovial cells at passage 1 (p.1) and 5 (p.5) were analyzed for different phenotypical markers by flow cytometric analysis, inflammatory factors by multiplex immunoassay, anabolic and degradative factors by qRT-PCR. P.1 and p.5 synovial cells as different cell models were co-cultured with adipose stem cells (ASC) to define SM effects.

Results: Synovial tissue showed a higher percentage of CD68 marker in moderate compared with low-grade synovitis. Isolated synovial cells at p.1 were positive to typical markers of SM (CD14, CD16, CD68, CD80 and CD163) and SF (CD55, CD73, CD90, CD105, CD106), whereas p.5 synovial cells were positive only to SF markers and showed a higher percentage of CD55 and CD106. At p.1 synovial cells released a significantly higher amount of all inflammatory (IL6, CXCL8, CCL2, CCL3, CCL5) and some anabolic (IL10) factors than those of p.5. Moreover, p.1 synovial cells also expressed a higher amount of some degradative factors (MMP13, S100A8, S100A9) than p.5 synovial cells. Co-culture experiments showed that the amount of SM in p.1 synovial cells differently induced or down-modulated some of the inflammatory (IL6, CXCL8, CCL2, CCL3, CCL5) and degradative factors (ADAMTS5, MMP13, S100A8, S100A9).

Conclusions: We found that p.1 (mix of SM and SF) and p.5 (only SF) synovial cells represent two cell models that effectively reproduce the low- or moderate-grade synovitis environment. The presence of SM in culture specifically induces the modulation of the different factors analyzed, confirming that SM are key effector cells.

Keywords: Osteoarthritis, Synovial fibroblasts, Synovial macrophages, Inflammatory factors, Degradative factors

Background

Osteoarthritis (OA) is defined as a disease of the whole joint because it affects not only the cartilage but the subchondral bone and the synovial tissue that undergo structural and metabolic modifications [1, 2]. Different reports have recognized the importance of synovial inflammation as a key factor associated with the pain and symptoms of OA, even in the early phase of the disease [3–5]. New imaging techniques (ultrasound and magnetic resonance imaging) demonstrate synovitis with effusion in 95 % of patients with OA and synovitis without effusion in 70 % of patients [6]. A recent report has identified a gene expression pattern of cells from inflamed and non-inflamed areas of synovial tissue in OA [7].

Synovial inflammation is a process characterized by synovial thickening (hypertrophy and hyperplasia) and cell infiltration (lymphocytes and macrophages) [8, 9]. Histological analysis of synovium in OA shows an increased number of lining cells and infiltrating cells, mainly

* Correspondence: gina.lisignoli@ior.it

[1]SC Laboratorio di Immunoreumatologia e Rigenerazione Tissutale, Istituto Ortopedico Rizzoli, Via di Barbiano 1/10, Bologna 40136, Italy

[2]SD Laboratorio RAMSES, Istituto Ortopedico Rizzoli, Bologna 40136, Italy

Full list of author information is available at the end of the article

consisting of macrophages [8, 10] with a very low percentage of B and T cells [11]. Synovial inflammation is now accepted as an important feature of the symptoms and progression of OA [6].

Normal synovial layers in OA are composed of synovial fibroblasts (SF) and inflammatory leukocytes (lymphocytes and macrophages) [12]. SF are mesenchymal cells that display many characteristics of fibroblasts, including vimentin, CD55, CD90, cadherin-11, vascular adhesion molecule-1 (VCAM-1) and intracellular adhesion molecule-1 (ICAM-1) [13–15]. SF constitutively produce IL6, chemokine (C-X-C motif) ligand (CXCL)8/IL8, chemokine (C-C motif) ligand (CCL)2/monocyte chemotactic protein (MCP-1), transforming growth factor (TGF)β, and fibroblast growth factor [13]. Moreover, synovium was recently reported to contain cells that, after isolation and cell-culture expansion, display a mesenchymal stem cell (MSC) phenotype indistinguishable from SF [15]. Synovial macrophage-like (SM) cells in OA show a phenotype similar to other resident cell macrophages, including CD11b, CD14, CD16 and CD68, and they produce the main inflammatory mediators, such as IL1, IL6, TNFα, matrix metalloproteinases (MMPs) and aggrecanases (ADAMTS), which contribute to articular matrix degradation [16]. Isolated synovial cells in OA are mainly composed of SF with 7 % SM, less than 0.5 % neutrophils and less than 0.1 % T cells [17]. It has been shown that depletion of CD14-positive SM results in a decline in IL1β and TNFα, thus indicating that these cells play a role in inflammation [17]. In the early stage of OA, a unique chemokine signature has been associated with synovial inflammation [3, 18]. CCL5/RANTES and CCL19/macrophage inflammatory protein (MIP)3β chemokines are mainly associated with inflammation [19].

Up to now there has been no in-depth characterization of the synovium and isolated synovial cells in OA. Recent papers [20, 21] have highlighted the importance of better characterization of synovial cells to elucidate the relationship between the different cell types to better define an in vitro cell model. This characterization might lead to better understanding of the interplay between cells in inflammatory and non-inflammatory conditions, to define a synovial cell model as a foundation for devising tailored therapeutic intervention.

To gain new insight into this topic we first analyzed synovial tissue biopsies for the expression of typical markers of SF, SM and endothelial cells and then we followed their expression in isolated synovial cells both at passage 1 (mix of SF and SM), and passage 5 (SF). Subsequently, we performed in-depth analysis of isolated cells for different phenotypical markers, inflammatory, anabolic and degradative factors. Finally, as inflammation induces adipose stem cells (ASC) to exert anti-inflammatory effects [22], we used these cells to test whether in co-culture experiments the presence of SM in synovial cells differently induced or down-modulated some of the inflammatory (IL6, CXCL8/IL8, CCL2/MCP-1, CCL3/MIP1-α, CCL5/RANTES) and degradative factors (ADAMTS5, MMP13, S100A8, S100A9) analyzed. We found that SM in culture induces the specific modulation of the different factors analyzed, thus confirming that SM are key effector cells.

Methods

Patient characterization

Synovial tissues were obtained from 26 patients with OA (14 women and 12 men, mean age 66 ± 11.10 years, body mass index 28 ± 4.45 Kg/m^2, disease duration 7 ± 4.8 years) and Kellgren/Lawrence grade 3/4 [23], who were undergoing total knee replacement surgery. Subcutaneous abdominal fat was obtained from six healthy patients undergoing liposuction. The study was approved by the Rizzoli Orthopaedic Institute ethical committee and all patients provided informed consent (Protocol number 15274).

Synovial tissue characterization

Synovial tissue specimens were fixed in B5 solution (freshly prepared 9:1 mixture of mercuric-chloride/40 % formaldehyde) at room temperature for 2 h and embedded in paraffin, and serial tissue sections (4 µm thick) from each specimen were prepared and routinely stained with hematoxylin-eosin. The histopathological features of each synovial tissue specimen were evaluated according to the synovitis inflammation scoring system described by Krenn [24], which rank each of the alteration evaluated (hyperplasia of the synovial lining layer, inflammatory infiltrate and stromal cell density) on a scale from 0 to 3. The parameters of synovitis inflammation scoring system were summarized as follows: 0–1 no synovitis; 2–3 low-grade synovitis; 4–6 moderate-grade synovitis; and 7–9 high-grade synovitis. The scoring was performed by two independent observers (CM and GL).

Immunohistochemical analysis of synovial tissue

Serial sections were incubated overnight at 4 °C with monoclonal anti-human-CD55 (2.5 µg/ml, Millipore, Temecula, CA, USA), –CD68 (10 µg/ml, Dako Cytomation, Denmark), –Factor VIII (10 µg/ml Dako), –CCL3/MIP1α (2.5 µg/ml R&D Systems, Minneapolis, MN, USA) and -S100A8 (4.5 µg/ml R&D) diluted in Tris-buffered saline (TBS) containing 0.1 % bovine serum albumin (BSA). Samples were then rinsed in TBS and sequentially incubated at room temperature for 20 minutes with multilinker biotinylated secondary antibody (Biocare Medical, Walnut Creek, CA, USA) and alkaline phosphatase-conjugated streptavidin (Biocare Medical). The reactions were developed using fast red substrate (Biocare Medical), counterstained with hematoxylin, and mounted in glycerol gel. Negative controls were performed using isotype control (Dako Cytomation). Semiquantitative analysis of immuno-histochemically stained slides were performed on 20 microscopic fields (×200 magnification) for each section. The analysis was performed using Red/Green/Blue (RGB) with Software NIS-Elements and Eclipse 90i microscope (Nikon Instruments Europe BV). Briefly, we acquired the total number of blue-stained nuclei and the total number of positive-stained red cells. The data were expressed as percentage of positive cells for CD55 and CD68, respectively. For Factor VIII analysis we counted the number of positive vessels in 20 microscopic fields. The data were expressed as the mean number of positive vessels/5 mm^2 area.

Isolation and characterization of synovial cells from non-digested fragments

Synovial cells were isolated following a standardized procedure as previously described [25] and were used for the experiments at both passages 1 and 5. Briefly, synovial tissue was fragmented and the pieces cultured for 7 days. Cultured synovial fragments were removed and fixed as described above. Synovial cells were grown in OPTIMEM culture medium (Life Technologies Italia, Monza, Italy) supplemented with 100 U/ml penicillin and 100 μg/ml streptomycin in a humidified atmosphere, at 37 °C with 5 % CO_2.

Synovial cells at both passages 1 (p.1) and 5 (p.5) were characterized by flow cytometry using the following markers expressed by SF (CD55 (2.5 μg/ml, Millipore), CD73, CD90, and CD105 (5 μg/ml, BD Pharmingen, San Jose, CA, USA), CD106 (10 μg/ml, Millipore), SM (CD14 and CD16 (5 μg/ml, Dako), CD68 (5 μg/ml, BD), CD80 (2 μg/ml, GeneTex Inc., Irvine, CA, USA), and CD163 (10 μg/ml, Abcam, Cambridge, UK)), and by endothelial (CD31, 2 μg/ml, R&D) and mononuclear cells (CD3, CD34, and CD45 (5 μg/ml, Dako). Briefly, after harvesting cells upon detachment, they were washed twice with PBS, centrifuged, and washed in a flow cytometry buffer (PBS supplemented with 2 % BSA and 0.1 % sodium azide).

Aliquots of 1×10^5 cells were then incubated with primary antibodies at 4 °C for 30 minutes, washed twice with a flow cytometry buffer, and incubated with polyclonal rabbit anti-mouse immunoglobulins/fluorescein isothiocyanate (FITC) conjugate (Dako Cytomation) at 4 °C for 30 minutes. After two final washes, the cells were analyzed using a fluorescence-activated cell sorting (FACS) CantoII Cytometer (Becton Dickinson). For isotype control, non-specific mouse IgG was substituted for the primary antibody.

Passage 1 and 5 synovial cells as specific cell models for cell co-culture

Synovial cells at both passages 1 and 5 (100,000 cells/well) were seeded in the lower chamber of a 6-well plate and co-cultured with clinical grade ASC (100,000 cells in Transwells®) for 7 days (medium was changed at day 2) in complete DMEM using a defined cell ratio (1:1) that assures no cell proliferation, as we previously reported [22]. ASC were isolated from subcutaneous abdominal fat according to Good Manufacturing Practice (GMP) [26], and were grown in αMEM supplemented with platelet lysate (PLP) and characterized for the CD markers CD14, CD34, CD45, CD73, CD90 (5 μg/ml, BD Pharmingen) and CD13 (1 μg/ml, eBioscience, San Diego, CA, USA) as we previously described [22, 26] (data not shown). Control cells were mono-cultures of ASC and synovial cells at both passages 1 and 5. The cells were harvested on day 7 for quantitative RT-PCR analysis and supernatant stored at −80 °C. The concentrations of IL6, CXCL8/IL8, CCL2/MCP-1, CCL3/MIP1-α, and CCL5/RANTES were analyzed in the supernatant for all conditions tested as described above.

Cytokine and chemokine release in supernatants

The concentrations of IL1β, IL4, IL6, CXCL8/IL8, IL10, CCL2/MCP-1, CCL3/MIP1α, CCL5/RANTES, TGFβ, and TNFα were simultaneously evaluated in the supernatants of ASC, synovial cells at both passages (1 and 5) in mono- and co-cultures, using multiplex bead-based sandwich immunoassay kits (BioRad Laboratories Inc., Segrate, Italy) following the manufacturer's instructions. Briefly, we added 50 μl to each well of the diluted standards (fourfold dilution series), controls, and samples in triplicate and added 50 μl of coupled beads, and the plate was incubated at room temperature for 30 minutes. The plate was then washed three times with 100 μl of wash buffer and incubated with 25 μl of detection antibodies for 30 minutes. Finally, the plate was washed three times and incubated with 50 μl of streptavidin-PE for 30 minutes and measured in a reader (Luminex Bioplex system, Bio-Rad Laboratories Inc.).

Real-time quantitative reverse transcription polymerase chain reaction (qRT-PCR) analysis

Total RNA was extracted from human ASC, synovial cells in mono- and co-cultures, using RNA PURE reagent (Euroclone Spa, Pero, Italy) according to the manufacturer's instructions, and then was treated with DNase I (DNA-free Kit, Life Technologies). Reverse transcription was performed using SuperScript VILO (Life Technology) reverse transcriptase and random hexamers, following the manufacturer's protocol.

Forward and reverse oligonucleotides for PCR amplification of ADAMTS4, ADAMTS5, MMP13, S100A8, and S100A9 are described in Table 1, and real-time PCR was run as previously described [22]. All primer efficiencies were confirmed to be high (>90 %) and comparable (Table 1). For each target gene, messenger RNA (mRNA)

Table 1 Oligonucleotide primers used for real-time polymerase chain reaction

Target gene	Primers (forward and reverse)	Product size (bp)	GenBank accession number	Primer efficiency (%)
RPS9	GATTACATCCTGGGCCTGAA ATGAAGGACGGGATGTTCAC	161	NM_001013	94.5
ADAMTS4	CTGCCTACAACCACCG GCAACCAGAACCGTCC	293	NM_005099.4	99.1
ADAMTS5	GCACTTCAGCCACCATCAC AGGCGAGCACAGACATCC	187	NM_007038.3	92.4
MMP13	TCACGATGGCATTGCT GCCGGTGTAGGTGTAGA	277	NM_002427	94.5
S100A8	TAGAGACCGAGTGTCCTCA CGCCCATCTTTATCACCAGA	126	NM_002964.4	93.4
S100A9	CCATCATCAACACCTTCCACCA CTGCTTGTCTGCATTTGTGTCC	179	NM_002965.3	91.4

levels were calculated, normalized to RPS9 according to the formula $2^{-\Delta Ct}$, and expressed as a percentage of the reference gene, as this was expressed in the same amount in all conditions tested.

Statistical analysis

Statistical analysis was performed using non-parametric tests because the data did not have a normal distribution (Kolmogorov-Smirnov test). Friedman's analysis and Dunn's post hoc test was used to analyze more than two groups of paired data, the Mann–Whitney U test was used to analyze unpaired two-group data and the Wilcoxon test was used to analyze paired two-group data. Groups with small samples were evaluated using the exact method. Values were expressed as the median and interquartile range. CSS Statistica Statistical Software (Statsoft Inc., Tulsa, OK, USA) was used for analysis and values of $p < 0.05$ were considered significant.

Results

OA synovial tissue explant characterization

Synovial tissue explants from 26 patients with OA were first scored on hematoxylin-eosin-stained slides, as reported by Krenn [24] and we found low-grade synovitis in 4 samples and moderate-grade synovitis in 22 samples. Vessel proliferation was also evaluated on Factor VIII-stained slides and there were fewer positive vessels ($90 \pm 35/5$ mm^2 area) in low-grade than in moderate-grade synovitis ($222 \pm 79/5$ mm^2 area). Then, for in-depth analysis of the main synovial cell populations present in the synovial tissue, we analyzed CD68 and CD55 to establish the percentage of synovial macrophages and synovial fibroblasts, in both low- and moderate-grade synovitis. As shown in Fig. 1a, CD68 was mainly positive on synovial macrophages located in the lining layer and on a few in the sublining layer (Additional file 1). There were approximately 13 % and 27 % of CD68-positive cells in low- and moderate-grade synovitis, respectively (Fig. 1b). The CD55 typical marker of synovial fibroblast was positive both on the sublining and lining layers (Fig. 1a) (Additional file 1) and was approximately 70 % positive in both low- and moderate-grade synovitis (Fig. 1b).

Synovial cells characterization

The cells outgrowing from cultured-synovium tissue fragments (Fig. 2a) were then morphologically and phenotypically analyzed. As shown in Fig. 2a, at p.0 cells started outgrowth from synovial tissue fragments; at p.1 we found two cell types, one spindle-shaped (defined as synovial fibroblasts, SF) and one with polygonal-star morphology (defined as synovial macrophages, SM), whereas at p.5 all cells had only spindle-shaped morphology. Moreover, to confirm that SM and SF had these peculiar cell morphologies, we immunocytochemically stained the isolated p.1 and p.5 cells with anti-CD68 and anti-CD55, typical markers of SM and SF, respectively (data not shown).

These cells at both passages (p.1 and p.5), were then characterized by flow cytometry for markers expressed by SF (CD55, CD73, CD90, CD105, and CD106), SM (CD14, CD16, CD68, CD80, and CD163), endothelial cells (CD31), and mononuclear cells (CD3, CD34, and CD45). As shown in Fig. 2b, p.1 synovial cells had a very low percentage (<3 %) of CD3, CD31, CD34, and CD45, an intermediate percentage (10–20 %) of CD14, CD16, CD68, CD80, CD106 and CD163, and a high percentage (60–100 %) of CD55, CD73, CD90, and CD105. Interestingly, CD80 and CD163 were expressed (approximately 12 %) only by p.1 synovial cells. Conversely, p.5 synovial cells had a very low or negative percentage of all the markers analyzed except for CD55, CD73, CD90, CD105 and CD106. In particular, CD55 and CD106 were the only markers more highly expressed by p.5 synovial cells.

Factors released by OA synovial cells

We subsequently evaluated inflammatory factors (IL1β, TNFα, IL6, CXCL8/IL8, CCL2/MCP-1, CCL3/MIP1α, and CCL5/RANTES) and anabolic factors (TGFβ, IL4, and IL10) released by p.1 and p.5 OA synovial cells. As shown in Fig. 3, p.1 synovial cells produced significantly more IL6, CXCL8/IL8, CCL2/MCP-1, CCL3/MIP1α, CCL5/RANTES, and IL10 than those at p.5. IL1β, TNFα, TGFβ and IL4 were not detected at either passage (p.1 or p.5). In particular, p.1 synovial cells released more IL6, CXCL8/IL8, and CCL2/MCP-1 than CCL3/MIP1α, CCL5/RANTES, and IL10. Interestingly, CCL2/MCP-1

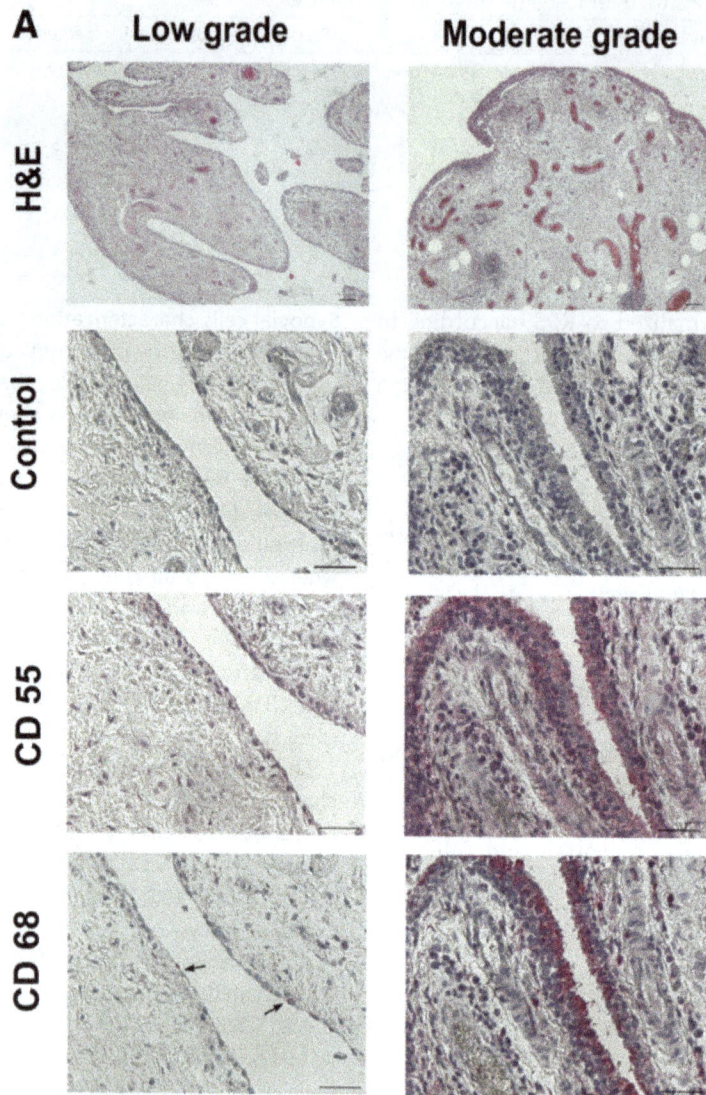

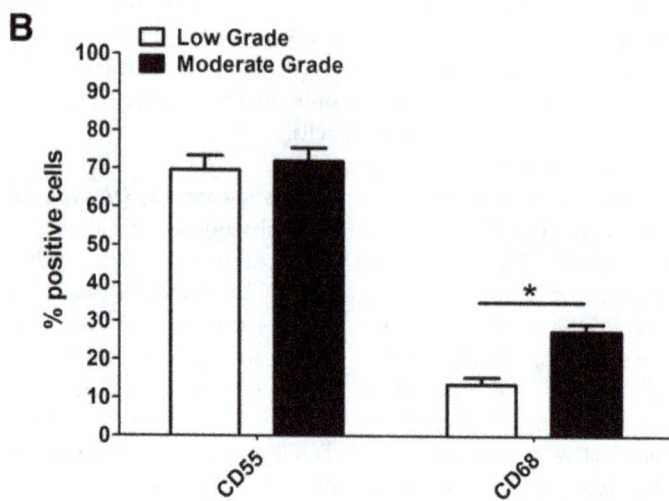

Fig. 1 (See legend on next page.)

(See figure on previous page.)
Fig. 1 Characterization of synovial tissue in osteoarthritis (OA). **a** Representative samples with low-grade (*left*) and moderate-grade (*right*) OA synovitis, stained with hematoxylin-eosin (*H&E*). *Bars* 100 μm (magnification × 40). Immunohistochemical analysis of CD55 and CD68 on representative cases with low-grade (*left*) and moderate-grade (*right*) synovitis in OA. Negative control for CD55 and CD68 (*Control*). *Bars* 50 μm. **b** Percentage of positive cells to CD55 and CD68 analyzed in both low-grade (n = 4) and moderate-grade (n = 22) synovitis in OA. Data are expressed as the median and interquartile range. *Significant differences between low-grade and moderate-grade synovitis: $p < 0.005$

was the most abundant factor released by p.5 synovial cells, whereas there was less IL6, CXCL8/IL8, and CCL5/RANTES. IL10 and CCL3/MIP1α from p.5 synovial cells were at the limit of detection or not detected, respectively.

OA synovial cell degradative factors

Then we analyzed different factors (ADAMTS4, ADAMTS5, MMP13, S100A8, S100A9) involved in the degradation of joint tissue. As shown in Fig. 4, both synovial cells at p.1 and p.5 expressed the same level of

ADAMTS4, whereas there was significantly more ADAMTS5 expressed in p.5 than in p.1 synovial cells. Conversely, MMP13, S100A8, and S100A9 were highly expressed in p.1 synovial cells, but there was very low expression of in MMP13 in p.5 synovial cells, and S100A8 and S100A9 were not detected.

Synovial macrophages influence cell co-culture effects

The presence of SM in p.1 synovial cells significantly increased the release of inflammatory, anabolic and

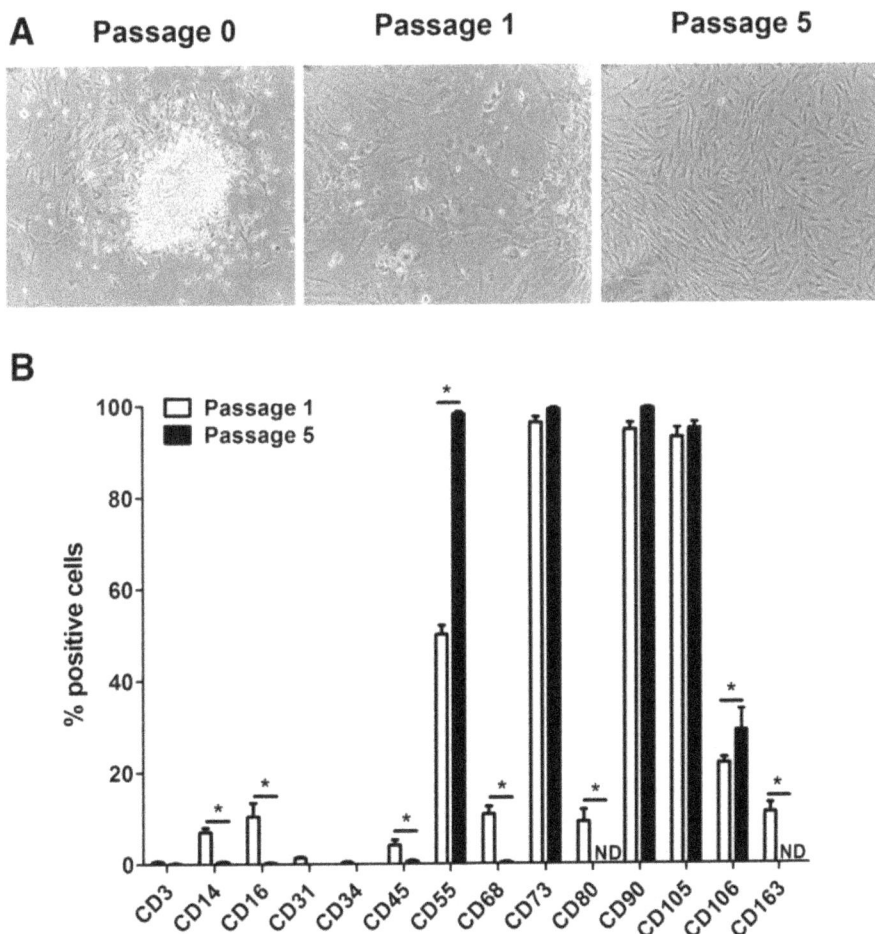

Fig. 2 Evaluation of isolated passage 1 and passage 5 synovial cells from moderate-grade synovitis in osteoarthritis. **a** Outgrowth of synovial cells from synovial non-digested fragments (*Passage 0*). Passage 1 synovial cells characterized by a mix of cells with a spindle and a polygonal-star shape. Passage 5 synovial cells characterized only by spindle-shaped morphology. **b** CD3,CD14, CD16, CD31, CD34, CD45, CD55, CD68, CD73, CD80, CD90, CD105, CD106, and CD163 immunocytochemical staining on passage 1 and passage 5 synovial cells analyzed by flow cytometry. Data are expressed as the median and interquartile range (n = 22). *Significant differences between passage 1 and passage 5 synovial cells: $p < 0.005$. *ND* not detected

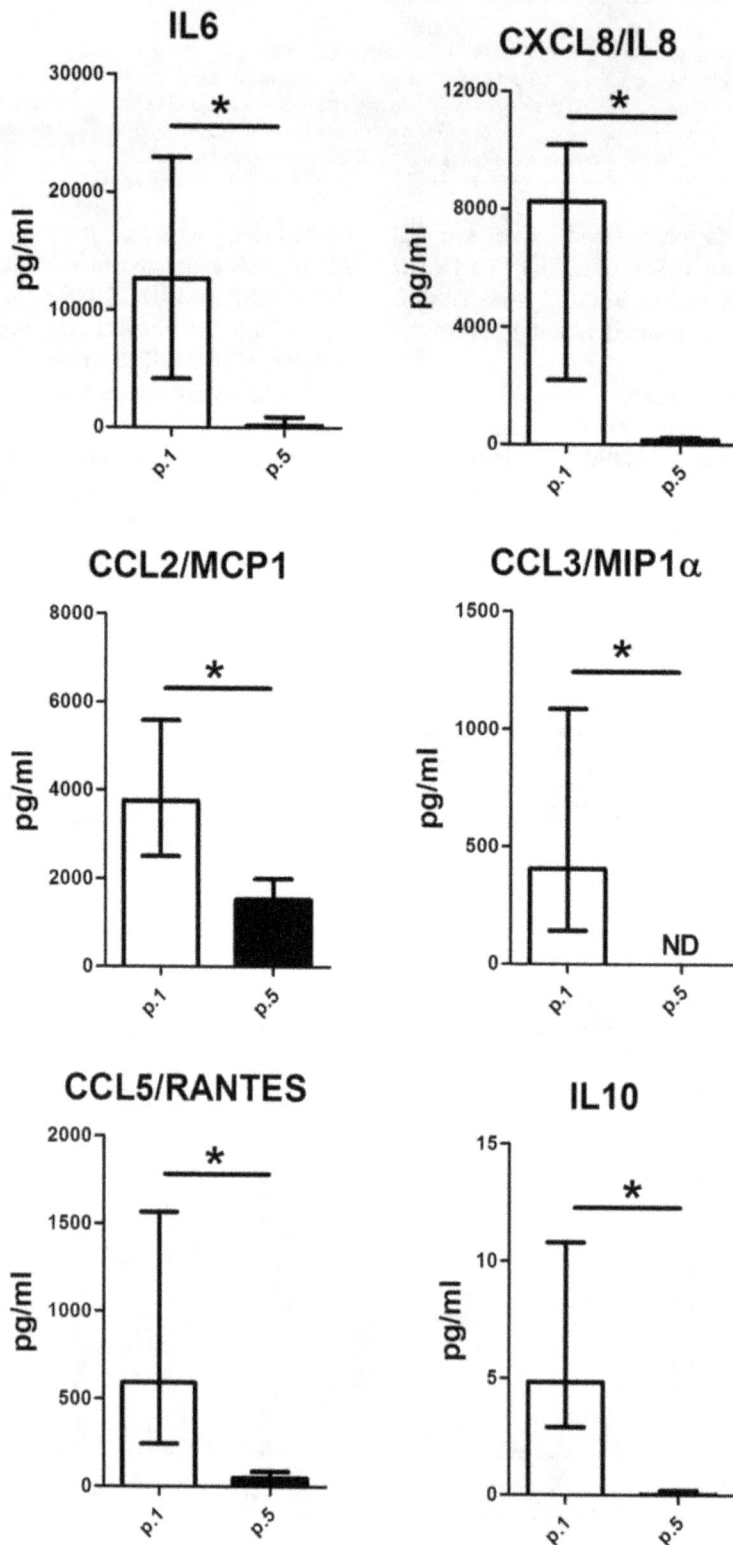

Fig. 3 Evaluation of inflammatory and anabolic factors released by passage 1 (*p.1*) and passage 5 (*p.5*) synovial cells from osteoarthritic moderate-grade synovitis. IL6, CXCL8/IL8, CCL2/monocyte chemotactic protein 1 (*MCP-1*), CCL3/macrophage inflammatory protein 1α (*MIP1α*), CCL5/RANTES, and IL10 were evaluated in the supernatant of both p.1 and p.5 synovial cells as described in "Methods". Data are expressed as the median and interquartile range (n = 22). *Significant differences between synoviocytes at p.1 and p.5: $p < 0.005$

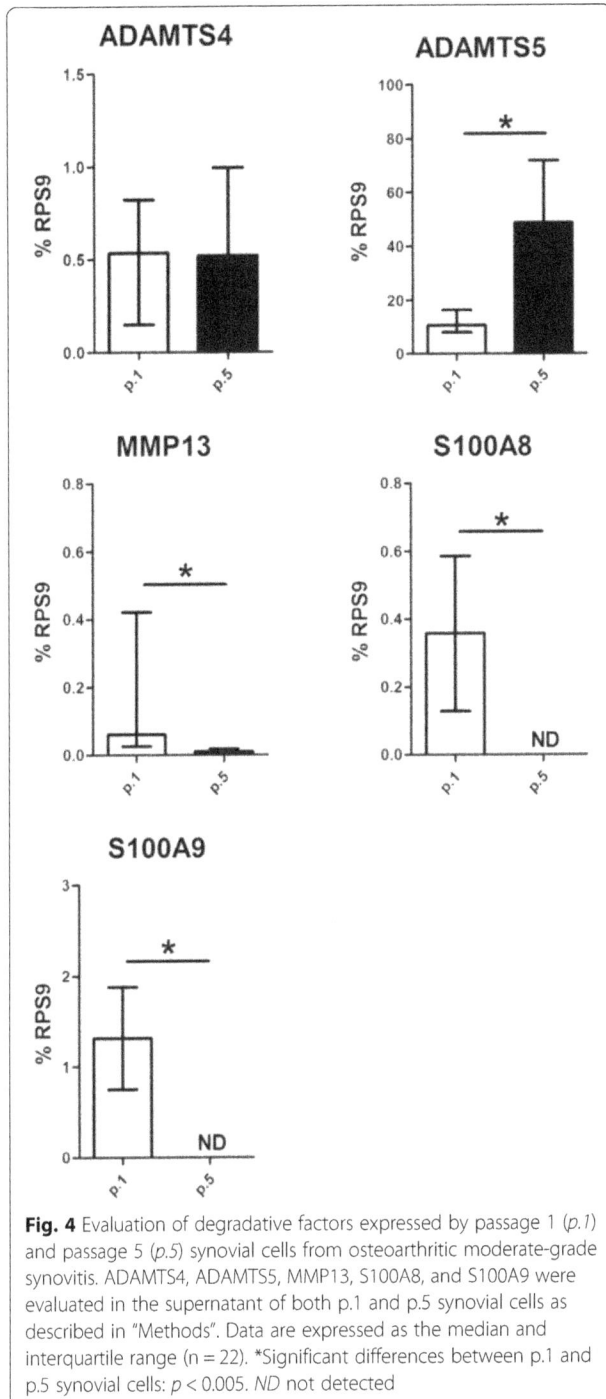

Fig. 4 Evaluation of degradative factors expressed by passage 1 (*p.1*) and passage 5 (*p.5*) synovial cells from osteoarthritic moderate-grade synovitis. ADAMTS4, ADAMTS5, MMP13, S100A8, and S100A9 were evaluated in the supernatant of both p.1 and p.5 synovial cells as described in "Methods". Data are expressed as the median and interquartile range (n = 22). *Significant differences between p.1 and p.5 synovial cells: $p < 0.005$. *ND* not detected

degradative factors, thus creating a significantly different milieu from p.5 synovial cells. Therefore, as p.1 and p.5 synovial cells represent two different cell culture models, we tested whether they could differently affect another cell type in co-culture. We chose adipose stem cells (ASC) as the cell model because they are reportedly activated by an inflammatory environment [22]. We analyzed inflammatory and degradative factors, previously tested in basal conditions in p.1 and

p.5 synovial cells (Figs. 3 and 4), after co-culture with ASC. We did not test IL10 because ASC express and release large amounts of this cytokine, but did not express the other factors analyzed (data not shown). As we previously reported [22], we confirmed that ASC in co-culture with p.1 synovial cells reduced the release of IL6, CXCL8/IL8, CCL2/MCP-1, CCL3/MIP1α, and CCL5/RANTES (Fig. 5a). Conversely, as shown in Fig. 5b, the co-culture of ASC with p.5 synovial cells (only SF) differently affected the release of the factors evaluated, thus indicating direct dependence by the presence of SM in culture. In particular, ASC when co-cultured with p.5 synovial cells were able to increase the release of IL6 and CXCL8/IL8, however they were unable to affect or significantly decreased, the release of macrophage-like chemokines, such as CCL2/MCP-1 and CCL5/RANTES, respectively. Interestingly, as shown in Fig. 5b, on p.5 synovial cells the ASC were unable to modulate CCL3/MIP1α that was still not released or expressed (data not shown) by SF. Moreover, as shown in Fig. 5c the analysis of degradative factors revealed that ASC on p.1 synovial cells decreased the expression of ADAMTS5, S100A8, and S100A9, but ADAMTS4 and MMP13 were not affected. Conversely, ASC on p.5 synovial cells induced the expression of MMP13 and did not modulate the other factors analyzed (Fig. 5d).

Moreover, to confirm that the effects observed were directly dependent on the amount of SM in synovial cells p.1 we also evaluated all the inflammatory and degradative factors in p.1 synovial cells isolated from low-grade synovial explants, which, as shown in Fig. 1b, contain a very low percentage of SM (CD68 positive). As shown in Fig. 5e-f, ASC were unable to reduce the inflammatory and degradative factors in p.1 synovial cells from low-grade synovitis, except for CCL5/RANTES and ADAMTS5, but MMP13 was induced.

Immunohistochemical analysis of CD68, CCL3/MIP1α and S100A8 on synovial tissue

Furthermore, to confirm that CCL3/MIP1α and S100A8 were specific markers of SM, we also immunostained serial sections of synovial tissue from patients with moderate synovitis using the positive control macrophage marker CD68. As shown in Fig. 6, we confirmed that SM positive to CD68 were also positive to CCL3/MIP1α and S100A8, which we also detected only on p.1 synovial cells. Positive cells were mainly located on the lining layer and around the vessels.

Discussion

Synovitis is a typical feature in a high percentage of patients with OA, even in the early phase of the disease [3]. Hyperplasia in the synovium is associated with an increased number of synovial lining cells in OA,

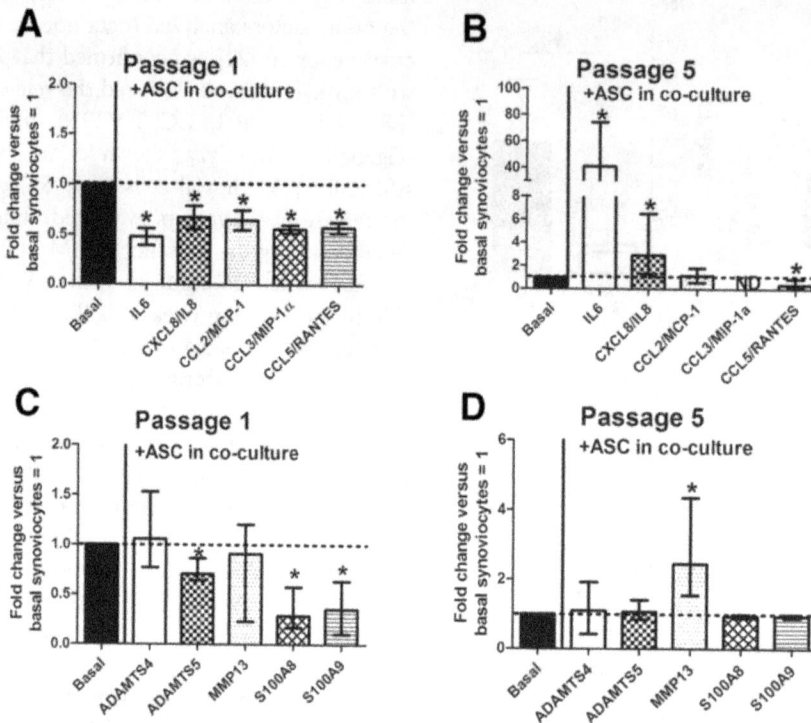

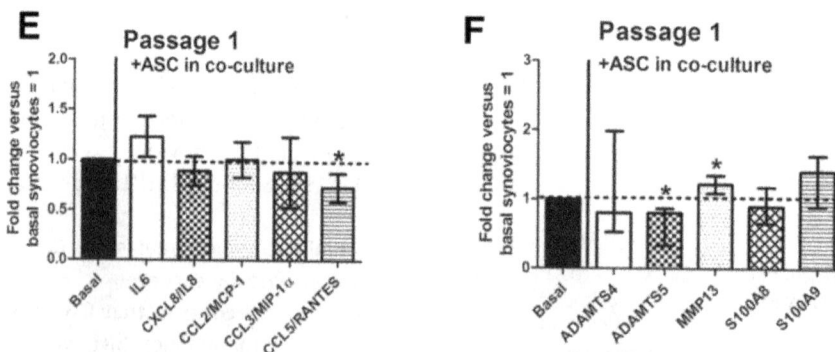

Fig. 5 Evaluation of the role of macrophage in cell co-cultures. **a-d** Co-culture of adipose stem cells (*ASC*) with passage 1 (p.1) (**a, c**) and passage 5 (p.5) (**b, d**) synovial cells from osteoarthritic moderate-grade synovitis and evaluation of released inflammatory (IL6, CXCL8/IL8, CCL2/MCP-1, CCL3/MIP1α, and CCL5/RANTES) and expressed degradative factors (ADAMTS4, ADAMTS5, MMP13, S100A8, and S100A9). Data are represented as fold changes versus basal synoviocytes = 1 and expressed as the median and interquartile range (n = 22). *Significant differences between p.1 and p.5 synovial cells: *p* < 0.005. **e-f** Co-culture of ASC with p.1 synovial cells from low-grade osteoarthritic synovitis and evaluation of released inflammatory (IL6, CXCL8/IL8, CCL2/MCP-1, CCL3/MIP1α, and CCL5/RANTES) (**e**) and expressed degradative factors (ADAMTS4, ADAMTS5, MMP13, S100A8, and S100A9) (**f**). Data are represented as fold changes versus basal synoviocytes = 1 and expressed as the median and interquartile range (n = 4). *Significant differences between p.1 and p.5 synovial cells: *p* < 0.005

accompanied by infiltration of inflammatory cells mainly consisting of macrophages [8]. Synovial tissue is a complex structure mainly composed of SF and SM, and in vitro cell models have mainly focused on SF. Therefore, we characterized synovial tissue from low-grade and moderate-grade synovitis and synovial cell outgrowth from cultured non-digested synovial fragments. These cells were analyzed at two cell passages (p.1, a mix of SF and SM and p.5, only SF) to define their phenotype, inflammatory and degradative factors and their functional role.

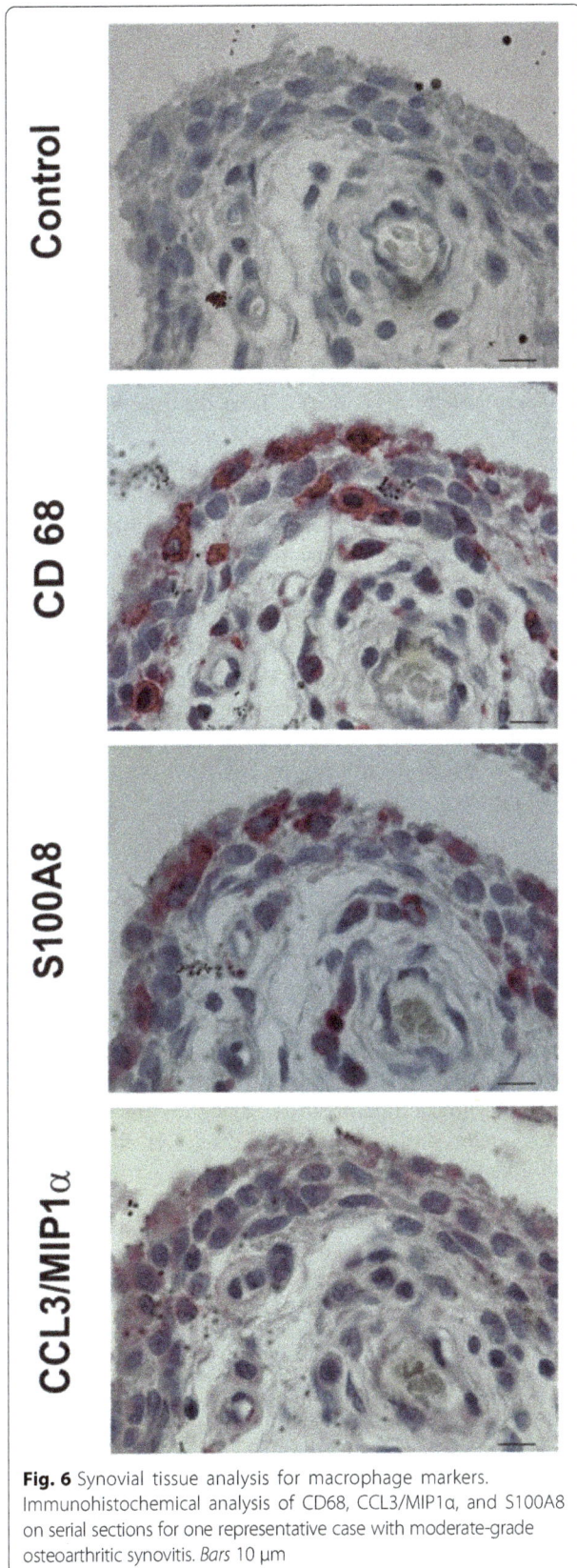

Fig. 6 Synovial tissue analysis for macrophage markers. Immunohistochemical analysis of CD68, CCL3/MIP1α, and S100A8 on serial sections for one representative case with moderate-grade osteoarthritic synovitis. *Bars* 10 μm

Our data show that synovium from patients with OA and moderate synovitis had approximately 27 % CD68 (SM) and 70 % CD55 (SF) positive cells, which are well-standardized markers for SM and SF, respectively. The synovial cells outgrowing in culture were evaluated at both p.1 and p.5. SF (p.5) were not positive to typical endothelial (CD31), hematopoietic (CD3, CD34, and CD45) and macrophage-like markers (CD14, CD16, CD68, CD80, and CD163) but they expressed more CD55 and CD106, which are considered relative specific markers of SF [13]. Moreover, SF at both p.1 and p.5 also expressed increased amounts of CD73, CD90 and CD105, which are considered typical markers for identifying mesenchymal stem cells (MSC). In line with several reports [14], the isolation of MSC and SF from the synovium is mainly based on the adhesion properties of the mononuclear cell fraction in vitro, from which they can be cultured-expanded as SF. However, detailed studies, as recently underlined by De Bari [15], are necessary to determine whether synovium-MSC are SF or different subsets, as in culture they are indistinguishable and no markers permit their selective identification. Only p.1 synovial cells were positive to typical macrophage markers, such as CD14, CD16, and CD68 and to some specific M1 or M2 macrophage markers, such as CD80 and CD163, thus showing the contemporary presence of pro-inflammatory M1 type and anti-inflammatory/regenerative M2 type in the OA synovium. Moreover, in contrast to other reports, we found the presence of macrophages in p.1 synovial cell culture, which has been reported to be reduced or absent in synovium-derived cells from digested fragments, and this confirms that enzymatic digestion affects the recovery of the different cell populations present in the synovium [14, 20]. Interestingly, p.1 synovial cells express only very small amounts of CD31, a typical endothelial marker, thus suggesting that this in vitro procedure does not ensure their isolation.

We found that p.1 synovial cells (mix of SF and SM) release significantly more IL6, CXCL8/IL8, CCL2/MCP-1, CCL3/MIP1α, CCL5/RANTES, and IL10 than those of p.5 (SF), thus suggesting that the absence of SM significantly reduces inflammation and does not induce the anabolic factor IL10. It has been shown that CCL2/MCP1 enhances CD106 [27]; our data show an increased number of positive CD106 on p.5 synovial cells that might be induced by CCL2/MCP1. In fact, even if CCL2/MCP1 is reduced compared to that of p.1 synovial cells, it is released in a greater quantity by p.5 synovial cells.

Bondeson et al. [17] reported that depletion of CD14-positive SM was associated with a decline in inflammation associated with decreased IL6, CXCL8/IL8, and CCL2/MCP-1, which is in line with our data in vitro. Among the factors analyzed, we found that S100A8, S100A9, and CCL3/MIP1α were the only undetectable factors (both at molecular and protein level) in p.5 synovial cells, a cell culture characterized by the absence of SM, thus confirming that they are specific markers of SM.

Synovial cells p.1 and p.5 represent two different in vitro cell models characterized by the presence and absence of SM, respectively, which are directly responsible for the low- and high-level inflammatory/degradative milieu. Different studies [28, 29] have used SF (p.5 synovial cells) as a cell model to test drugs or the effects of other cell types, without taking into consideration that synovial tissue is mainly composed of at least two cell types, SM and SF. It is has been known that OA SM are those mainly responsible for synovial inflammation [5, 16, 30] and it has been reported that inflammation induces ASC to exert an anti-inflammatory effect [22, 31, 32]. Therefore, to better define how the presence or absence of SM in cell culture influences the effects observed we evaluated the effects of ASC on inflammation and degradative factors co-cultured with the synovial p.1 and p.5 cell models. We found that in contrast with the anti-inflammatory effects found on p.1 synovial cells from moderate-grade OA, on p.5 synovial cells the ASC modulated the analyzed inflammatory factors differently. In particular, ASC significantly induced IL6 and CXCL8/IL8, decreased CCL5/RANTES, and did not modulate CCL2/MCP-1 or CCL3/MIP1α, which were still not expressed or released, thus demonstrating and confirming a specific dependence of this chemokine on SM and not on SF. Moreover, it is interesting to note that among the inflammatory factors analyzed, the CCL5/RANTES chemokine, mainly associated with a signature of synovial inflammation, was the only one that was still down-modulated in the presence of ASC, both in co-culture with p.1 with low- or moderate-grade synovitis, and with p.5 synovial cells, thus highlighting that this was an effect independent of the presence of SM.

It has been shown that CCL3/MIP1α has an important role in the recruitment of infiltrating leukocytes in the arthritic joint. Moreover, the CCL3-null mouse arthritis model is associated with a reduction of infiltrating cells and normal appearance of the synovium and cartilage, and the absence of pannus or bone resorption, thus confirming the important role of this chemokine in OA [33]. This evidence is also corroborated by a report of increased expression and secretion of CCL3-MIP1α when SF were co-cultured with activated leukocytes (monocytes or polymorphonuclear neutrophils) [34].

Our data show that ASC in co-culture with p.1 synoviocytes from moderate-grade OA decreased the typical inducible factors ADAMTS5, S100A8, and S100A9, and did not affect ADAMTS4 and MMP13. Conversely, in co-culture with p.5 synovial cells they only induced the expression of MMP13, thus suggesting that in the absence of SM, SF appear to acquire a characteristic more typical of SM, such as increased expression of MMP13. Interestingly, we also found that S100A8 and S100A9, the main catabolic factors produced by activated macrophages, were not detected in p.5 synovial cells co-cultured with ASC, thus confirming their specific expression on SM. These data were also confirmed on moderate-grade OA synovial tissue, where we found that S100A8 and CCL3/MIP1α were co-expressed with CD68, the typical macrophage marker.

Moreover, we found that S100A8 and S100A9 inhibition in p.1 synovial cells was also associated with IL6 and CXCL8/IL8 inhibition, which, as already reported [35], are strictly dependent. These data are also in line with a recent report that in a murine collagenase-induced OA model, ASC inhibited synovial activation mainly by reducing S100A8 and S100A9 [36]. Furthermore, large quantities of these catabolic factors have also been found in the synovial tissue of patients with OA, and they predict the development of cartilage destruction [37]. Interestingly, we also confirmed that in contrast to p.1 synovial cells obtained from patients with moderate-grade synovitis, p.1 synovial cells from patients with low-grade synovitis are unable to guide the anti-inflammatory and anti-catabolic effects of ASC, as found for p.5 synovial cells, as SM were present in very small numbers.

Conclusions

In summary, our data from in vitro analysis show the importance of using the correct in vitro cell models to recreate a milieu that closely resembles OA synovial tissue as the target tissue organ. The availability of in vitro cell models (p.1 and p.5 synovial cells) with large or small numbers of SM effectively reflects the different degrees of OA, which are characterized by different degrees of synovial inflammation, giving the opportunity of testing cells, anti-inflammatory drugs, or factors in a well-defined milieu.

Abbreviations

ADAMTS4: ADAM metallopeptidase with thrombospondin type 1 motif, 4; ADAMTS5: ADAM metallopeptidase with thrombospondin type 1 motif, 5; ASC: adipose stem cells; BSA: bovine serum albumin; CCL2/MCP1: chemokine (C-C motif) ligand 2/monocyte chemotactic protein 1; CCL3/MIP1α: chemokine (C-C motif) ligand 3/macrophage inflammatory protein 1α; CCL5/RANTES: chemokine (C-C motif) ligand 5; CD: cluster of differentiation; CXCL8/IL8: chemokine (C-X-C motif) ligand 8/interleukin 8; DMEM: Dulbecco's modified Eagle's medium; GMP: good manufacturing practice; ICAM-1: intracellular adhesion molecule-1; IL10: interleukin 10; IL4: interleukin 4; IL6: interleukin 6; MMP13: matrix metalloproteinase 13; OA: osteoarthritis; PBS: phosphate-buffered saline; PLP: platelet lysate; RGB: red/green/blue; RPS9: ribosomal protein S9; S100A8: S100 calcium binding protein A8; S100A9: S100 calcium binding protein A9; SF: synovial fibroblast; SM: synovial macrophage; TGFβ: transforming growth factor-β; TNFα: tumor necrosis factor-α; VCAM-1: vascular adhesion molecule-1.

Competing interests
The authors declare that they have no competing interests.

Authors' contributions
CM conceived and participated in the study design, performing scoring systems, image analyses, interpretation of data, and drafting the article. FP participated in the study design, carried out cell isolation, contributed to data collection and analysis, and helped to revise the manuscript. EG carried out mRNA preparations, conducted real-time PCR experiments, analyzed the data, and revised the manuscript. YS carried out the immunoassays, participated in histological assessment, and revised the manuscript. LG carried out immunohistochemical analysis, analyzed the data, and revised the manuscript. LC carried out flow cytometry analysis, collected the data, and revised the manuscript. GF participated in the provision of study materials, acquired clinical data, obtained written consent from patients, and revised the manuscript. SF-P provided GMP-ASC and revised the manuscript. GL conceived the study, performed statistical analysis, and gave final approval of the manuscript. All authors read and approved the final version of the manuscript.

Acknowledgements
The authors wish to thank Mr. Keith Smith for editing. This study was partially supported by the European Seventh Framework Programme (project ADIPOA; Health-2009-1.4-3, 241719) and partially by Horizon 2020 (project ADIPOA2; PHC-15-2014, 643809).

Author details
[1]SC Laboratorio di Immunoreumatologia e Rigenerazione Tissutale, Istituto Ortopedico Rizzoli, Via di Barbiano 1/10, Bologna 40136, Italy. [2]SD Laboratorio RAMSES, Istituto Ortopedico Rizzoli, Bologna 40136, Italy. [3]Clinica Ortopedica e Traumatologica II, Istituto Ortopedico Rizzoli, Bologna 40136, Italy. [4]EFS-Pyrénéés-Méditerranéé, Toulouse F-31300, France.

References
1. Loeser RF, Goldring SR, Scanzello CR, Goldring MB. Osteoarthritis: a disease of the joint as an organ. Arthritis Rheum. 2012;64:1697–707.
2. Krasnokutsky S, Attur M, Palmer G, Samuels J, Abramson SB. Current concepts in the pathogenesis of osteoarthritis. Osteoarthritis Cartilage. 2008; 16 Suppl 3:S1–3.
3. Scanzello CR, Goldring SR. The role of synovitis in osteoarthritis pathogenesis. Bone. 2012;51:249–57.
4. Sellam J, Berenbaum F. The role of synovitis in pathophysiology and clinical symptoms of osteoarthritis. Nat Rev Rheumatol. 2010;6:625–35.
5. De Lange-Brokaar BJE, Ioan-Facsinay A, van Osch GJ, Zuurmond AM, Schoones J, et al. Synovial inflammation, immune cells and their cytokines in osteoarthritis: A review. Osteoarthritis and Cartilage. 2012;20:1484–99.
6. Henrotin Y, Lambert C, Richette P. Importance of synovitis in osteoarthritis: Evidence for the use of glycosaminoglycans against synovial inflammation. Semin Arthritis Rheum. 2014;43(5):579–87.
7. Lambert C, Dubuc JE, Montell E, Vergés J, Munaut C, Noël A, et al. Gene expression pattern of cells from inflamed and normal areas of osteoarthritis synovial membrane. Arthritis Rheumatol. 2014;66(4):960–8.
8. Benito MJ, Veale DJ, FitzGerald O, van den Berg WB, Bresnihan B. Synovial tissue inflammation in early and late osteoarthritis. Ann Rheum Dis. 2005;64:1263–7.
9. Goldenberg DL, Egan M, Cohen AS. Inflammatory synovitis in degenerative joint disease. J Rheumatol. 1982;9:204–9.
10. Farahat MN, Yanni G, Poston R, Panayi GS. Cytokine expression in synovial membranes of patients with rheumatoid arthritis and osteoarthritis. Ann Rheum Dis. 1993;52:870–5.
11. Bondeson J, Foxwell B, Brennan F, Feldmann M. Defining therapeutic targets by using adenovirus: blocking NF-kappaB inhibits both inflammatory and destructive mechanisms in rheumatoid synovium but spares anti-inflammatory mediators. Proc Natl Acad Sci USA. 1999;96:5668–73.
12. Smith MD. The Normal Synovium. Open Rheumatol J. 2011;5:100–6.
13. Bartok B, Firestein GS. Fibroblast-like synoviocytes: Key effector cells in rheumatoid arthritis. Immunol Rev. 2010;233:233–55.
14. De Bari C, Dell'Accio F, Tylzanowski P, Luyten FP. Multipotent mesenchymal stem cells from adult human synovial membrane. Arthritis Rheum. 2001;44:1928–42.
15. De Bari C. Are mesenchymal stem cells in rheumatoid arthritis the good or bad guys? Arthritis Res Ther. 2015;17(1):113.
16. Bondeson J, Blom AB, Wainwright S, Hughes C, Caterson B, van den Berg WB. The role of synovial macrophages and macrophage-produced mediators in driving inflammatory and destructive responses in osteoarthritis. Arthritis Rheum. 2010;62:647–57.
17. Bondeson J, Wainwright SD, Lauder S, Amos N, Hughes CE. The role of synovial macrophages and macrophage-produced cytokines in driving aggrecanases, matrix metalloproteinases, and other destructive and inflammatory responses in osteoarthritis. Arthritis Res Ther. 2006;8:R187.
18. Scanzello CR, McKeon B, Swaim BH, DiCarlo E, Asomugha EU, Kanda V, et al. Synovial inflammation in patients undergoing arthroscopic meniscectomy: Molecular characterization and relationship to symptoms. Arthritis Rheum. 2011;63:391–400.
19. Tang CH, Hsu CJ, Fong YC. The CCL5/CCR5 axis promotes interleukin-6 production in human synovial fibroblasts. Arthritis Rheum. 2010;62:3615–24.
20. Van Landuyt KB, Jones EA, McGonagle D, Luyten FP, Lories RJ. Flow cytometric characterization of freshly isolated and culture expanded human synovial cell populations in patients with chronic arthritis. Arthritis Res Ther. 2010;12:R15.
21. Chang CB, Han SA, Kim EM, Lee S, Seong SC, Lee MC. Chondrogenic potentials of human synovium-derived cells sorted by specific surface markers. Osteoarthritis Cartilage. 2013;21:190–9.
22. Manferdini C, Maumus M, Gabusi E, Piacentini A, Filardo G, Peyrafitte JA, et al. Adipose-derived mesenchymal stem cells exert antiinflammatory effects on chondrocytes and synoviocytes from osteoarthritis patients through prostaglandin E2. Arthritis Rheum. 2013;65:1271–81.
23. Kellgren JH, Lawrence JS. Radiological assessment of osteo-arthrosis. Ann Rheum Dis. 1957;16:494–502.
24. Krenn V, Morawietz L, Häupl T, Neidel J, Petersen I, König A. Grading of chronic synovitis–a histopathological grading system for molecular and diagnostic pathology. Pathol Res Pract. 2002;198:317–25.
25. Lisignoli G, Grassi F, Piacentini A, Cocchini B, Remiddi G, Bevilacqua C, et al. Hyaluronan does not affect cytokine and chemokine expression in osteoarthritic chondrocytes and synoviocytes. Osteoarthritis Cartilage. 2001;9:161–8.
26. Bourin P, Peyrafitte JA, Fleury-Cappellesso S. A first approach for the production of human adipose tissue-derived stromal cells for therapeutic use. Methods Mol Biol. 2011;702:331–43.
27. Lin YM, Hsu CJ, Liao YY, Chou MC, Tang CH. The CCL2/CCR2 axis enhances vascular cell adhesion molecule-1 expression in human synovial fibroblasts. PLoS One. 2012;7, e49999.
28. Eymard F, Pigenet A, Citadelle D, Flouzat-Lachaniette CH, Poignard A, Benelli C, et al. Infrapatellar fat pad induces an inflammatory and a pro-degradative phenotype in autologous fibroblast-like synoviocytes from patients with knee OA. Arthritis Rheumatol. 2014;66(8):2165–74.
29. Sieghart D, Liszt M, Wanivenhaus A, Bröll H, Kiener H, Klösch B, et al. Hydrogen sulphide decreases IL-1β-induced activation of fibroblast-like synoviocytes from patients with osteoarthritis. J Cell Mol Med. 2015;19:187–97.
30. Han SA, Lee S, Seong SC, Lee MC. Effects of CD14 Macrophages and proinflammatory cytokines on chondrogenesis in osteoarthritic synovium-derived stem cells. Tissue Eng Part A. 2014;20:2680–91.
31. ter Huurne M, Schelbergen R, Blattes R, Blom A, de Munter W, Grevers LC, et al. Antiinflammatory and chondroprotective effects of intraarticular injection of adipose-derived stem cells in experimental osteoarthritis. Arthritis Rheum. 2012;64:3604–13.
32. Manferdini C, Maumus M, Gabusi E, Paolella F, Grassi F, Jorgensen C, et al. Lack of anti-inflammatory and anti-catabolic effects on basal inflamed osteoarthritic chondrocytes or synoviocytes by adipose stem cell-conditioned medium. Osteoarthritis Cartilage. 2015;23(11):2045–57.
33. Chintalacharuvu SR, Wang JX, Giaconia JM, Venkataraman C. An essential role for CCL3 in the development of collagen antibody-induced arthritis. Immunol Lett. 2005;100:202–4.
34. Hanyuda M, Kasama T, Isozaki T, Matsunawa MM, Yajima N, Miyaoka H, et al. Activated leucocytes express and secrete macrophage inflammatory protein-1 upon interaction with synovial fibroblasts of rheumatoid arthritis via a 2-integrin/ICAM-1 mechanism. Rheumatology. 2003;42:1390–7.

S100A8/A9 increases the mobilization of pro-inflammatory Ly6C^{high} monocytes to the synovium during experimental osteoarthritis

Niels A. J. Cremers[1], Martijn H. J. van den Bosch[1], Stephanie van Dalen[1], Irene Di Ceglie[1], Giuliana Ascone[1], Fons van de Loo[1], Marije Koenders[1], Peter van der Kraan[1], Annet Sloetjes[1], Thomas Vogl[2], Johannes Roth[2], Edwin J. W. Geven[1], Arjen B. Blom[1] and Peter L. E. M. van Lent[1]*

Abstract

Background: Monocytes are dominant cells present within the inflamed synovium during osteoarthritis (OA). In mice, two functionally distinct monocyte subsets are described: pro-inflammatory Ly6C^{high} and patrolling Ly6C^{low} monocytes. Alarmins S100A8/A9 locally released by the synovium during inflammatory OA for prolonged periods may be dominant proteins involved in stimulating recruitment of Ly6C^{high} monocytes from the circulation to the joint. Our objective was to investigate the role of S100A8/A9 in the mobilization of Ly6C^{high} and Ly6C^{low} monocytic populations to the inflamed joint in collagenase-induced OA (CiOA).

Method: S100A8 was injected intra-articularly to investigate monocyte influx. CiOA was induced by injection of collagenase into knee joints of wild-type C57BL/6 (WT), and S100a9$^{-/-}$ mice. Mice were sacrificed together with age-matched saline-injected control mice (n = 6/group), and expression of monocyte markers, pro-inflammatory cytokines, and chemokines was determined in the synovium using ELISA and RT-qPCR. Cells were isolated from the bone marrow (BM), spleen, blood, and synovium and monocytes were identified using FACS.

Results: S100A8/A9 was highly expressed during CiOA. Intra-articular injection of S100A8 leads to elevated expression of monocyte markers and the monocyte-attracting chemokines CCL2 and CX3CL1 in the synovium. At day 7 (d7) after CiOA induction in WT mice, numbers of Ly6C^{high}, but not Ly6C^{low} monocytes, were strongly increased (7.6-fold) in the synovium compared to saline-injected controls. This coincided with strong upregulation of CCL2, which preferentially attracts Ly6C^{high} monocytes. In contrast, S100a9$^{-/-}$ mice showed a significant increase in Ly6C^{low} monocytes (twofold) within the synovium at CiOA d7, whereas the number of Ly6C^{high} monocytes remained unaffected. In agreement with this finding, the Ly6C^{low} mobilization marker CX3CL1 was significantly higher within the synovium of S100a9$^{-/-}$ mice. Next, we studied the effect of S100A8/A9 on release of Ly6C^{high} monocytes from the BM into the circulation. A 14% decrease in myeloid cells was found in WT BM at CiOA d7. No decrease in myeloid cells in S100a9$^{-/-}$ BM was found, suggesting that S100A8/A9 promotes the release of myeloid populations from the BM.

Conclusion: Induction of OA locally leads to strongly elevated S100A8/A9 expression and an elevated influx of Ly6C^{high} monocytes from the BM to the synovium.

Keywords: S100, Mobilization, Ly6C high/low monocytes, Systemic effects, Collagenase-induced osteoarthritis

* Correspondence: Peter.vanlent@radboudumc.nl
[1]Experimental Rheumatology, Department of Rheumatology, Radboud University Medical Center, PO Box 9101, Nijmegen 6500 HB, The Netherlands
Full list of author information is available at the end of the article

Background

Osteoarthritis (OA) is a chronic degenerative disease of the joints and currently its high prevalence increases even further due to aging and an increasingly obese population [1–3]. Current treatment options focus on targeting the symptoms and are limited to analgesics and anti-inflammatory drugs, with many patients eventually having to undergo joint replacement surgery [4–6]. Novel therapies that focus on preventing joint damage are warranted. A better insight into the etiology and disease progression is therefore needed [3, 4].

The etiology of OA is multi-factorial, and it is considered to be a disease of the whole joint in which the synovium also plays an important role [7–9]. Synovial activation is clearly present in more than 50% of patients with OA and contributes to the pathophysiology and clinical symptoms [6–10]. Systemic and local synovial inflammation is increasingly recognized to be involved in joint pathologic change [6, 11, 12]. Although most types of leucocytes have been described to be present within the inflamed OA synovium, monocytes and macrophages are thought to be the predominant cell types driving the pathologic change [13–15]. OA is characterized by joint damage, which leads to the release of proteins or alarmins such as S100A8/A9 promoting activation of monocytes/macrophages within the synovium followed by an inherent release of inflammatory cytokines, such as IL-1β, TNF-α and additional release of S100 alarmins [7, 9, 10, 16]. The most prominent proteins from the S100 family that are released during OA are S100A8 (myeloid-related proteins: MRP8) and S100A9 (MRP14), which belong to the group of damage-associated molecular patterns proteins (DAMPs) or alarmins, and play a crucial role in innate immunity [17–19]. S100A8 and S100A9 form heterodimers under low calcium conditions within the cell and assemble into $(S100A8/A9)^2$ hetero-tetramers in the presence of calcium [20]. When myeloid cells are stressed S100A8/A9 is secreted and binds to the toll-like receptor (TLR)4 receptor promoting pro-inflammatory effects [19, 21]. We previously described that S100A8/A9 proteins are expressed for prolonged periods in collagenase-induced OA (CiOA), a model driven by synovial inflammation, and that they are important stimulators of tissue pathology [22–24]. In addition, patients with OA are characterized by high levels of S100A8/A9 in blood and synovium, and baseline serum levels of patients with symptomatic OA predict development of joint destruction 2 years thereafter [22, 23]. Moreover, S100A8/A9 promotes the migration of monocytes, which when activated, are also important producers of S100A8/A9 thereby forming a positive feedback loop [25, 26].

Monocytes are recruited from the bone marrow (BM) towards the site of inflammation via a combined action of adhesion molecules, e.g. LFA-1 and VCAM, and chemokines, such as (C-C motif) ligand 2 (CCL2) that is known to bind the C-C chemokine receptor type 2 (CCR) [27–30]. In mice, two functionally distinct monocyte subpopulations are described. The pro-inflammatory Ly6C^{high} monocytes, which express high levels of CCR2, are involved in removing debris, and the Ly6C^{low} monocytes, which express high levels of CX3CR1, are suggested to be involved in repair processes as they release anabolic factors like vascular endothelial growth factor (VEGF) and transforming growth factor (TGF)-β [31, 32]. Ly6C^{high} monocytes reside in the BM and upon release from the BM into the circulation can either stay in their state or transform into Ly6C^{low} monocytes [32, 33]. Once in the blood, both Ly6C^{high} as Ly6C^{low} monocytes can be mobilized to the peripheral tissue in response to chemokines [34]. Ly6C^{high} monocytes are mainly attracted by CCL2 and Ly6C^{low} monocytes by CX3CL1, which can bind to CCR2 and CX3CR1, respectively [35]. When the monocytes arrive at the injured site, they can differentiate into M1-like pro-inflammatory or M2-like anti-inflammatory macrophages, dependently on the environmental cues [33]. The aim of our study is to investigate whether local production of S100A8/A9 in the inflamed joint and their subsequent release into the circulation is involved in recruitment of the different monocyte cell populations to the joint in inflammatory CiOA.

Methods
Animals

The Committee for Animal Experiments of the Dutch Central Commission on Animal Experiments approved all procedures involving animals (CCD# 2015-0014). One hundred fifty-eight female mice (strain: 106 C57BL/6 and 52 S100a9$^{-/-}$), 8–12 weeks of age, and weighing 21 ± 1.5 g (minimum 19 g, maximum 26 g) were provided with standard diet and water *ad libitum* and maintained on a 12-h light/dark cycle under specific pathogen-free housing conditions at the Central Animal Facility Nijmegen. More details on the housing conditions have been previously described [36]. S100a9$^{-/-}$ mice were originally generated at the University of Münster as previously described [37]. An overview of the animals used for the different experiments and analyzed time-points can be found in Table 1. No animals died during the experiments and no animals were excluded during the experiments or data analysis. All mice were randomly divided over the experiments and different conditions. All outcomes were measured by an observer who was blinded to the allocation of the animals to the experimental groups, when possible. The mice were anesthetized with 5% isoflurane in O_2/N_2O and killed by exsanguination, followed by cervical dislocation. At the end of the experiment, at day 7, 21, or 42 after induction of CiOA, different tissues (synovium, blood, and contralateral femur) were collected and used for histologic evaluation,

Table 1 Overview of animals used in experiments

Experiment	Readout	Time point	Number of animals per group and strains
CiOA/control	Monocyte populations and RNA expression synovium and BM	Day 7	6 CiOA/6 control C57BL/6
			6 CiOA/6 control S100a9$^{-/-}$
CiOA/control	BM count	Day 7, 21, and 42	6 CiOA/7 control C57BL/6 (day 7)
			6 CiOA/7 control C57BL/6 (day 21)
			7 CiOA/7 control C57BL/6 (day 42)
CiOA/control	Monocyte populations and BM count	Day 7	5 CiOA/5 control C57BL/6
			5 CiOA/5 control S100a9$^{-/-}$
CiOA	Immunohistologic evaluation (and serum for protein analysis)	Day 7, 21, and 42	10 per time-point C57BL/6 (day 7)
			10 per time-point S100a9$^{-/-}$ (day 7)
			10 per time-point C57BL/6 (day 21)
			10 per time-point S100a9$^{-/-}$ (day 21)
			10 per time-point C57BL/6 (day 42)
			10 per time-point S100a9$^{-/-}$ (day 42)
i.a. injection with S100A8/BSA	Immunohistologic evaluation	Day 1	8 C57BL/6
i.a. injection with S100A8/BSA	RNA expression	Day 1	6 C57BL/6

CiOA collagenase-induced osteoarthritis, *i.a.,* intra-articular, *BM* bone marrow

collection of serum for protein analysis, measurement of messenger RNA (mRNA) expression, and determination of different cell populations.

Collagenase induced OA model and tissue isolation

CiOA was unilaterally induced in wild-type (WT) C57BL/6 mice by injection of one unit of collagenase type VII from *Clostridium histolyticum* (Sigma Chemical Co., St. Louis, MO, USA) in a volume of 6 μL twice on alternate days in the right knee joint, as previously described [38]. An equal volume of saline was injected into the right knee of age-matched mice and served as the treated control. Mice were killed at different time points (day 7, 21, or 42) after CiOA induction, and the different readouts as described in Table 1 were determined. In short, mRNA expression (reverse transcription quantitative PCR (RT-qPCR)) and protein levels (Luminex/ELISA) of mobilization markers and pro-inflammatory cytokines, including S100A8 and S100A9, were measured in the synovium and BM cells isolated from the contralateral femur. Synovial biopsies were taken using a 3-mm-diameter biopsy punch. The absolute number of cells in the contralateral BM per femur was determined by crushing the complete femur with a mortar and pestle, intensive lavation with PBS, and counting of the cells. Monocyte subpopulations of BM cells present in the contralateral femur, and CiOA-affected synovial tissue were analyzed by FACS. Tissue sections were stained with hematoxylin and eosin (HE) and histologically scored for synovial activation (number of cell layers of synovial intima lining), and immunohistochemically stained for S100A8, S100A9 and Ly6C.

Intra-articular injection of S100A8 protein

Mice were injected intra-articularly with a volume of 6 μL PBS containing 5 μg of S100A8 recombinant protein in the right knee and 5 μg bovine serum albumin (BSA) protein as a control in the left knee, after which the mice were killed and synovium was isolated for histologic evaluation and for RT-qPCR analysis as described in Table 1.

RNA isolation and RT-qPCR

Total RNA from BM cells was isolated using TRIzol reagent according to the manufacturer's protocol (Invitrogen). Cells of the synovial tissue were lyzed and homogenized using ceramic MagNa Lyser Green Beads (Roche) and the MagNa Lyser (Roche) three times for 20 s at 6000 rpm with 1 min interspersed cooling. RNA of the synovium was further extracted with the RNeasy Fibrous Tissue mini kit (Qiagen, catalog (cat) # 74704, Venlo, The Netherlands). DNase treatment (Qiagen: RNase-Free DNase Set) was performed between the first washing steps with RW1 buffer. RNA concentration was determined using the nanodrop 2000 spectrophotometer (Thermo Scientific). For the reverse transcriptase treatment, 1 μg sample RNA was linearized in a volume of 11 μL water for 15 min at 65 °C and then together with total reverse transcriptase mix (containing 100 μM DTT, 10 mM dNTP each, 0.2 μg oligodT primer, 20 units RNA inhibitor (RNAsin: Promega cat # N251A), and 200 units reverse transcriptase (Invitrogen 28025-013)) in a total volume of 20 μL incubated for 5 min at 25 °C, 60 min at 39 °C and 5 min at 94 °C. Hereafter the complementary DNA (cDNA) was diluted × 20 and used for

RT-qPCR, using the StepOnePlus Real-Time PCR System (Applied Biosystems). The reaction was performed in a volume of 10 μL containing 3 μL cDNA, 0.6 μM primers, 5 μL iQ SYBR Green Supermix (Bio-Rad Laboratories). After incubation of 3 min, amplification was carried out for 40 cycles of 15 s at 95 °C and 30 s at 60 °C. The melting temperature of the products was defined to indicate amplification specificity. All values were normalized to the reference gene *Gapdh*, which is often used in CiOA experiments and showed stable expression during this model, and was presented as $-\Delta$ cycle threshold ($-\Delta Ct$) [39]. We decided to present the negative ΔCt (Ct of the reference gene minus the Ct of the gene of interest) to improve the ease of interpretation (higher values in the graphs representing higher expression). Fold change can be calculated as the difference in $-\Delta Ct$ (giving $\Delta\Delta Ct$) between saline vs CiOA or WT vs S100a9$^{-/-}$ groups, and then $2^{\Delta\Delta Ct}$. Primers are summarized in Table 2. All primers were custom-designed using Primer-BLAST (https://www.ncbi.nlm.nih.gov/tools/primer-blast/) at standard settings with a product size of 70–150 bp, spanning an exon-exon junction, max poly-X at 4, max GC in primer 3' end at 3, and primer GC content between 20 and 80%, and subsequently validated in serial dilutions of mice cDNA to test the amplification efficiency of the RT-qPCR. For an efficiency of 100%, the slope is $- 3.32$; all our primers passed the minimal efficiency requirements of 90–110%, corresponding with a slope between $- 3.58$ and $- 3.1$. All primers were checked for specificity by performing a melt curve, confirming a single product after the PCR assay and no formation of aspecific by-products.

Histologic evaluation of total knee joints

Dissected total knee joints were fixed in 4% formalin, decalcified in 5% formic acid, and subsequently embedded in paraffin. Coronal knee joint sections of 7 μm thickness were made and mounted on superfrost glass slides (SuperFrost® Plus, Menzel-Glaser, Germany). Deparaffinized sections were stained with HE. Synovial activation was evaluated by two blinded observers scoring the thickening of the synovial lining layer (number of cell layers of the intima) and the cellular influx as described previously [40].

Immunohistochemical staining of S100A8, S100A9, and Ly6C

Knee joints sections were stained for S100A8, S100A9, and Ly6C as described previously [22]. In short, antigen retrieval was performed by incubating for 15 min in citrate buffer at 60 °C. Thereafter, sections were incubated for 1 h with the primary antibodies directed against

Table 2 Primer sequences of mouse inflammatory and mobilization markers

	Sense	Antisense
Reference gene		
Gapdh	5'-ggcaaattcaacggcaca-3'	5'-gttagtggggtctcgctcctg-3'
Inflammation marker		
S100A8	5'-tgtcctcagtttgtgcagaatataaat-3'	5'-tttatcaccatcgcaaggaactc-3'
S100A9	5'-ggcaaaggctgtgggaagt-3'	5'-ccattgagtaagccattcccttta-3'
Mobilization markers		
CCL2	5'-ttggctcagccagatgca-3'	5'-cctactcattgggatcatcttgct-3'
CX3CL1	5'-gtgccattgtcctggagac-3'	5'-catttctccttcgggtcag-3'
KC	5'-tggctgggattcacctcaa-3'	5'-gagtgtggctatgacttcggttt-3'
MIP-1a	5'-caagtcttctcagcgccatatg-3'	5'-tcttccggctgtaggagaagc-3'
Cell markers		
CX3CR1	5'-gagtatgacgattctgctgagg-3'	5'-cagaccgaacgtgaagacgag-3'
CCR2	5'-ctatctgctcaacttggccatct-3'	5'-tgagcccagaatggtaatgtga-3'
Ly6C	5'-gcagtgctacgagtgctatgg-3'	5'-actgacgggtctttagtttcctt-3'
F4/80	5'-aatcctgtgaagatgtgg-3'	5'-gagtgttgatgcaaatgaag-3'
Adhesion molecules		
LFA1	5'-gaatgtatgaagggcaaagtc-3'	5'-gcagcaaactggtaggaag-3'
VCAM	5'-ccaagtctctccaaaagatatacagctt-3'	5'-atgacggtgtgtccctct-3'
L-selectin	5'-actgctctgttgtgacttcc-3'	5'-tgtatggcgactaaatctgtg-3'
PECAM1	5'-tccctgggaggtcgtccat-3'	5'-gaacaaggcagcggggttta-3'
VE-cadherin	5'-tcctcttgcatcctcactatcaca-3'	5'-gtaagtgaccaactgctcgtgaat-3'

mouse S100A8 (host, rabbit), mouse S100A9 (host, rabbit) (both were made at our own facilities [41], and used at a concentration of 1 µg/mL), or mouse Ly6C (host, rat) (Abcam cat # 15627, at a concentration at 2 µg/mL). Rabbit (for S100A8 and S100A9) or rat (for Ly6C) IgG antibody was used as a control. After washing, S100A8 and S100A9 sections were incubated with horseradish peroxidase (HRP)-conjugated goat anti-rabbit IgG (Dako, Glostrup, Denmark) for 30 min. For the Ly6C staining, after incubation with the primary antibody, and washing, sections were incubated with secondary rabbit anti rat IgG biotin-labeled antibody for 30 min, followed by washing and a 30-min incubation with VECTASTAIN elite ABC HRP kit (Peroxidase, Rabbit IgG) (Vector laboratories, Burlingame, CA, USA, cat # PK6101). Sections were peroxidase-stained using diaminobenxidine and counterstained using Mayer's hemotoxylin (Biochemica, Amsterdam, the Netherlands).

Determination of monocyte subpopulations using flow cytometry

Cells isolated from the BM and synovial tissues were analyzed for monocyte subpopulations by seven-color staining and flow cytometry using the Gallios flow cytometer (Beckman Coulter, Indianapolis, IN, USA). The antibodies and fluorophores that were used are summarized in Table 3. First, single cells were selected using the side scatter and pulse width. Next, viable cells were gated using the side scatter and negative for the SYTOX blue viability staining. Myeloid cells, were gated negative for the dump channel (CD90/B220/CD49b/NK1.1) to deplete T cells, B cells, and natural killer (NK) cells, and positively selected for CD11b. Cells were next plotted for Ly6G and Ly6C to distinguish neutrophils and monocytes, respectively. Monocytes were selected and finally plotted for F4/80 and Ly6C. Herein, Ly6C^{high} and Ly6C^{low} monocytes and macrophages could be selected dependent on the tissue. Monocyte subsets were identified as (B220/CD90/CD49b/NK1.1/Ly6G)^{low}CD11b^{high}(F4/80/

MHCII/CD11c)^{low} and further distinguished by their Ly6C expression, using Kaluza flow cytometry analysis software (Beckman Coulter).

Statistics

Data were analyzed using GraphPad Prism 5.01 software (San Diego, CA, USA). Outliers were tested using Grubbs' test, but no outliers were found. Data were analyzed using the two-sided t test to compare two variables or one-way analysis of variance when comparing multiple variables. Bonferroni's multiple comparison post hoc test was applied as correction for multiple comparisons when investigating multiple dependent research questions. Results were considered significantly different at $p < 0.05$ (with significance level denoted as $^*p < 0.05$, $^{**}p < 0.01$, and $^{***}p < 0.001$).

Results

Increased numbers of monocytes in the synovium after induction of CiOA coincides with high levels of S100A8/A9

We first investigated whether monocytes are attracted to the inflamed joint in experimental inflammatory OA. At day 7 after induction of CiOA, the number of cell layers in the intima-lining layer was increased and mainly consisted of leucocytes with monocyte morphology. Most of the cells within the synovial lining strongly expressed Ly6C, a protein characteristic of monocytes, as shown by immuno-localization (Fig. 1a vs control b).

Next we studied whether S100A8/A9 expression was related to this increase in monocyte numbers within the inflamed joint. mRNA levels of S100A8 and S100A9 were strongly enhanced (35-fold and 60-fold, respectively) at CiOA day 7, when compared to saline-injected controls (Fig. 1e). Immuno-localization shows that S100A8/A9 protein was strongly expressed by monocytes within the inflamed synovial lining (Fig. 1c vs control d). At later time points after CiOA, S100A8/A9 levels were still high whereas

Table 3 Antibodies used to detect monocyte subsets using flow cytometry

Marker	Fluorophore	Manufacturer (catalog number)
CD11b	FITC	BD Biosciences (553310)
Ly6C	APC-Cy7	BD Biosciences (560596)
Ly6G	APC	Biolegend (127614)
CD90.2	PE	BD Biosciences (553006)
B220/antiCD45	PE	BD Biosciences (553090)
CD49b	PE	BD Biosciences (553858)
NK1.1	PE	BD Biosciences (553165)
F4/80	PE-Cy7	Biolegend (123114)
MHCII	PE-Cy7	Biolegend (116420)
CD11c	PE-Cy7	BD Biosciences (558079)
SYTOX Blue Dead Cell Stain	SYTOX blue	Thermo Fisher Scientific (S34857)

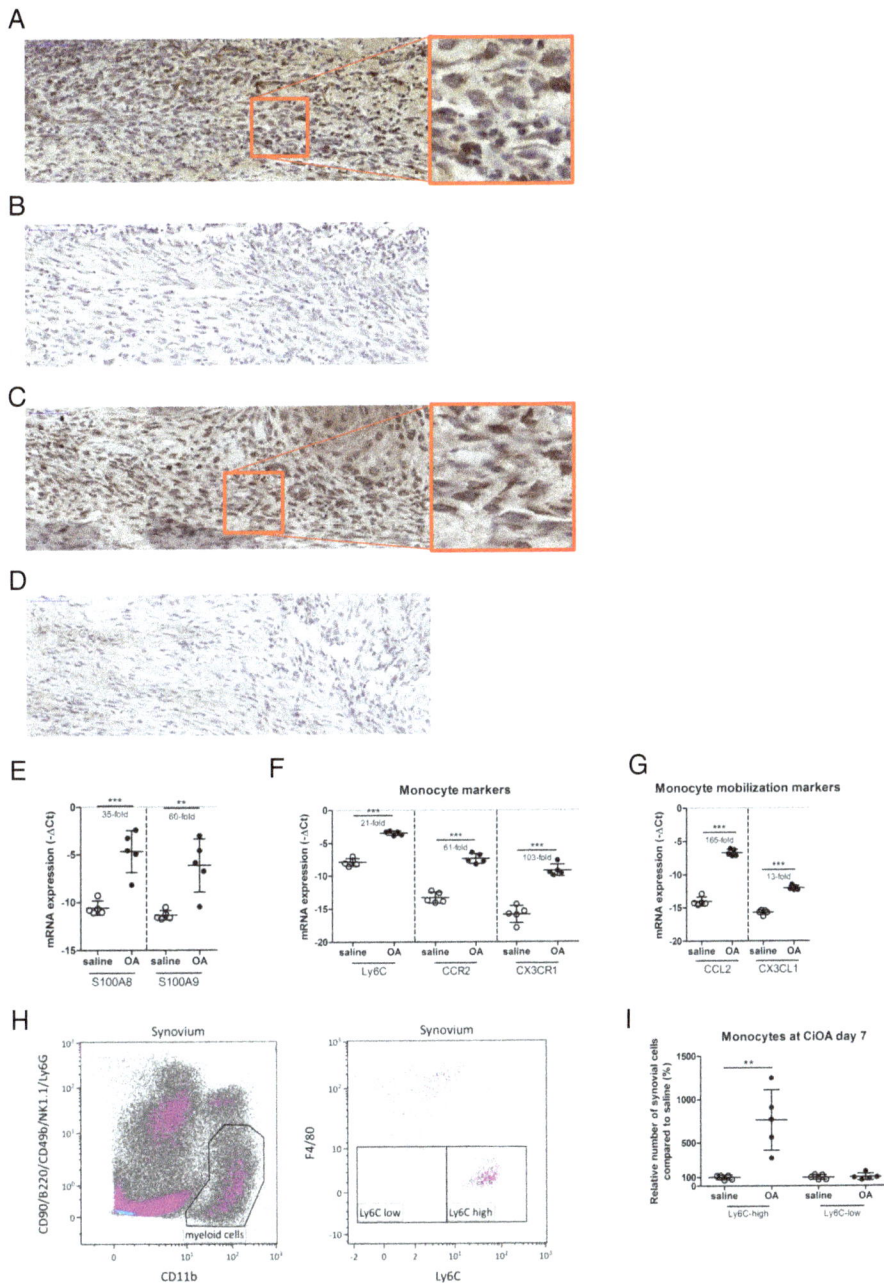

Fig. 1 S100A8/A9 mRNA and protein expression is strongly increased in the synovium at day 7 of collagenase-induced osteoarthritis (CiOA), leading to elevated Ly6C[high] monocytes locally into the joint. **a** Monocytes are strongly infiltrated during early CiOA as shown by highly expressed Ly6C protein staining and based on cell morphology in the synovial lining layer of the knee joints at CiOA day 7. **b** IgG control staining for the Ly6C antibody of the same joint shows no aspecific staining. **c** S100A9 protein is expressed in synovial monocytes at CiOA day 7 as shown by immuno-localization. **d** IgG control staining for the S100A9 antibody of the same joint shows no aspecific staining. **e** S100A8 and S100A9 mRNA expression is strongly induced in the synovium at CiOA day 7 when compared to saline-injected controls. **f**, **g** Monocyte marker Ly6C, and the more monocyte-subset-specific markers, CCR2 (Ly6C[high]) and CX3CR1 (Ly6C[low]) are strongly induced (**f**), together with the monocyte attracting chemokines CCL2 (Ly6C[high]) and CX3CL1 (Ly6C[low]) (**g**) in synovium at CiOA day 7, when compared to saline-injected controls. **h** Monocyte gating strategy for flow cytometric analysis: single viable cells were plotted for B220/CD90/CD49b/NK1.1/Ly6G and CD11b, in which myeloid cells were selected, and next the monocyte subsets could be identified based on their F4/80/MHCII/CD11c and Ly6C expression. **i** The relative number of Ly6C[high] monocytes were increased, whereas Ly6C[low] monocyte subpopulations remained unaffected locally in the joint at CiOA day 7 compared to saline-injected controls, as observed using flow cytometry. Data represent mean ± SD of five individual mice. *Significantly different from saline-injected control (**$p < 0.01$, ***$p < 0.001$). Ct cycle threshold

in contrast IL-1β, TNF-α and IL-6 rapidly decreased [22], suggesting that synovial inflammation in CiOA is dominated by S100A8/A9 production.

To analyze the presence of pro-inflammatory Ly6C^{high} monocytes and reparative Ly6C^{low} monocyte subsets, we next investigated mRNA expression within the inflamed synovium of chemokine receptors associated with specific monocyte subsets (Fig. 1f). Ly6C^{high} monocytes are characterized by expression of mainly CCR2 and to a lesser extent CX3CR1, whereas Ly6C^{low} monocytes predominantly express CX3CR1. mRNA expression levels of Ly6C, CCR2, and CX3CR1 were all strongly increased within the inflamed synovium of early-phase CiOA (day 7) (21-fold, 61-fold, and 103-fold, respectively) (Fig. 1f). Next we analyzed monocyte-subset-attracting chemokines (Fig. 1g). CCL2 (MCP-1) is dominant for Ly6C^{high} monocytes, whereas CX3CL1 particularly attracts Ly6C^{low} monocytes. mRNA expression levels of CCL2 were strongly increased (165-fold), whereas CX3CL1 was only increased 13-fold (Fig. 1g). The strongly increased expression of both CCR2 and its ligand CCL2 within the inflamed synovium suggests an elevated presence of Ly6C^{high} monocytes.

Specifically, Ly6C^{high} monocytes are increased in the synovium after induction of CiOA

To analyze more accurately which monocyte subsets are indeed preferentially increased within the inflamed synovium during the first phase of CiOA, we treated synovial tissue obtained from mice with CiOA and saline-injected control mice with collagenase and analyzed the cell composition by flow cytometry. Single viable cells were selected, after which myeloid cells were identified as CD11b^{high} and B220/CD90/CD49b/NK1.1/Ly6G^{low} to exclude B cells, T cells, NK -cells, and neutrophils. Next, monocytes subsets can be further divided based on their Ly6C expression (Fig. 1h). In synovium at CiOA day 7, the number of Ly6C^{high} monocytes was significantly increased (764% increase) in contrast to Ly6C^{low} monocytes, which were not different in synovium obtained from saline-injected control mice (Fig. 1i).

Intra-articular injection of S100A8 protein induces expression of monocyte markers in the synovium

Since influx of Ly6C^{high} monocytes coincides with high S100A8/A9 levels, we next investigated whether S100A8/A9 is able to regulate monocyte influx. We injected S100A8 (5 μg), which is described to be the most dominant form of the S100A8/A9 complex in mice [21], or BSA as control, into the knee joint of naive mice and determined the expression of several markers involved in monocyte attraction in the synovium after 24 h, using RT-qPCR (Fig. 2a-f). To get an impression whether monocytes are present, we first measured

mRNA levels of Ly6C and F4/80. Significant upregulation of both Ly6C and F4/80 (2.1-fold and 3.7-fold, respectively) was observed (Fig. 2a and b).

mRNA levels of the Ly6C^{high} monocyte-attracting chemokine CCL2 and its receptor CCR2 were significantly elevated (7.8-fold and 4.1-fold, respectively) after S100A8 injection (Fig. 2c and d). In contrast, mRNA levels of the Ly6C^{low}-attracting chemokine CX3CL1 and its receptor CX3CR1 were lower and were not statistically significant (1.8-fold and 2.1-fold, respectively) (Fig. 2e and f). To verify that monocytes are indeed recruited to the joint in response to S100A8 injection, we stained sections of the joints with HE 24 h after S100A8 injection. Figure 2g clearly shows the strong presence of inflammatory cells exhibiting typical monocyte morphology, which resided particularly in the synovial lining layer. This influx of inflammatory cells was absent in BSA-injected controls (Fig. 2h).

Locally induced CiOA leads to a significant S100A8/A9-driven decrease of Ly6C^{high} monocytes in the BM, but not in the blood and spleen

As injection of S100A8 into the mouse knee joint leads to attraction of Ly6C^{high} monocytes particularly, we next investigated the role of S100A8/A9 on monocyte subpopulations during early CiOA in more detail. To this end, we used S100a9$^{-/-}$ mice, which functionally are double knockout for S100A8 and S100A9, since S100A8 is missing at protein level as well [37].

Locally induced inflammation in the joint may have an impact on migration of monocytes from the BM into the blood, and subsequently to the inflamed joint. Local induction of CiOA resulted in elevated levels of S100A8/A9 (up to 882 ng/mL and on average 502 ng/mL) in the blood at day 7 (Additional file 1: Figure S1) and induced systemic effects within the BM of WT mice. Measuring the total number of myeloid cells within a complete femur at several time points after induction of OA in WT mice demonstrated a reduction in myeloid cell number of 14% ($p = 0.0210$), 14% ($p = 0.0205$), and 15% ($p = 0.1335$) at day 7, 21, and 42 after CiOA induction, respectively (Fig. 3a), corresponding to release of Ly6C^{high} monocytes at day 7 ($p = 0.0616$), day 21 ($p = 0.0036$), and day 42 ($p = 0.3982$) (Fig. 3b), which only was significant at day 21, as determined by flow cytometry (Fig. 3c). In contrast, no changes in absolute myeloid cell numbers or Ly6C^{high} monocytes were observed in the femurs of S100a9$^{-/-}$ mice at CiOA day 7 when compared to their saline-injected controls. This suggests that S100A8/A9 stimulates the efflux of monocytes from the BM into the blood. However the increase of monocytes into the blood at this time-point had no effect on the ratio of Ly6C^{high} and Ly6C^{low} subsets in both the blood (Fig. 3d) and in the spleen (Fig. 3e). No difference was

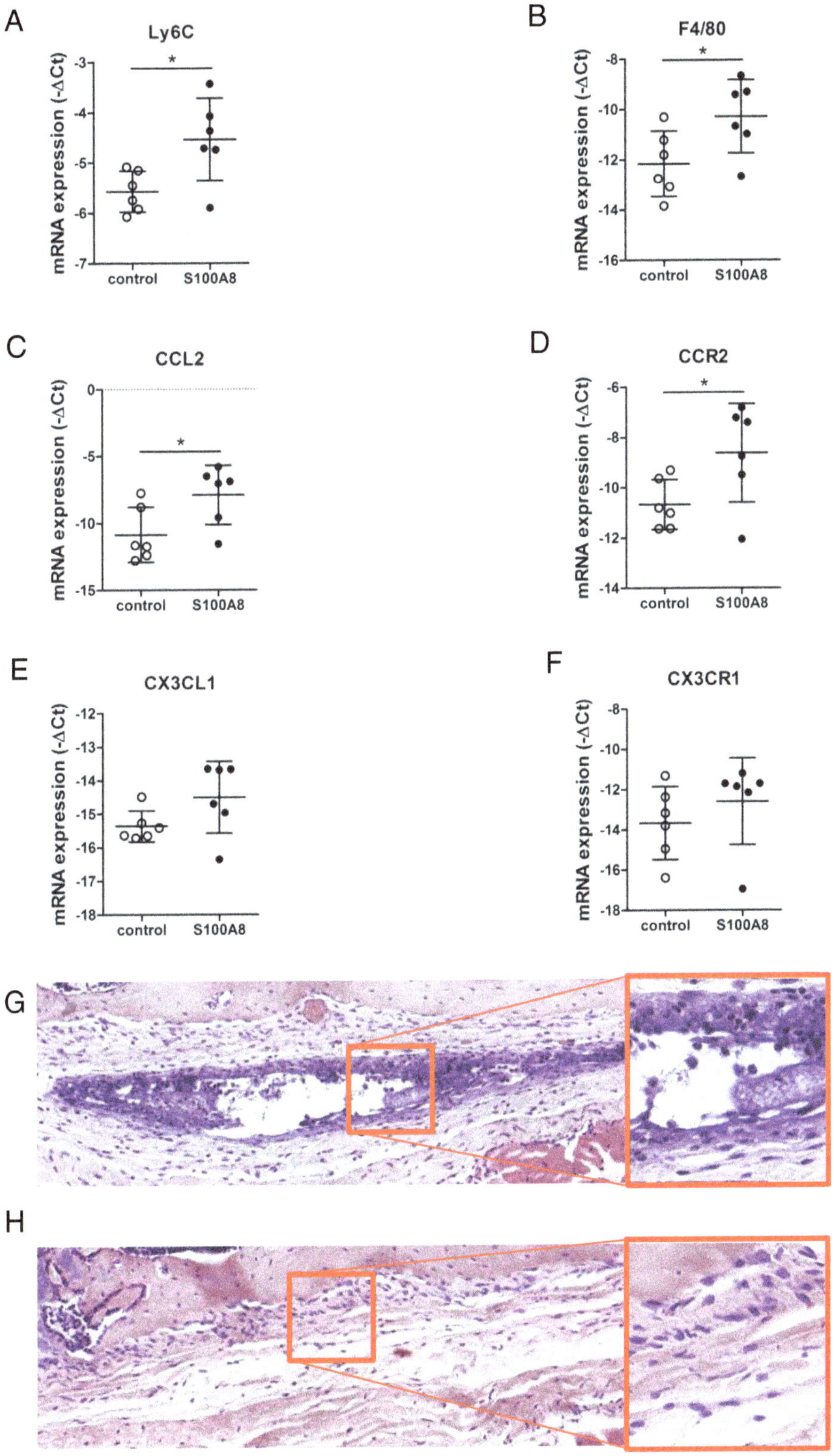

Fig. 2 (See legend on next page.)

Fig. 2 Intra articular injection of S100A8 leads to local induction of monocytes in the synovium. **a-f** mRNA expression of monocyte marker Ly6C (**a**), macrophage marker F4/80 (B), Ly6C^{high} chemokine CCL2 (**c**), and Ly6C^{high} chemokine receptor CCR2 (**d**) are increased in the synovium of mice 24 h after intra articular injection with S100A8, compared to BSA-injected controls, whereas Ly6C^{low} chemokine CX3CL1 (**e**), and Ly6C^{low} chemokine receptor CX3CR1 (**f**) are not affected after S100A8 administration, as analyzed using RT-qPCR. Data represent mean ± SD of six individual mice. *Significantly different from treated control (*$p < 0.05$). **g, h** HE staining on histological sections of the joint 24 h after intra-articular (i.a.) injection with S100A8 demonstrated strong presence of inflammatory cells with monocyte-like morphology in the synovial lining layer of the knee joints (**g**), whereas BSA injection as control resulted in less pronounced presence of inflammatory cells (**h**). Ct cycle threshold

found at day 7 CiOA when compared to saline injected controls, and also not between WT and S100a9$^{-/-}$ mice (see Fig. 3f and g for the monocyte gating strategy of the blood and spleen, respectively, using flow cytometry).

Increased numbers of Ly6C^{low}, but not Ly6C^{high} monocytes in the synovium of day 7 CiOA in S100a9$^{-/-}$ mice

As we observed differences in BM efflux between WT and S100a9$^{-/-}$ mice, we additionally studied whether there also was a difference in cell influx into the synovium between these two strains. At day 7 after induction of CiOA in S100a9$^{-/-}$, a lower number of inflammatory cells with monocyte morphology was observed in histological sections within the synovium when compared to WT mice (Fig. 4a vs WT b). We next studied mRNA expression of monocyte subset chemokine receptors and their ligands within the CiOA synovium of S100a9$^{-/-}$ mice (Fig. 4c). Expression levels of Ly6C^{high} monocyte chemokine CCL2 and its receptor CCR2 were similar in S100a9$^{-/-}$ and WT mice at CiOA day 7. In contrast, Ly6C^{low} chemokine CX3CL1 was significantly increased (1.9-fold) in S100a9$^{-/-}$ mice at CiOA day 7, whereas the mRNA expression of Ly6C^{low} monocyte chemokine receptor CX3CR1 was similar in WT and S100A9 mice at CiOA day 7.

Finally, synovium obtained from S100a9$^{-/-}$ mice at CiOA day 7 was shortly treated with collagenase and the numbers of Ly6C^{high} and Ly6C^{low} monocytes in the synovium were analyzed by flow cytometry (Fig. 4d). At day 7 CiOA in WT mice we found a significant rise in Ly6C^{high} monocytes, whereas Ly6C^{low} were not altered when compared to saline-injected WT mice. Interestingly, in S100a9$^{-/-}$ mice, levels of Ly6C^{high} monocytes were not altered when compared to saline-injected controls, whereas there was a significant increase in Ly6C^{low} monocytes (205%).

Taken together, locally induced S100A8/A9 production in early OA causes influx of Ly6C^{high} monocytes particularly, which are responsible for early production of cytokines and tissue damage. Moreover, inhibition of S100A8/A9 might give preference to influx of Ly6C^{low} monocytes, thereby regulating repair.

Discussion

Recent studies have shown that synovitis significantly contributes to the development of pathologic change in

the joint during inflammatory osteoarthritis [6]. Previously, we demonstrated that the alarmin S100A8/A9 plays an important role in synovitis and joint pathologic change in CiOA [22]. In the present study, we further explored the involvement of S100A8/A9 in the recruitment of monocyte subpopulations towards the synovium in CiOA. Our findings suggest that prolonged S100A8/A9 production during induction of inflammatory OA locally leads to strongly elevated mobilization of predominantly Ly6C^{high} monocytes into the joint in OA and from the BM.

The monocyte is the major inflammatory cell type within the synovium throughout the course of inflammatory OA [13–15]. In the mouse, two types of monocytes have been described. Ly6C^{high} monocytes, expressing high levels of CCR2 and guided by chemokine CCL2 are involved in removing tissue debris and produce mainly pro-inflammatory cytokines like IL-1β and S100A8/A9. In contrast, Ly6C^{low} monocytes, expressing high levels of CX3CR1 and attracted by CX3CL1, release anabolic factors like VEGF and TGF-β, involved in repairing joint tissue [31, 32].

The relative number and the interplay between Ly6C^{high} and Ly6C^{low} monocytes within the synovium determine the severity of inflammation and regulate further development of pathologic change in the tissues. Previous studies in our laboratory showed that selective removal of resident lining macrophages prior to induction of CiOA largely inhibited monocyte cell influx and development of joint destruction [40, 42].

In OA, resident synovial macrophages that cover the surface of the synovium are the first cells cleaning the extracellular matrix (ECM) fragments released by damaged joint tissue [43]. These fragments are recognized by TLRs and scavenger receptors, leading to activation of synovial macrophages thereby releasing high levels of CCL2. This elevates influx of Ly6C^{high} monocytes favoring further removal of tissue debris.

On the other hand, a shift towards higher numbers of Ly6C^{high} monocytes within the inflamed synovium may foster pathologic change in the joint by elevated release of pro-inflammatory cytokines. However, only low levels of cytokines like TNF-α, IL-1β, and IL-6 were observed during the first phase of CiOA and probably are only marginally involved in driving pathologic change in the joint. Induction of CiOA in mice lacking IL-1α/β had no

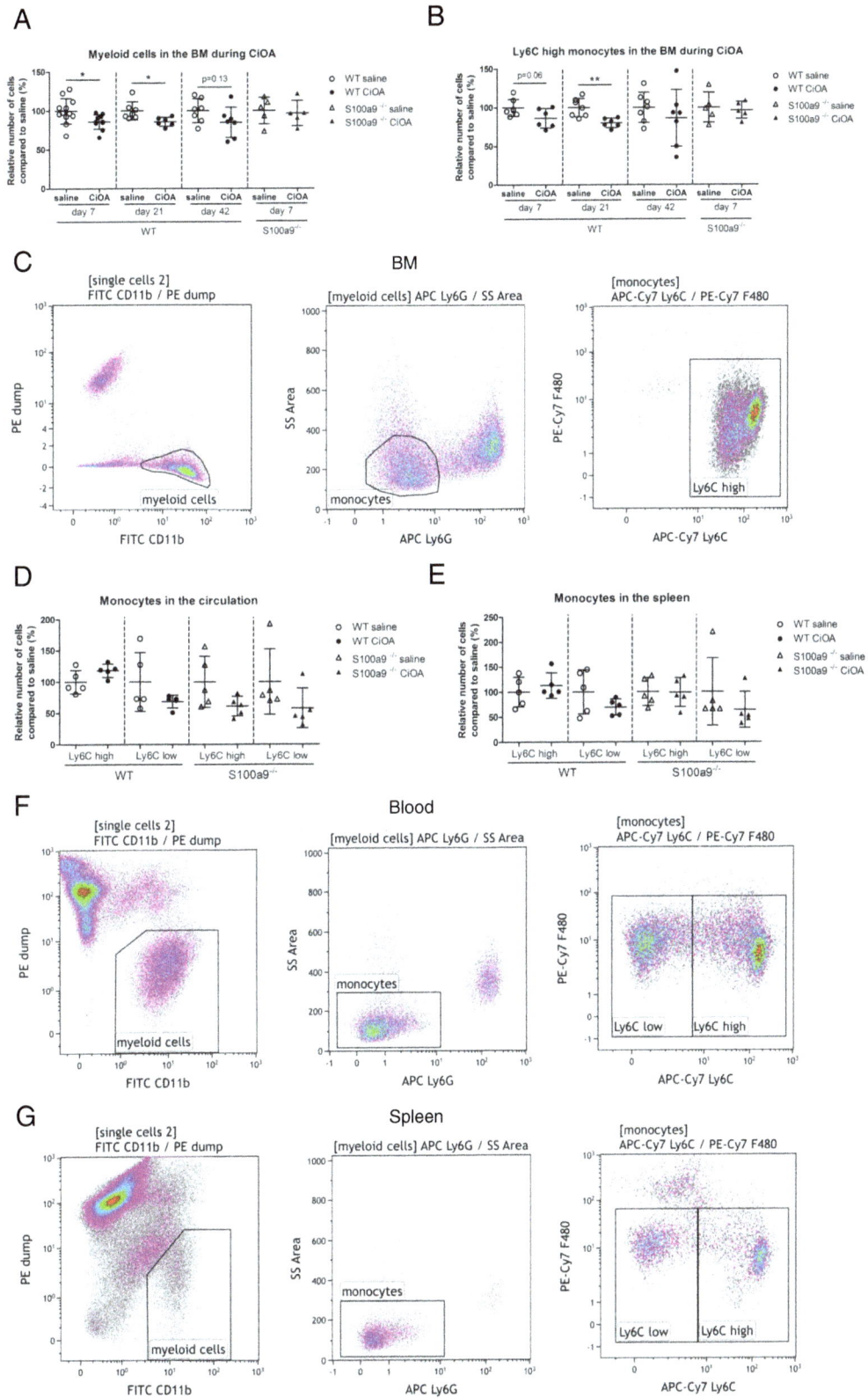

Fig. 3 (See legend on next page.)

(See figure on previous page.)

Fig. 3 The number of Ly6C^high monocytes decreases during collagenase-induced osteoarthritis (CiOA) in the bone marrow (BM) of wild-type (WT) but not S100a9^-/- mice, but not in the blood and spleen of WT or S100a9^-/- mice. **a** The relative number of myeloid cells in the complete contralateral femur of WT mice was decreased early during CiOA compared to saline-injected controls, whereas no effects were found in S100a9^-/- mice at CiOA day 7. **b** The relative number of Ly6C^high monocytes in the complete contralateral BM of WT mice was also decreased early during CiOA compared to saline-injected control animals, whereas no effect was observed in S100A9^-/- mice. **c** Gating strategy of monocyte subsets in the BM, using flow cytometry. **d, e** The relative number of Ly6C^high and Ly6C^low monocyte subpopulations was not affected in the peripheral blood (**d**), and spleen (**e**) at CiOA day 7 in WT or S100a9^-/- mice when compared to saline-injected control animals. **f, g** Gating strategy of monocyte subsets in the peripheral blood (**f**) and spleen (**g**), measured using flow cytometry. Data represent mean ± SD of 5–7 individual mice per group (except for WT mice on day 7 where n = 11–12 animals). *Significantly different from saline-injected control (*$p < 0.05$, **$p < 0.01$, ***$p < 0.001$)

effect on either synovitis or on joint pathology [44]. The outcome was similar using IL-6^-/- and TNF-α^-/- mice (manuscript in preparation). In contrast, alarmin S100A8/A9 was very strongly upregulated within the synovium and measured in significant amounts for prolonged periods up till day 42 after CiOA induction. The heterodimer is released by monocytes and activated macrophages and stimulates nearby synovial cells via TLR4 to release chemokines that attract monocyte populations [45, 46].

In the present study we found that levels of CCL2, attracting Ly6C^high monocytes, are much higher in day 7

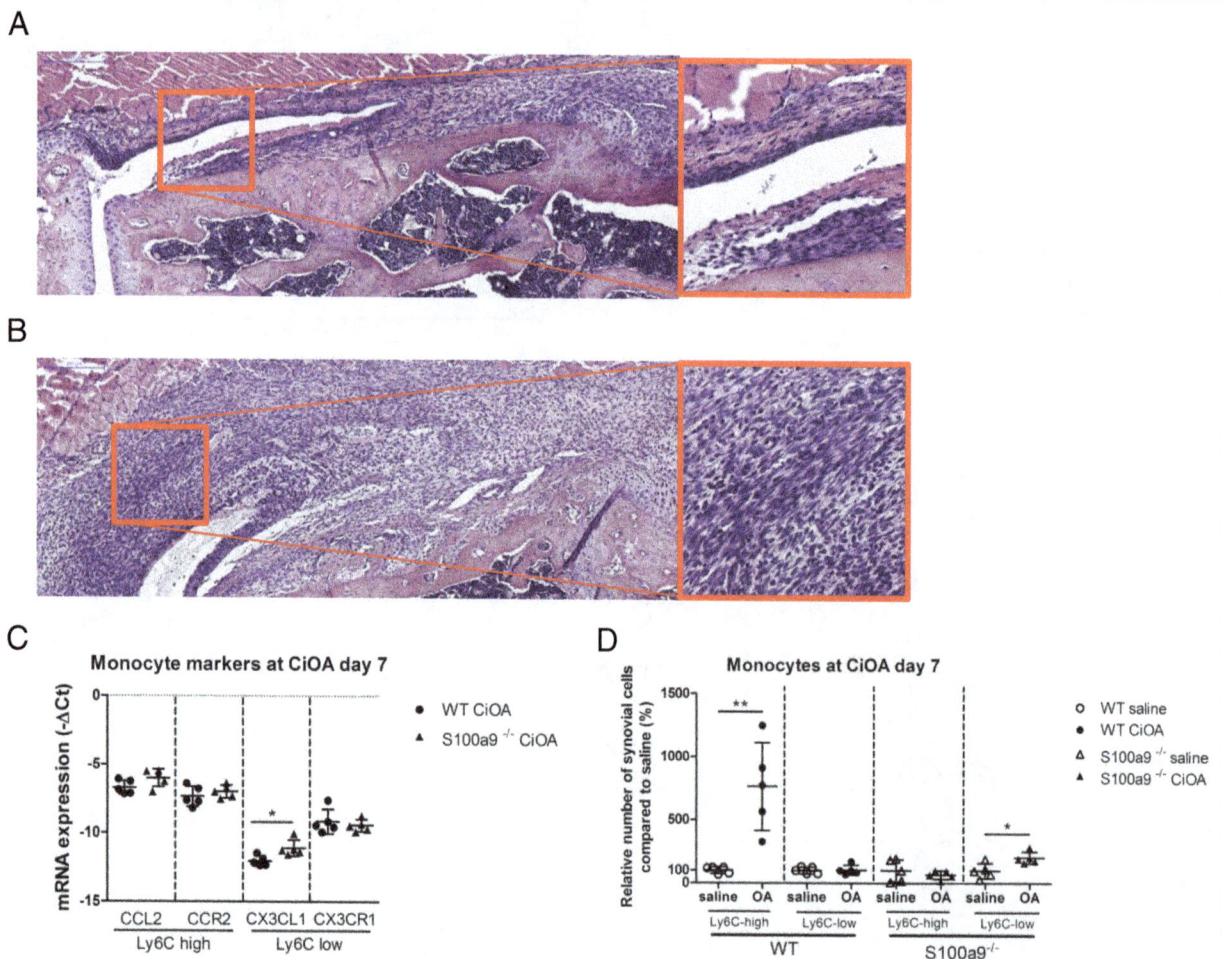

Fig. 4 S100a9^-/- mice have locally more Ly6C^low monocytes in early collagenase-induced osteoarthritis (CiOA), compared to wild-type (WT) mice at CiOA day 7. **a, b** Less influx of inflammatory cells in S100a9^-/- (**a**) mice compared to WT mice (**b**) at CiOA day 7, as shown by HE staining. **c** mRNA expression of the Ly6C^low monocyte-subset-attracting chemokine CX3CL1 is increased in the synovium of S100a9^-/- mice compared to WT mice at CiOA day 7, while Ly6C^high monocyte-subset-attracting chemokine CCL2 and both monocyte subset cell markers CCR2 (Ly6C^high) and CX3CR1 (Ly6C^low) were not different between the two strains. **d** Relative number of Ly6C^high monocytes are increased locally in the joint of WT mice, whereas Ly6C^low monocytes are increased in S100a9^-/- mice, compared to saline-injected controls, as analyzed by flow cytometry. Data represent mean ± SD of five individual mice per group. *Significantly different from saline-injected control (*$p < 0.05$, ***$p < 0.001$)

CiOA compared to saline-injected controls in WT mice, resulting in increased presence of Ly6C^{high} monocytes in the synovium. In addition, CCL2 expression was strongly enhanced in the synovium after i.a. injection of S100A8, pointing towards an important role for S100A8/A9 in this process. Whereas in synovium at day 7 CiOA, expression of CCR2/CCL2, characteristic of Ly6C^{high} monocytes, was comparable in both WT and S100a9$^{-/-}$ mice, the Ly6C^{low}-attracting chemokine CX3CL1 and Ly6C^{low} monocyte population was raised in the synovium of S100a9$^{-/-}$ mice. Since Ly6C^{high} monocytes were not elevated in S100a9$^{-/-}$ synovium, but the Ly6C^{low} monocytes were, S100A8/S100A9 may favor the presence of Ly6C^{high} monocytes within the inflamed synovium, not only by chemotactic attraction but also by suppressing their differentiation into the Ly6C^{low} population thereby maintaining the monocyte population into a more pro-inflammatory state.

Recently it was shown that monocytes have a memory, which is triggered by TLR4 ligands like lipopolysaccharide (LPS) [47]. This memory is initiated by epigenetic programming and may drive monocytes into a cell type that sustains its pro-inflammatory characteristics [48]. S100A8/A9 is an important TLR4 ligand released in high levels for prolonged periods in the joint in OA and may be a major mediator driving this epigenetic programming. Ly6C^{high} monocytes are high producers of S100A8/A9, which may form a positive feedback loop. Finally Ly6C^{high} and Ly6C^{low} monocytes are possibly able to differentiate into M1-like and M2-like macrophages, respectively [49, 50]. The local environment within the synovium strongly influences the signature of the monocytes and their differentiation into their mature forms [50, 51].

BM and spleen form important reservoirs for Ly6C^{high} monocytes, which become available under inflammatory conditions. Local induction of CiOA causes high levels of S100A8/A9 within the synovium for prolonged periods; up to 5 μg/mL have been measured in synovial washouts of CiOA synovium [52]. These proteins leak from the joint into the blood and elevated levels of S100A8/A9 levels were measured throughout the course of OA until the endpoint at day 42. Other pro-inflammatory cytokines like IL-1β, TNF-α, or IL-6 were not detected within the blood.

Interestingly local induction of CiOA in the knee joints of WT mice induced a significant efflux of Ly6C^{high} monocytes from the BM into the blood when compared to saline-injected WT mice, which was absent at CiOA day 7 in S100a9$^{-/-}$ mice. This indicates that low-grade local joint inflammation in OA is able to initiate release of Ly6C^{high} monocytes from the BM. This is in agreement with an earlier study showing that locally induced low-grade inflammation in the heart in myocardial infarction [32, 53] induced efflux from the BM resulting in elevated local influx of Ly6C^{high} monocytes within the lesions. Which mechanisms that are initiated within the inflamed joint drive monocyte efflux from the BM is momentarily under investigation. In contrast to conventional pro-inflammatory cytokines, which were undetectable in the blood, S100A8/A9 levels were very high during the course of CiOA. S100A8/A9 in the blood is not only transported as a free protein but also inside extracellular vesicles (EVs). EVs, released by activated immune cells like monocytes/neutrophils, have been shown to contain S100A8/A9 [54, 55]. They are released at local inflammatory sites and additionally transported to distant areas where they can affect other cells by either fusion with their membrane or when recognized by receptors [54, 55]. In addition, mechanisms like sympathetic nerve signaling may explain part of the systemic effects observed in the BM. Earlier studies suggested that myocardial infarction liberates monocytes from the BM due to sympathetic nerve signaling thereby boosting atherosclerosis in which pathologic change is highly regulated by the influx of monocyte sub-populations [53].

Myeloid precursors in the BM differentiate into Ly6C^{high} monocytes driven by growth factors like PU.1, and M-CSF. Local inflammation promotes the release of Ly6C^{high} monocytes from the BM into the circulation where they either remain in that state or are transformed into Ly6C^{low} monocytes [32]. Interestingly, S100a9$^{-/-}$ mice did not have elevated efflux of monocytes at CiOA day 7. S100A8/A9 is also abundantly expressed within the BM. Systemic inflammatory triggers and/or sympathetic nerve signaling may promote local release of S100A8/A9 heterodimer within the BM stimulating migration of Ly6C^{high} monocytes to the blood. This is supported by our findings that expression levels of LFA-1 (Integrin-β2), VCAM, L-selectin, PECAM1, and VE-cadherin were significantly decreased in the BM of S100a9$^{-/-}$ mice (Additional file 1: Figure S2). It is described that all these adhesion molecules contribute to leucocyte adhesion and migration in the BM [34, 56]. S100A8/A9 alarmins are strong activators of the beta-2 integrin on myeloid cells and have been shown to be important in transendothelial migration of phagocytes [26, 57–59]. Moreover, previous studies have already shown that S100A8/A9 drives primary BM expansion of myeloid-derived suppressor cells (MDSC) driven by the S100A9/CD33 pathway thereby altering hematopoiesis [60].

Apart from the BM the spleen also forms an important reservoir for storage of Ly6C^{high} monocytes [61] and may contribute to sustaining synovitis in OA. Although it is described that acute inflammation promotes monocyte release from the spleen [62], we did not find any effect on the ratio of monocyte populations in the spleen of mice at CiOA day 7. This is in agreement with an earlier study in which it was found that in a more severe model of arthritis, splenectomized mice did not differ in ankle swelling or clinical score compared to non-splenectomized mice [63], suggesting that monocytes released from the spleen do not contribute to synovial inflammation in arthritis.

Although BM efflux of monocytes was significantly raised at CiOA day 7, no effect on the ratio of monocyte subsets was observed within the blood. Although the data as presented in this manuscript strongly suggest a role for S100A8/A9 in the efflux of cells from the BM and into the inflamed joint, we cannot prove a causal relation for this mechanism. Monocytes are released from the BM as Ly6C^{high} monocytes and the ratio of Ly6C^{high} and Ly6C^{low} may be rapidly balanced by systemic factors. Tracking studies using fluorescent-labeled monocytes are in progress and will answer to what extent Ly6C^{high} monocytes released from the BM are able to reach the joint in OA.

OA is characterized by cartilage and bone destruction, which is related to synovitis [6]. A privileged presence of Ly6C^{high} monocytes within the synovium leads to prolonged production of inflammatory cytokines (particularly S100A8/A9) and proteases, which may contribute to joint destruction. Earlier studies showed that S100A8/A9 is crucial in mediating cartilage and bone destruction within the CiOA model [22]. S100A8/A9 stimulates chondrocytes to produce matrix metalloproteinases (MMPs) thereby degrading the surrounding ECM [64], which drives synovitis in a positive feedback loop. In addition, S100A8/A9 directly stimulated osteoclastogenesis and strongly increased osteoclast-mediated bone destruction. The human analogs of Ly6C^{high} and Ly6C^{low} in the mouse are classical CD14++CD16- and non-classical CD14 + CD16+, respectively. Investigating the balance of these monocyte subsets within inflammatory OA in synovium and BM may give more insight into how synovitis and joint destruction are connected to this crippling disease.

In summary we found that S100A8/A9 is a crucial alarmin involved in favoring recruitment of Ly6C^{high} monocytes into the CiOA knee joint. Local production of S100A8/A9 attracts Ly6C^{high} monocytes and may suppress their differentiation into Ly6C^{low} monocytes. Moreover production of S100A8/A9 within the bone marrow may further promote efflux of Ly6C^{high} monocytes into the circulation. Ly6C^{high} monocytes are potent producers of S100A8/A9 keeping the monocyte population in a pro-inflammatory state and forming a positive feedback loop. Understanding the underlying inflammatory process in the synovium in OA may lead to new therapeutic targets and inhibiting S100A8/A9 may be an interesting therapeutic target to improve the outcome of OA pathology.

Conclusions

Induction of OA leads to the elevation of S100A8/A9 locally in the joint and systemically in the circulation, and leads to the mobilization of Ly6C^{high} monocytes from the BM to the joint. S100A8/A9 has an important role in driving OA pathology, probably by regulating the local environment in the joint determining whether Ly6C^{high} or Ly6C^{low} monocytes are recruited.

Additional file

Additional file 1: Figure S1. S100A8/A9 protein levels are systemically elevated in the serum during early CiOA. Systemic levels of S100A8/A9 protein in serum of WT mice are increased early during CiOA compared to saline-injected control mice, measured using ELISA. Data represent mean ± SD of five individual mice per group per time point. *Significantly different from saline-injected control (*$p < 0.05$, **$p < 0.01$, ***$p < 0.001$). **Figure S2.** Expression of adhesion molecules is lower in the BM of WT mice, compared to S100a9$^{-/-}$ mice, at CiOA day 7. mRNA expression of several adhesion molecules is lower in the BM of S100a9$^{-/-}$ mice compared to WT mice at CiOA day 7. Data represent mean ± SD of five individual mice. *Significantly different from saline-injected control (*$p < 0.05$, **$p < 0.01$, ***$p < 0.001$). (PPT 142 kb)

Abbreviations

bp: Base pair (s); BM: Bone marrow; BSA: Bovine serum albumin; cDNA: Complementary DNA; CCL2: (C-C motif) ligand; CCR2: C-C chemokine receptor type 2; CiOA: Collagenase-induced osteoarthritis; Ct: Cycle threshold; DAMPs: Damage-associated molecular patterns proteins; ELISA: Enzyme-linked immunosorbent assay; EVs: extracellular vesicles; FACS: Fluorescence-activated cell sorting; HE: Haematoxylin and eosin; IL: interleukin; MRP: Myeloid related proteins; NK: Natural killer; OA: Osteoarthritis; PBS: Phosphate-buffered saline; RT-qPCR: Reverse-transcription quantitative PCR; TGF: Transforming growth factor; TLR: Toll-like receptor; TNF: Tumor necrosis factor; VEGF: Vascular endothelial growth factor; WT: Wild-type

Acknowledgements

Not applicable.

Funding

This study was supported by grants from the Radboud University Medical Center (UMC) and the Dutch Arthritis Foundation (#13-3-402). The funding sources had no role in study design, collection, analysis, or interpretation of the data, or in writing the manuscript or the decision to submit the manuscript.

Authors' contributions

NAJC, MvdB, EJWG, ABB, and PLEMvL conceived and designed the experiments; NAJC, MvdB, SvD, IDC, GA, and AS performed the experiments; NAJC, MvdB, EJWG, ABB, and PLEMvL analyzed the data; TV and JR contributed reagents/materials/analysis tools; NAJC, MvdB, FvdL, MK, PvdK, ABB, and PLEMvL wrote the paper; all authors read and approved the final manuscript.

Consent for publication

Not applicable.

Competing interests

The authors declare that they have no competing interests.

Author details
[1]Experimental Rheumatology, Department of Rheumatology, Radboud University Medical Center, PO Box 9101, Nijmegen 6500 HB, The Netherlands. [2]Institute of Immunology, University of Munster, Munster, Germany.

References

1. Zhang Y, Jordan JM. Epidemiology of osteoarthritis. Clin Geriatr Med. 2010;26:355–69.
2. Palazzo C, Nguyen C, Lefevre-Colau MM, Rannou F, Poiraudeau S. Risk factors and burden of osteoarthritis. Ann Phys Rehabil Med. 2016;59:134–8.
3. Bijlsma JW, Berenbaum F, Lafeber FP. Osteoarthritis: an update with relevance for clinical practice. Lancet. 2011;377:2115–26.
4. Thysen S, Luyten FP, Lories RJ. Targets, models and challenges in osteoarthritis research. Dis Model Mech. 2015;8:17–30.
5. Berenbaum F. New horizons and perspectives in the treatment of osteoarthritis. Arthritis Res Ther. 2008;10 Suppl 2:S1.
6. Sokolove J, Lepus CM. Role of inflammation in the pathogenesis of osteoarthritis: latest findings and interpretations. Ther Adv Musculoskelet Dis. 2013;5:77–94.
7. Krasnokutsky S, Attur M, Palmer G, Samuels J, Abramson SB. Current concepts in the pathogenesis of osteoarthritis. Osteoarthritis Cartilage. 2008; 16 Suppl 3:S1–3.
8. Benito MJ, Veale DJ, FitzGerald O, van den Berg WB, Bresnihan B. Synovial tissue inflammation in early and late osteoarthritis. Ann Rheum Dis. 2005;64:1263–7.
9. Scanzello CR, Goldring SR. The role of synovitis in osteoarthritis pathogenesis. Bone. 2012;51:249–57.
10. Sellam J, Berenbaum F. The role of synovitis in pathophysiology and clinical symptoms of osteoarthritis. Nat Rev Rheumatol. 2010;6:625–35.
11. Haywood L, McWilliams DF, Pearson CI, Gill SE, Ganesan A, Wilson D, Walsh DA. Inflammation and angiogenesis in osteoarthritis. Arthritis Rheum. 2003;48:2173–7.
12. Spector TD, Hart DJ, Nandra D, Doyle DV, Mackillop N, Gallimore JR, Pepys MB. Low-level increases in serum C-reactive protein are present in early osteoarthritis of the knee and predict progressive disease. Arthritis Rheum. 1997;40:723–7.
13. Raghu H, Lepus CM, Wang Q, Wong HH, Lingampalli N, Oliviero F, Punzi L, Giori NJ, Goodman SB, Chu CR, et al. CCL2/CCR2, but not CCL5/CCR5, mediates monocyte recruitment, inflammation and cartilage destruction in osteoarthritis. Ann Rheum Dis. 2017;76:914–22.
14. Van Lent PL, Blom A, Holthuysen AE, Jacobs CW, Van De Putte LB, Van Den Berg WB. Monocytes/macrophages rather than PMN are involved in early cartilage degradation in cationic immune complex arthritis in mice. J Leukoc Biol. 1997;61:267–78.
15. van den Bosch MH, Blom AB, Schelbergen RF, Koenders MI, van de Loo FA, van den Berg WB, Vogl T, Roth J, van der Kraan PM, van Lent PL. Alarmin S100A9 induces proinflammatory and catabolic effects predominantly in the M1 macrophages of human osteoarthritic synovium. J Rheumatol. 2016;43:1874–84.
16. Kandahari AM, Yang X, Dighe AS, Pan D, Cui Q. Recognition of immune response for the early diagnosis and treatment of osteoarthritis. J Immunol Res. 2015;2015:192415.
17. Perera C, McNeil HP, Geczy CL. S100 Calgranulins in inflammatory arthritis. Immunol Cell Biol. 2010;88:41–9.
18. Kang KY, Woo JW, Park SH. S100A8/A9 as a biomarker for synovial inflammation and joint damage in patients with rheumatoid arthritis. Korean J Intern Med. 2014;29:12–9.
19. Schiopu A, Cotoi OS. S100A8 and S100A9: DAMPs at the crossroads between innate immunity, traditional risk factors, and cardiovascular disease. Mediators Inflamm. 2013;2013:828354.
20. Vogl T, Gharibyan AL, Morozova-Roche LA. Pro-inflammatory S100A8 and S100A9 proteins: self-assembly into multifunctional native and amyloid complexes. Int J Mol Sci. 2012;13:2893–917.
21. Vogl T, Tenbrock K, Ludwig S, Leukert N, Ehrhardt C, van Zoelen MA, Nacken W, Foell D, van der Poll T, Sorg C, Roth J. Mrp8 and Mrp14 are endogenous activators of Toll-like receptor 4, promoting lethal, endotoxin-induced shock. Nat Med. 2007;13:1042–9.
22. van Lent PL, Blom AB, Schelbergen RF, Sloetjes A, Lafeber FP, Lems WF, Cats H, Vogl T, Roth J, van den Berg WB. Active involvement of alarmins S100A8 and S100A9 in the regulation of synovial activation and joint destruction during mouse and human osteoarthritis. Arthritis Rheum. 2012;64:1466–76.
23. Schelbergen RF, de Munter W, van den Bosch MH, Lafeber FP, Sloetjes A, Vogl T, Roth J, van den Berg WB, van der Kraan PM, Blom AB, van Lent PL. Alarmins S100A8/S100A9 aggravate osteophyte formation in experimental osteoarthritis and predict osteophyte progression in early human symptomatic osteoarthritis. Ann Rheum Dis. 2016;75:218–25.
24. Schelbergen RF, Geven EJ, van den Bosch MH, Eriksson H, Leanderson T, Vogl T, Roth J, van de Loo FA, Koenders MI, van der Kraan PM, et al. Prophylactic treatment with S100A9 inhibitor paquinimod reduces pathology in experimental collagenase-induced osteoarthritis. Ann Rheum Dis. 2015;74:2254–8.
25. Gross SR, Sin CG, Barraclough R, Rudland PS. Joining S100 proteins and migration: for better or for worse, in sickness and in health. Cell Mol Life Sci. 2014;71:1551–79.
26. Pruenster M, Kurz AR, Chung KJ, Cao-Ehlker X, Bieber S, Nussbaum CF, Bierschenk S, Eggersmann TK, Rohwedder I, Heinig K, et al. Extracellular MRP8/14 is a regulator of beta2 integrin-dependent neutrophil slow rolling and adhesion. Nat Commun. 2015;6:6915.
27. Lin YM, Hsu CJ, Liao YY, Chou MC, Tang CH. The CCL2/CCR2 axis enhances vascular cell adhesion molecule-1 expression in human synovial fibroblasts. PLoS One. 2012;7:e49999.
28. Deshmane SL, Kremlev S, Amini S, Sawaya BE. Monocyte chemoattractant protein-1 (MCP-1): an overview. J Interferon Cytokine Res. 2009;29:313–26.
29. Jung H, Mithal DS, Park JE, Miller RJ. Localized CCR2 activation in the bone marrow niche mobilizes monocytes by desensitizing CXCR4. PLoS One. 2015;10:e0128387.
30. Imhof BA, Aurrand-Lions M. Adhesion mechanisms regulating the migration of monocytes. Nat Rev Immunol. 2004;4:432–44.
31. Thomas G, Tacke R, Hedrick CC, Hanna RN. Nonclassical patrolling monocyte function in the vasculature. Arterioscler Thromb Vasc Biol. 2015;35:1306–16.
32. Dutta P, Nahrendorf M. Monocytes in myocardial infarction. Arterioscler Thromb Vasc Biol. 2015;35:1066–70.
33. Sheel M, Engwerda CR. The diverse roles of monocytes in inflammation caused by protozoan parasitic diseases. Trends Parasitol. 2012;28:408–16.
34. Shi C, Pamer EG. Monocyte recruitment during infection and inflammation. Nat Rev Immunol. 2011;11:762–74.
35. Amsellem V, Abid S, Poupel L, Parpaleix A, Rodero M, Gary-Bobo G, Latiri M, Dubois-Rande JL, Lipskaia L, Combadiere C, Adnot S. Roles for the CX3CL1/CX3CR1 and CCL2/CCR2 chemokine systems in hypoxic pulmonary hypertension. Am J Respir Cell Mol Biol. 2017;56(5):597–608.
36. Cremers NA, Suttorp M, Gerritsen MM, Wong RJ, van Run-van Breda C, van Dam GM, Brouwer KM, Kuijpers-Jagtman AM, Carels CE, Lundvig DM, Wagener FA. Mechanical stress changes the complex interplay between HO-1, inflammation and fibrosis, during excisional wound repair. Front Med (Lausanne). 2015;2:86.
37. Manitz MP, Horst B, Seeliger S, Strey A, Skryabin BV, Gunzer M, Frings W, Schonlau F, Roth J, Sorg C, Nacken W. Loss of S100A9 (MRP14) results in reduced interleukin-8-induced CD11b surface expression, a polarized microfilament system, and diminished responsiveness to chemoattractants in vitro. Mol Cell Biol. 2003;23:1034–43.
38. van der Kraan PM, Vitters EL, van de Putte LB, van den Berg WB. Development of osteoarthritic lesions in mice by "metabolic" and "mechanical" alterations in the knee joints. Am J Pathol. 1989;135:1001–14.
39. van den Bosch MH, Blom AB, Kram V, Maeda A, Sikka S, Gabet Y, Kilts TM, van den Berg WB, van Lent PL, van der Kraan PM, Young MF: WISP1/CCN4 aggravates cartilage degeneration in experimental osteoarthritis. Osteoarthritis Cartilage. 2017. doi: 10.1016/j.joca.2017.07.012. [Epub ahead of print].
40. Blom AB, van Lent PL, Holthuysen AE, van der Kraan PM, Roth J, van Rooijen N, van den Berg WB. Synovial lining macrophages mediate osteophyte formation during experimental osteoarthritis. Osteoarthritis Cartilage. 2004;12:627–35.
41. Goebeler M, Roth J, Burwinkel F, Vollmer E, Bocker W, Sorg C. Expression and complex formation of S100-like proteins MRP8 and MRP14 by macrophages during renal allograft rejection. Transplantation. 1994;58:355–61.
42. Blom AB, van Lent PL, Libregts S, Holthuysen AE, van der Kraan PM, van Rooijen N, van den Berg WB. Crucial role of macrophages in matrix metalloproteinase-mediated cartilage destruction during experimental osteoarthritis: involvement of matrix metalloproteinase 3. Arthritis Rheum. 2007;56:147–57.

43. Rengel Y, Ospelt C, Gay S. Proteinases in the joint: clinical relevance of proteinases in joint destruction. Arthritis Res Ther. 2007;9:221.

44. van Dalen SC, Blom AB, Sloetjes AW, Helsen MM, Roth J, Vogl T, van de Loo FA, Koenders MI, van der Kraan PM, van den Berg WB, et al. Interleukin-1 is not involved in synovial inflammation and cartilage destruction in collagenase-induced osteoarthritis. Osteoarthritis Cartilage. 2017;25:385–96.

45. Fassl SK, Austermann J, Papantonopoulou O, Riemenschneider M, Xue J, Bertheloot D, Freise N, Spiekermann C, Witten A, Viemann D, et al. Transcriptome assessment reveals a dominant role for TLR4 in the activation of human monocytes by the alarmin MRP8. J Immunol. 2015;194:575–83.

46. Sunahori K, Yamamura M, Yamana J, Takasugi K, Kawashima M, Yamamoto H, Chazin WJ, Nakatani Y, Yui S, Makino H. The S100A8/A9 heterodimer amplifies proinflammatory cytokine production by macrophages via activation of nuclear factor kappa B and p38 mitogen-activated protein kinase in rheumatoid arthritis. Arthritis Res Ther. 2006;8:R69.

47. Bekkering S, Joosten LA, van der Meer JW, Netea MG, Riksen NP. The epigenetic memory of monocytes and macrophages as a novel drug target in atherosclerosis. Clin Ther. 2015;37:914–23.

48. Bekkering S, Blok BA, Joosten LA, Riksen NP, van Crevel R, Netea MG. In vitro experimental model of trained innate immunity in human primary monocytes. Clin Vaccine Immunol. 2016;23:926–33.

49. Auffray C, Fogg D, Garfa M, Elain G, Join-Lambert O, Kayal S, Sarnacki S, Cumano A, Lauvau G, Geissmann F. Monitoring of blood vessels and tissues by a population of monocytes with patrolling behavior. Science. 2007;317:666–70.

50. Italiani P, Boraschi D. From Monocytes to M1/M2 macrophages: phenotypical vs. functional differentiation. Front Immunol. 2014;5:514.

51. Liddiard K, Taylor PR. Understanding local macrophage phenotypes in disease: shape-shifting macrophages. Nat Med. 2015;21:119–20.

52. Schelbergen RF, van Dalen S, ter Huurne M, Roth J, Vogl T, Noel D, Jorgensen C, van den Berg WB, van de Loo FA, Blom AB, van Lent PL. Treatment efficacy of adipose-derived stem cells in experimental osteoarthritis is driven by high synovial activation and reflected by S100A8/A9 serum levels. Osteoarthritis Cartilage. 2014;22:1158–66.

53. Dutta P, Courties G, Wei Y, Leuschner F, Gorbatov R, Robbins CS, Iwamoto Y, Thompson B, Carlson AL, Heidt T, et al. Myocardial infarction accelerates atherosclerosis. Nature. 2012;487:325–9.

54. Burke M, Choksawangkarn W, Edwards N, Ostrand-Rosenberg S, Fenselau C. Exosomes from myeloid-derived suppressor cells carry biologically active proteins. J Proteome Res. 2014;13:836–43.

55. Maus RLG, Jakub JW, Nevala WK, Christensen TA, Noble-Orcutt K, Sachs Z, Hieken TJ, Markovic SN. Human melanoma-derived extracellular vesicles regulate dendritic cell maturation. Front Immunol. 2017;8:358.

56. Albelda SM, Buck CA. Integrins and other cell adhesion molecules. FASEB J. 1990;4:2868–80.

57. Newton RA, Hogg N. The human S100 protein MRP-14 is a novel activator of the beta 2 integrin Mac-1 on neutrophils. J Immunol. 1998;160:1427–35.

58. Donato R, Cannon BR, Sorci G, Riuzzi F, Hsu K, Weber DJ, Geczy CL. Functions of S100 proteins. Curr Mol Med. 2013;13:24–57.

59. Vogl T, Ludwig S, Goebeler M, Strey A, Thorey IS, Reichelt R, Foell D, Gerke V, Manitz MP, Nacken W, et al. MRP8 and MRP14 control microtubule reorganization during transendothelial migration of phagocytes. Blood. 2004;104:4260–8.

60. Chen X, Eksioglu EA, Zhou J, Zhang L, Djeu J, Fortenbery N, Epling-Burnette P, Van Bijnen S, Dolstra H, Cannon J, et al. Induction of myelodysplasia by myeloid-derived suppressor cells. J Clin Invest. 2013;123:4595–611.

61. Kim E, Yang J, Beltran CD, Cho S. Role of spleen-derived monocytes/macrophages in acute ischemic brain injury. J Cereb Blood Flow Metab. 2014;34:1411–9.

62. Swirski FK, Nahrendorf M, Etzrodt M, Wildgruber M, Cortez-Retamozo V, Panizzi P, Figueiredo JL, Kohler RH, Chudnovskiy A, Waterman P, et al. Identification of splenic reservoir monocytes and their deployment to inflammatory sites. Science. 2009;325:612–6.

63. Misharin AV, Cuda CM, Saber R, Turner JD, Gierut AK, Haines 3rd GK, Berdnikovs S, Filer A, Clark AR, Buckley CD, et al. Nonclassical Ly6C(-) monocytes drive the development of inflammatory arthritis in mice. Cell Rep. 2014;9:591–604.

64. Yammani RR. S100 proteins in cartilage: role in arthritis. Biochim Biophys Acta. 2012;1822:600–6.

The effects of resistance training on muscle strength, joint pain, and hand function in individuals with hand osteoarthritis

Nicoló Edoardo Magni[1*], Peter John McNair[1] and David Andrew Rice[1,2]

Abstract

Background: Hand osteoarthritis is a common condition characterised by joint pain and muscle weakness. These factors are thought to contribute to ongoing disability. Some evidence exists that resistance training decreases pain, improves muscle strength, and enhances function in people with knee and hip osteoarthritis. However, there is currently a lack of consensus regarding its effectiveness in people with hand osteoarthritis. Therefore, the aim of this systematic review and meta-analysis was to establish whether resistance training in people with hand osteoarthritis increases grip strength, decreases joint pain, and improves hand function.

Methods: Seven databases were searched from 1975 until July 1, 2016. Randomised controlled trials were included. The Cochrane Risk of Bias Tool was used to assess studies' methodological quality. The Grade of Recommendations Assessment, Development, and Evaluation system was adopted to rate overall quality of evidence. Suitable studies were pooled using a random-effects meta-analysis.

Results: Five studies were included with a total of 350 participants. The majority of the training programs did not meet recommended intensity, frequency, or progression criteria for muscle strengthening. There was moderate-quality evidence that resistance training does not improve grip strength (mean difference = 1.35; 95% confidence interval (CI) = −0.84, 3.54; I^2 = 50%; $p = 0.23$). Low-quality evidence showed significant improvements in joint pain (standardised mean difference (SMD) = −0.23; 95% CI = −0.42, −0.04; I^2 = 0%; $p = 0.02$) which were not clinically relevant. Low-quality evidence demonstrated no improvements in hand function following resistance training (SMD = −0.1; 95% CI = −0.33, 0.13; I^2 = 28%; $p = 0.39$).

Conclusion: There is no evidence that resistance training has a significant effect on grip strength or hand function in people with hand osteoarthritis. Low-quality evidence suggests it has a small, clinically unimportant pain-relieving effect. Future studies should investigate resistance training regimes with adequate intensity, frequency, and progressions to achieve gains in muscle strength.

Keywords: Hand osteoarthritis, Rehabilitation, Conservative treatment, Resistance training, Muscle strength, Grip strength, Pain, Function

* Correspondence: nico.magni@aut.ac.nz
[1]Health and Rehabilitation Research Institute, Auckland University of Technology, 90 Akoranga Drive, Northcote, Auckland 0627, New Zealand
Full list of author information is available at the end of the article

Background

Hand osteoarthritis (OA) is present in 26% of females and 13% of males over the age of 71 [1]. Despite its relevance in terms of pain, disability, and economic burden on society, OA has often been referred to as 'the forgotten disease' [2]. Compared with the knee and hip joints, there are far fewer studies that have focused on conservative treatment for this pathology. Current clinical management of hand OA is centered on medications, which have been shown to be associated with notable side effects (e.g., ulcers, bleeding, renal failure, opioid addiction) [3]. The need for more effective and safe conservative interventions has been advocated by a number of authors [2, 4, 5]. Among the conservative treatments available for OA, exercises have been shown to be cost-effective and useful in improving quality of life [6]. Exercise aims to reduce the magnitude of change observed in strength, joint range of motion, proprioception, and alignment, which are often impaired due to the natural course of the disease and disuse [7]. Such impairments lead to reductions in function and quality of life [8].

Resistance training is an exercise intervention that has been utilised to decrease symptoms, impairment, and improve function in individuals with OA at the knee and hip [9, 10]. Several studies have demonstrated its effectiveness and this treatment modality is included in the American College of Rheumatology 2012 treatment guidelines for knee and hip OA, but not for hand OA [11]. The EULAR 2007 recommendations for the management of hand OA suggested the use of education plus exercise for the treatment of this pathology [12]. However, findings from only one randomised controlled trial (RCT) were used to support this recommendation and there was no direct evidence for education or exercises alone for the treatment of hand OA.

A number of studies have highlighted reduced muscle strength in those with hand OA [1, 13–16]. Furthermore, it is well known that many tasks of work and daily living require notable force to be exerted to complete them successfully [17]. Therefore, one might expect greater attention to have been paid to limiting muscle strength deficits through interventions such as resistance training. Previous reviews on hand OA have highlighted the limited number of studies assessing the effect of exercise on people with hand OA [4, 5, 18, 19]. To date, no reviews have focused specifically on the efficacy of resistance training exercises for hand OA and examined the training regimes adopted in the intervention studies. Thus, the aim of the current study was to perform a systematic review and meta-analysis of the effect of resistance training on grip strength, joint pain, and hand function in people with hand OA. Based on findings from studies in other joints affected by OA [9], we hypothesised that resistance training would improve muscle strength, joint pain, and function in people with hand OA.

Methods
Design and search strategy

This systematic review was conducted in accordance with the Preferred Reporting Items for Systematic Reviews and Meta-Analyses (PRISMA) guidelines [20]. The search strategy was based on the Population, Intervention, Comparison and Outcome (PICO) format. The electronic databases EBSCO host (CINAHL, MEDLINE, SPORTDiscus), Allied and Complementary Medicine Database (AMED) via OVID, Cochrane Central Register of Controlled Trials via Wiley, Web of Science, and Scopus were searched between 1975 and July 2016. The search was limited to published studies including human participants older than 18 years and published in English, Italian, or Spanish. The keywords utilised for the search included: hand(s), thumb(s), carpometacarpal(s), trapeziometacarpal(s), wrist(s), osteoarthr(itis)(osis)(itic), OA, train(ining)(ed), strength(ening)(ened), exercis(e)(ed)(es)(ing), physiotherap(y)(ist), physical therap(y)(ist), rehab(ilitation)(ilitative), manual therap(y)(ies), RCT(s), random(ly)(ised), trial(s)(led), experiment(s)(al). An additional table explains the search strategy in more detail (See Additional file 1: Table S1). Each database was searched by two people.

Eligibility criteria

To be included in this review, studies must have been investigating the effects of resistance training in adults with hand OA. Eligible papers were published RCTs. Studies were considered if they included a between-group comparison after treatment in people with hand OA. Because this review was focused on the effect of resistance training, studies had to compare resistance training interventions with a nonexercising control intervention to be eligible for inclusion. Studies including multimodal intervention (e.g., splinting, manual therapy, ultrasound, yoga) were excluded. Studies including exercise without reference to resistance/strength training were not suitable for inclusion. The primary variables of interest were grip strength, joint pain, and hand function. Systematic, narrative reviews and experimental studies were identified and manual searches of their reference lists were undertaken to identify additional studies. Forward searches of included studies were completed in Google Scholar and Scopus.

Study inclusion

All of the studies identified were collected in bibliographic software (Endnote X7; Thomson Reuters), where the inclusion and exclusion criteria were applied by two individuals. All duplicated studies were eliminated before title and abstract screening. The retained articles were retrieved in full text and assessed for inclusion. Disagreement on study inclusion was first discussed and if consensus was not reached the opinion of a third person was sought. A search of the reference lists of the included studies was undertaken to identify further articles.

Risk of bias and overall quality of evidence

Using the risk of bias table suggested by the Cochrane Statistical Methods Group and the Cochrane Bias Methods Group [21], a critical appraisal of each study was performed by two researchers. The risk of bias table's seven items assessed the internal validity of the studies. Each item was scored as low risk, high risk, or unclear risk.

To evaluate the overall quality of the evidence, the Grade of Recommendations Assessment, Development, and Evaluation (GRADE) system was utilised [22]. The quality of evidence was downgraded by one point from high quality for each factor that we encountered: risk of bias (if it was deemed that the bias may affect trial outcomes); inconsistency of results (wide variance of effect sizes or significant or large heterogeneity between trials: $p < 0.05$, $I^2 > 50\%$); indirectness (application of intervention, intervention, or outcomes that differed from what we indicated in our PICO research question); and imprecision (optimal information size not met). A GRADE profile was completed for each pooled estimate. Two reviewers judged whether these factors were present for each outcome and in cases of disagreement a third reviewer was involved. The quality of evidence was defined as: high (the authors are confident that the true effect is close to the one estimated); moderate (the authors are moderately confident in the effect estimate); low (the true effect may be significantly different from the estimated); and very low (the true effect is most likely different from the estimated) [23].

Data extraction

Descriptive statistics (means, standard deviations) for demographic and pre–post outcome dependent variables were extracted and cross-checked. When appropriate, the postintervention values for the exercise and control groups were used to calculate the mean difference (MD) or the standardised mean difference (SMD), which was the difference between groups values, divided by the pooled SD, with adjustment for small sample sizes (Hedges g: SMD). If more information was required for the quantitative analysis, authors were contacted to obtain further data.

Data synthesis and analysis

Meta-analysis was performed in Review Manager (RevMan) software (version 5.3; Cochrane Collaboration) using the inverse variance method. We assumed that the studies' variability, beyond subject-level sampling error, was random and consequently we adopted a random-effect model [20, 24]. Effect sizes of 0.2, 0.5, and 0.8 were considered small, medium, and large, respectively [25]. Publication bias was assessed by visually inspecting funnel plots [23]. Statistical heterogeneity was assessed using chi-square tests and the I^2 statistic, the latter providing a measure of the proportion of the observed variance that would remain if the sampling error was eliminated [26]. Where this proportion is of further interest, Borenstein et al. [26] have suggested that 95% prediction intervals should be calculated to appreciate the variability of the true effect size within the population under study.

Results

The initial search identified 2072 papers. After duplicate elimination, 1470 studies underwent title and abstract screening, resulting in 42 studies considered suitable for inclusion. Following full paper review, five articles met the criteria for inclusion. Figure 1 outlines the RCTs selection through the review. No additional papers were retrieved from previous reviews, reference searches, or forward searches of included studies. Table 1 presents a comprehensive description of each trial included in the paper. A summary of findings and GRADE quality ratings are reported in Table 2.

Study characteristics

The participants' count was based on the participants retained at the follow-up period (see Table 1). Out of the 350 participants, 305 (87%) were female. Mean age ranged from 61 to 81 years old. The primary outcome measures were grouped into grip strength, joint pain, and self-reported hand function. Grip strength was assessed through a dynamometer [27–31]. Joint pain measurements included the AUSCAN pain subscale [30], the Numerical Rating Scale (NRS) [27, 29, 31], and a six-point Likert scale [28]. Self-reported measures of hand function included the AUSCAN function subscale [27, 30] and the Functional Index of Hand Osteoarthritis (FIHOA) [29, 31].

Experimental intervention

Duration and supervision

Dziedzic et al. [27] had an ongoing exercise program with no set ending date. The remaining studies adopted training programs of 6–16 weeks [28–31]. Outcome measures were assessed at the end of the exercise period, except Dziedzic et al. [27] who measured grip strength at 24 weeks after participants' inclusion in the trial. Two studies supervised participants individually over one session, followed by a home exercise program (HEP) [30, 31]. Two studies supervised participants over four

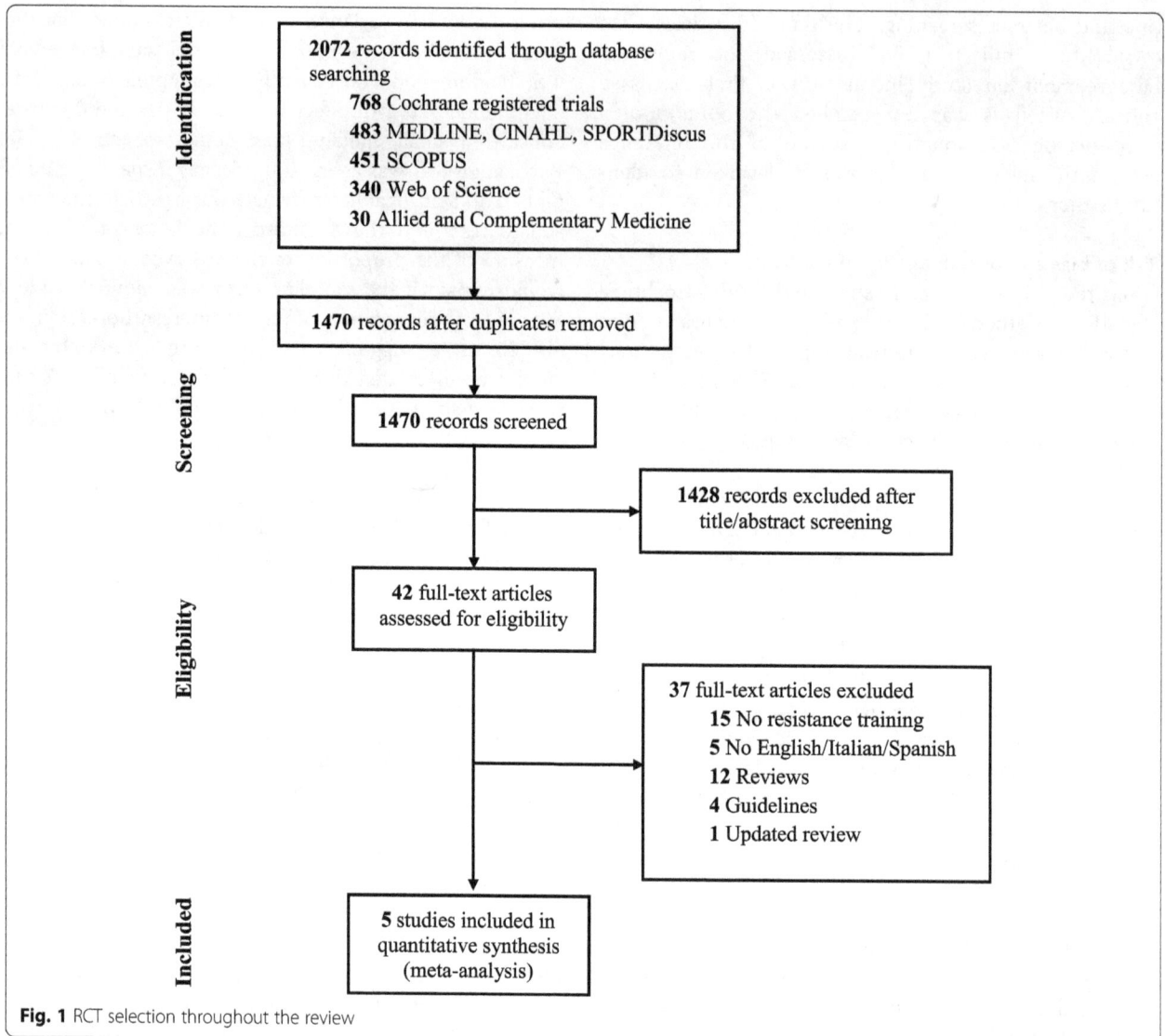

Fig. 1 RCT selection throughout the review

group sessions [27, 29]. Østerås et al. [29] provided group sessions over the first 3 weeks and towards the end of the trial (week 8). The timing of participant attendance in the group sessions of the study by Dziedzic et al. [27] was not clear. Lefler and Armstrong [28] reported that participants were supervised over 6 weeks, three times a week (18 sessions). However, it is not clear whether the sessions were individual or group sessions.

Training modality and frequency

Gripping and forearm flexor exercises were performed in all studies through different exercises (see Table 1). Three studies included specific exercises to improve thumb extension and abduction strength [27, 29, 31]. Finger and wrist extensor strengthening exercises were performed by two studies [27, 28]. Shoulder strengthening exercises were performed in only one study [29]. Two studies required participants to exercise every day

[27, 30] and three studies to exercise three times per week [28, 29, 31]. Repetitions at the beginning of training for each exercise ranged from three [27] to 10 [28–31].

Exercise intensity and progression

Only one study reported the percent of maximum voluntary contraction (40% of MVC) at which participants exercised [28]. Three other studies [29–31] presented enough data to infer an exercise load. Hennig et al. [31] and Østerås et al. [29] reported that participants were asked to 'squeeze as hard as possible' (100% of MVC) while performing gripping exercises. Rogers and Wilder [30] had participants perform exercises between 16 and 19% of MVC. We were unable to calculate the exercise intensity for Dziedzic et al. [27] because there was not enough information available. All studies progressed the exercises by increasing the number of repetitions up to a

Table 1 Characteristics of included studies and intervention

Study	Participants	Interventions	Outcome (follow-up time): statistical significance	Baseline differences
Dziedzic et al. (2015) [27]	RGb = 65 CGb = 65 N = 104 66% F 66 (9.1) years old	RG (n = 55): supervision = 1 group session/week (for 4 weeks). exercise = elastic bands fingers e/f, Play-Doh finger e/f (? % MVC), 0.5–0.75 kg wrist e/f dosage = 3 reps/day, every day progression = up to 10 reps/day CG (n = 49): leaflet and advice (extensive information)	Grip strength (24 wks): NS AUSCAN pain (12 wks): NS AUSCAN function (12 wks): NS	Strength (p = ?) Pain (p = 0.6) Function (p = 0.5)
Hennig et al. (2015) [31]	RGb = 40 CGb = 40 N = 71 100% F 60.8 (7) years old	RG (n = 37): supervision = 1 individual session with 8 follow-up calls exercise = elastic bands e/a thumb, rubber ball for grip strength (100% MVC) dosage = 10 reps (weeks 1 and 2), 3 days/week progression = 12 reps (weeks 3 and 4), 15 reps (weeks 5–12), 3 days/week CG (n = 34): leaflet and advice (limited information)	Grip strength (12 wks): S NRS pain (12 wks): S FIHOA (12 wks): S	Strength (p = 0.4) Pain (p = ?) Function (p = ?)
Lefler and Armstrong (2004) [28]	RGb = ? CGb = ? N = 19 90% F 81 (9) years old	RG (n = 9): supervised = every session (for 6 weeks); exercise = pinch grip lifting (isometric, 6-sec holds), wrist rolls (isotonic) (MVC = 40%) dosage = 10 reps, 3 days/week progression = up to 15 reps at 60% MVC isometric, 6–8 reps more than 60% MVC isotonic CG (n = 10): no intervention	Grip strength (6 wks): S Likert pain scale (6 wks): NS	Strength (p = 0.08) Pain (p = 0.53)
Østerås et al. (2014) [29]	RGb = 65 CGb = 65 N = 120 90% F 66 (9) years old	RG (n = 57): supervised = 4 group sessions (weeks 1–3 and 8) exercise = shoulder e/f, biceps curl, elastic band e/a thumb, pipe squeeze (100% MVC) dosage = 10 reps, moderate/vigorous intensity (weeks 1 and 2), 3 days/week progression = 15 reps (weeks 3–12) CG (n = 63): usual care (GP visit)	Grip strength (12 wks): NS NRS pain (12 wks): S FIHOA (12 wks): NS	Strength (p = 0.3) Pain (p = 0.4) Function (p = 0.26)
Rogers and Wilder (2009)[a] [30]	RGb = 76 CGb = 76 N = 46 87% F 75 (6.7) years old	RG (n = 46): supervised = 1 individual session exercise = gripping (16–19% MVC), key pinch, fingertip pinch all with rubber ball dosage = 10 reps (weeks 1, 2, 3 and 4), every day progression = 12 reps, 15 reps, 20 reps all increased every fourth week CG (n = 46): sham hand moisturiser	Grip strength (16 wks): NS AUSCAN pain (16 wks): NS AUSCAN function (16 wks): NS	Strength (p = 0.96) Pain (p = 0.84) Function (p = 0.87)

RGb participants allocated to the resistance training group, CGb participants allocated to the control group, N participants retained at follow-up, F female, RG resistance training group, n group sample size retained at follow-up, wks weeks, e/f extension/flexion, MVC maximum voluntary contraction, ? unable to calculate/unknown, reps repetitions, CG control group, AUSCAN Australian Canadian Osteoarthritis Hand Index, NS nonsignificant, e/a extension/abduction, NRS Numerical Rating Scale, FIHOA Functional Index of Hand Osteoarthritis, S significant
[a]Cross-over study design

maximum of 20. Only one study [28] included a progressive increase in exercise load (up to 60% of MVC).

Control intervention

Two studies provided the control group with a leaflet and advice over one session [27, 31]. Two studies did not provide any intervention to the control group [28, 29]. Østerås et al.'s [29] control group was allowed to receive usual care, which in Norway consisted of general practitioner visits only. Rogers and Wilder [30] crossed over the same participants from a placebo hand moisturiser to the resistance training group and vice versa, with a 16-week washout period.

Risk of bias

The risk of bias across the studies varied substantially (see Fig. 2). All of the studies failed to blind the treatment providers and participants due to the nature of the intervention. Dziedzic et al. [27], Hennig et al. [31], and Østerås et al. [29] presented the lowest risk of bias. Rogers and Wilder [30] and Lefler and Armstrong [28] presented the highest risk of bias.

Overall quality of evidence and meta-analyses

The results from the meta-analyses for grip strength, joint pain, and hand function are presented as forest plots in Fig. 3. Funnel plots for each outcome are provided in Fig. 4. Visual inspection did not reveal publication bias.

Grip strength

Out of the five studies included, only two studies showed a significant change in grip strength after resistance training compared with the control group [28, 31].

Table 2 Summary of findings: resistance training compared with no exercise for hand osteoarthritis

Outcomes	Anticipated absolute effects* (95% CI)		Number of participants (studies)	Quality of evidence (GRADE)	Comments
	Risk with no exercise	Risk with resistance training			
Grip strength (at study completion) assessed with: hand dynamometer. Follow-up: range 6–24 weeks	Mean grip strength (at study completion) in the control group was 17.7 kg	Mean grip strength (at study completion) in the intervention group was 1.35 kg higher (0.84 lower to 3.54 higher)	350 (5 RCTs)	⊕⊕⊕⊖ moderate[a]	MD 1.35 kg (95% CI = −0.84, 3.54). Relative increase 8% with resistance exercise (95% CI = −5% weaker, 20% stronger). MCID for grip strength is 20%[b]
Hand pain (at study completion) assessed with: AUSCAN pain, 11-point NRS, Likert scale. Lower scores mean less pain. Follow-up: range 6–16 weeks		Pain score in the resistance training groups was on average −0.23 SDs (−0.42 lower to −0.04 lower) lower than in the control groups.[e]	379 (5 RCTs)	⊕⊕⊖⊖ low[a,c]	These results can be interpreted as an improvement of 0.46 (95% CI = 0.08, 0.84) points on a 11-point NRS scale.[d] MCID for pain is 2 points [39]
Hand function (at study completion) assessed with: AUSCAN function, FIHOA. Lower scores mean better function. Follow-up: range 6–16 weeks		The function score in the resistance training groups was on average −0.10 SDs (−0.33 lower to 0.13 higher) lower than in the control groups.	363 (4 RCTs)	⊕⊕⊖⊖ low[a,c]	As a rule of thumb, 0.2 SDs represents a small difference, 0.5 a moderate difference, and 0.8 a large difference

Patient or population: hand osteoarthritis
Setting: general practice, community, retirement villages
Intervention: resistance training
Comparison: no exercise

CI confidence interval, AUSCAN Australian Canadian Osteoarthritis Hand Index, NRS Numerical Rating Scale, FIHOA Functional Index of Hand Osteoarthritis, RCT randomised controlled trial, MD mean difference, SD standard deviation, MCID minimal clinically important difference, GRADE Grade of Recommendations Assessment, Development, and Evaluation

* Risk in the intervention group (and its 95% CI) is based on the assumed risk in the comparison group and the relative effect of the intervention (and its 95% CI)

GRADE Working Group grades of evidence

High quality: We are very confident that the true effect lies close to that of the estimate of the effect

Moderate quality: We are moderately confident in the effect estimate (the true effect is likely to be close to the estimate of the effect, but there is a possibility that it is substantially different)

Low quality: Our confidence in the effect estimate is limited (the true effect may be substantially different from the estimate of the effect)

Very low quality: We have very little confidence in the effect estimate (the true effect is likely to be substantially different from the estimate of effect)

[a] Downgraded because few participants (imprecision)

[b] MCID for grip strength in people following a radial fracture [47]

[c] Downgraded because participants were not blinded to intervention (risk of bias)

[d] The control group pain mean (SD) 4.6 (2) was calculated by averaging the 11-point NRS scores of Dziedzic et al. [27], Hennig et al. [31], and Østerås et al. [29][e] This result was statistically significant (p = 0.02)

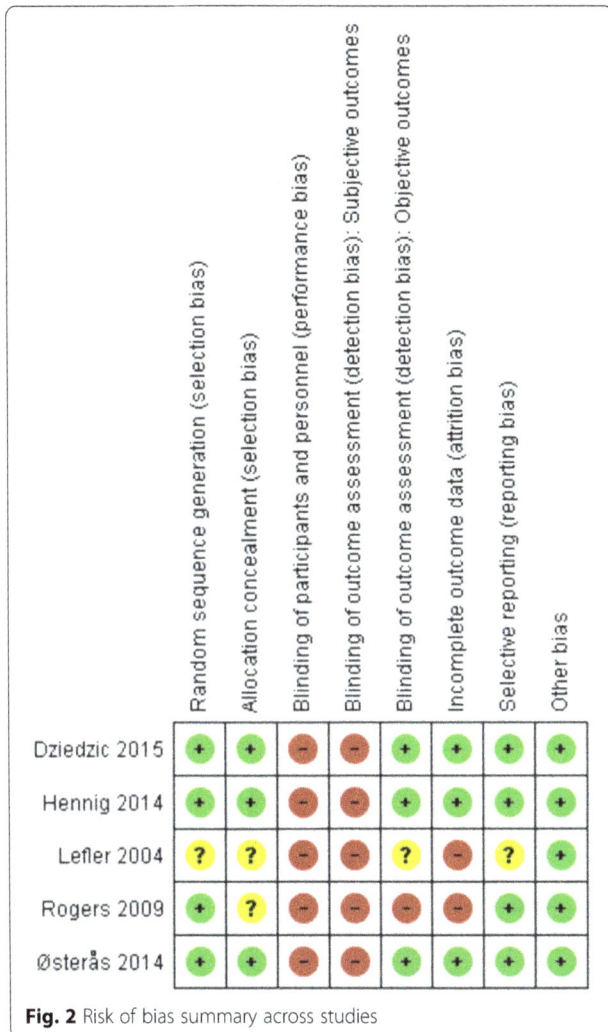

Fig. 2 Risk of bias summary across studies

The pooled results provide moderate-quality evidence that resistance exercises, as performed by these combined interventions, do not improve grip strength (MD 1.35 (95% CI = −0.84, 3.54), $p = 0.23$). The I^2 value was 50% ($\chi^2 = 7.97$, $p = 0.09$). The prediction indicated that 95% of the effect of resistance training would lie between −5.2 and 7.9 kg.

Joint pain
Most of the studies included in the present review showed a trend toward improvement in pain intensity for the resistance training group. However, only two studies reported statistically significant changes in pain [29, 31] compared with the control group. The pooled results provide low-quality evidence that resistance exercises provide pain relief (SMD −0.23 (95% CI = −0.42, −0.04), $p = 0.02$). The I^2 value was 0% ($\chi^2 = 1.69$, $p = 0.79$). The prediction interval indicated that 95% of effect sizes would lie between −0.54 and 0.08.

Hand function
Only one study reported significant differences in self-reported hand function after resistance training compared with the control group [31]. The pooled results provide low-quality evidence that resistance exercises do not improve hand function (SMD −0.1 (95% CI = −0.33, 0.13), $p = 0.39$). The I^2 value was 28% ($\chi^2 = 4.14$, $p = 0.25$). The prediction interval indicated that 95% of effect sizes would lie between −0.9 and 0.7.

Discussion
This meta-analysis assessed the effect of resistance training on grip strength, joint pain, and hand function in participants with hand OA. It was clear that there are very few experimental studies which have specifically addressed the effects of resistance training in this population. Previous reviews have highlighted this problem, and also emphasised the general scarcity of research involving conservative interventions for hand OA [2, 4, 5, 17, 18, 32]. These findings are surprising considering that resistance training has been used in other forms of OA with positive effects on pain, function, and patients' quality of life [7]. The five studies included had small sample sizes and the outcome data were not available for participants lost at follow-up.

There was 'moderate-quality evidence' that the resistance training utilised in the included studies did not improve grip strength. Of note, our overall finding concerning grip strength is in contrast to a recent review by Østerås et al. [32]. These authors noted that there was a strong trend for an improvement following training. This discrepancy most likely is related to the data analysed in the meta-analysis; that is, Østerås et al. [32] included findings from an abstract in their analysis, and furthermore, they were not able to include additional data concerning the findings of Rogers and Wilder's [30] work (which we were able to include after personal communication).

Nevertheless, our findings are surprising because all studies included in our analysis included gripping or forearm flexor exercises against resistance. The absence of grip strength improvement in the majority of the studies raises some questions regarding the appropriateness of the resistance training programs utilised. In addition, the technique used in the measurement of grip strength may not be congruent with the types of exercise undertaken in the intervention [33]. For instance, in the current review only two papers identified the hand position utilised for grip strength testing [29, 30], and in both instances the same position was utilised for all participants. This would limit the observation of strength gains if individuals trained at muscle lengths shorter or longer than the testing position (training specificity principle) [34].

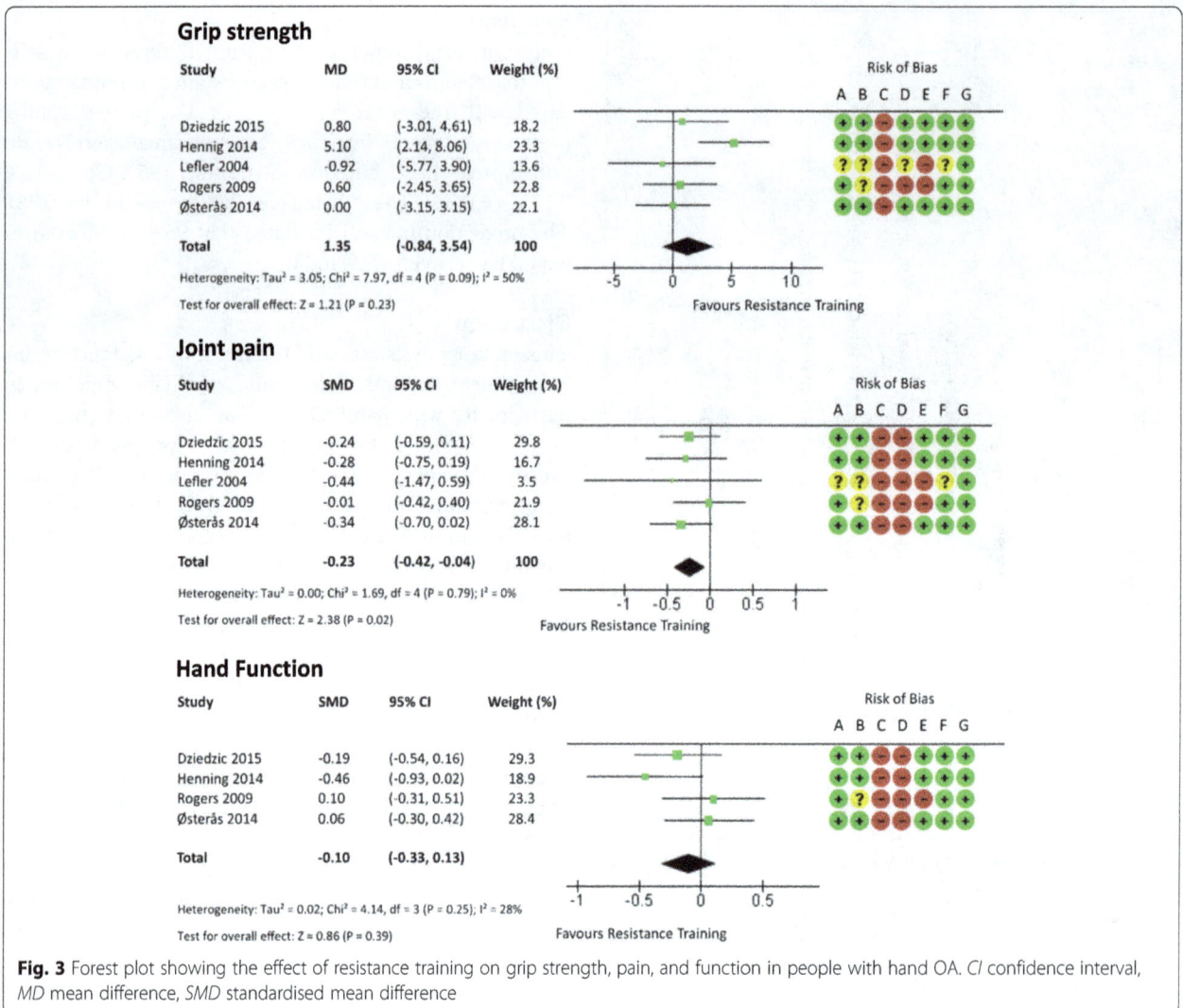

Fig. 3 Forest plot showing the effect of resistance training on grip strength, pain, and function in people with hand OA. *CI* confidence interval, *MD* mean difference, *SMD* standardised mean difference

Additionally, a key point in resistance training guidelines concerns the volume of exercise required. The majority of the studies adopted exercise frequency, intensity, sets, repetitions, and progression which are not sufficient to induce strength gains in older adults [35]. For instance, it was apparent that four studies progressed participants by increasing the number of repetitions rather than the exercise intensity [27, 29–31], and were therefore pursuing an approach that is more efficacious for enhancing muscle endurance as compared with strength [35]. With regard to absolute exercise intensity, it has been recommended that loads of at least 60% of MVC are utilised with intensity increasing as training progresses to levels approaching 80% of MVC [35]. Only two studies [29, 31] reported resistance training loads sufficient to induce increases in muscle strength (100% of MVC). Of these, Hennig et al. [31] reported significant changes in grip strength while Østerås et al. [29] reported only limited changes. In both cases, participants were instructed to squeeze an object as hard as possible. Because grip forces are unable to be measured using such a protocol, there is no way of being sure that participants were indeed working at 100% of MVC, as compared with exercising at resistance levels that can be quantified more accurately (e.g., on a hand-held dynamometer or weights).

Pain during exercise may have influenced load and intensity performed. In this regard, Hennig et al. [31] reported that participants' joint pain intensity immediately post exercise was high (NRS: 5.6 ± 2.2) while no data were available for the study by Østerås et al. [29]. It is possible that in the study by Østerås et al. [29], in which strength changes were small, participants self-limited the exercise intensity to avoid increases in joint pain. Similarly, the low exercise load utilised by the other included studies [28, 30] may reflect the intention to avoid high joint compressive forces and further damage to the articular cartilage. However, there is a growing body of

Grip strength

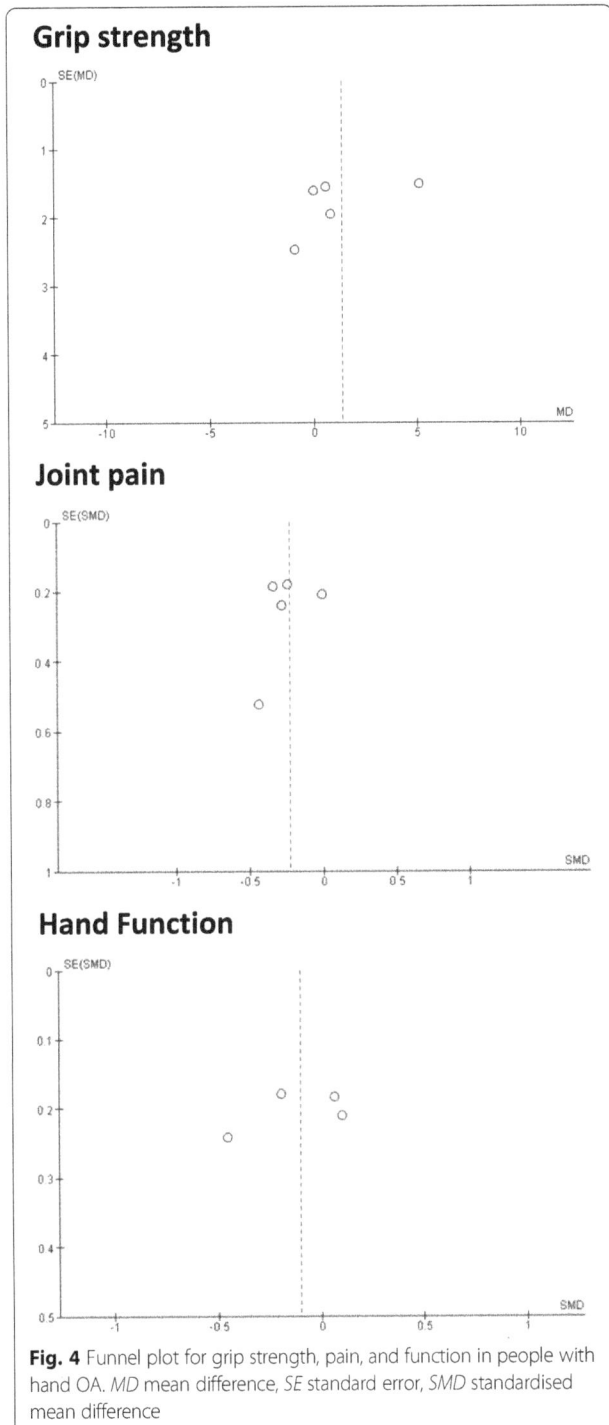

Joint pain

Hand Function

Fig. 4 Funnel plot for grip strength, pain, and function in people with hand OA. *MD* mean difference, *SE* standard error, *SMD* standardised mean difference

condition that pain intensity returns to baseline values within 24 hours of the previous session [31, 38].

There was low-quality evidence suggesting that resistance training reduces joint pain. Additionally, when the standardised mean difference calculated in the current study was transformed into absolute values on a 11-point NRS scale (see Table 2), the difference between groups was 0.46 points (95% CI = 0.08, 0.84), which does not reach the minimal clinically important difference of two points commonly used in OA trials [39]. At the knee joint, findings are more encouraging, with a RCT [37] reporting a mean reduction in pain of 2.3 points following high-intensity resistance exercises. There is no reason to suspect that such findings might not be possible at the hand given the mechanisms advanced for its success. These include muscle strengthening altering alignment and hence loading on damaged structures within a joint, reducing the potential for inflammation and hence pain. Other authors [40] have suggested that increased proprioceptive awareness leads to improved placement of joints during motion, reducing load. There is also a strong potential for an antinociceptive effect of resistance training through modulation of endogenous analgesia [41–43] and/or anti-inflammatory effects that may reduce peripheral and central sensitisation [44].

Low-quality evidence demonstrated that hand function was not improved following resistance training. Similar results were obtained by a recent review by Bertozzi et al. [18] which showed no significant effects of exercise interventions on hand function in people with thumb carpo-metacarpal joint OA. In contrast, Østerås et al. [32] found a trend (*p* = 0.07) toward exercise being beneficial for function. A number of factors may be associated with these findings. These include the assessment of function by questionnaires that do not include tasks that the participants find difficult to perform, questionnaires that focus primarily on tasks requiring fine motor control tasks, rather than strength tasks, and/or resistance training programs not targeting appropriate muscle groups. As suggested by van Baar et al. [10] and adopted by Hoeksma et al. [45], it may be that targeting the individual's specific needs is a solution. However, where researchers take this pathway, it is important that they provide descriptions of the criteria which lead them to focus on a specific type of exercise, and also provide the training parameters and improvements that occurred for those participants. Without such information, readers have no way of discerning how to prioritise types of exercise that would be most valuable for their patients. In future studies, the resistance training exercises utilised could be described in detail according to the Consensus on Exercise Reporting Template (CERT) [46].

It may be viewed as a limitation of the current study that we chose to focus on studies utilising resistance

evidence suggesting that high levels of pain during or immediately after resistance training sessions (up to 6 on a NRS scale) do not negatively affect outcomes, but rather improve overall levels of pain for the duration of the training program in people with hand and knee OA [31, 36, 37]. Such pain intensities have been previously considered acceptable in people with OA, on the training exercises only. We are aware that in clinical practice multimodal therapies are often utilised and a combination of conservative and pharmacological interventions are adopted. However, to optimise both the efficiency and cost-effectiveness of OA treatment it is important to understand which component(s) of an intervention offer the most benefit (or otherwise). Our focus on resistance training is also justified by the established effectiveness of this intervention in other joints such as knee OA [9]. Furthermore, a number of functional tasks at the hand require notable muscle forces to be generated and it has been suggested that 20–25 kg of grip strength is required for daily life activities [17]. An additional limitation of the present study is that a review protocol was not published before starting the search. We are aware that this is suggested by the PRISMA guideline. However, we prespecified the use of meta-analysis for all the outcomes chosen, which included strength, pain, and function. Another limitation is the small number of participants included in the meta-analysis. This was acknowledged and the overall quality of evidence was downgraded (see Table 2). Nevertheless, all of the studies except that by Lefler and Armstrong [28] performed power calculations, suggesting that the optimal information size was probably met. A per-protocol analysis was performed on the postintervention data reported in each study. Data for participants who dropped out were not available. Formal statistical analyses to assess publication bias were not performed due to the limited number of studies available. Visual inspection of funnel plots did not identify any clear indication of publication bias. In addition, the absence of clinically significant improvements in the main outcome variables makes the effects of any publication bias unlikely to change the main conclusions of our review. Finally, we need to acknowledge as a limitation the inclusion of studies published only in English, Spanish, or Italian.

Conclusions

There is no evidence indicating that resistance training increases grip strength or has a clinically significant benefit on hand OA pain and function. However, this may be related to the paucity of studies and low-quality study designs. Future studies should consider focusing exercise programs specifically on identified muscle deficits as well as optimising exercise training parameters to achieve clinically significant strength improvements in people with hand OA.

Abbreviations

AUSCAN: Australian Canadian Osteoarthritis Hand Index; CI: Confidence interval; CERT: Consensus on Exercise Reporting Template; FIHOA: Functional index of hand OA; GRADE: Grade of Recommendations Assessment, Development, and Evaluation; HEP: Home exercise program; MCID: Minimal clinically important difference; MD: mean difference; MVC: Maximum voluntary contraction; NRS: Numerical Rating Scale; OA: Osteoarthritis; PICO: Population, Intervention, Comparison and Outcome; PRISMA: Preferred Reporting Items for Systematic Reviews and Meta-Analyses; RCT: Randomised controlled trial; SD: standard deviation; SMD: Standardised mean difference

Acknowledgements
The authors wish to thank all researchers of the included studies who provided additional data.

Funding
None.

Authors' contributions
NEM, PJM, and DAR conceived and designed the study. NEM and DAR performed the literature search, data extraction, and assessed the risk of bias and overall quality of evidence. PJM resolved disagreement between NEM and DAR. NEM, PJM, and DAR performed and interpreted the data analysis. NEM drafted the manuscript. DAR and PJM revised the manuscript. All authors read and approved the final manuscript.

Authors' information
Nothing to report.

Competing interests
The authors declare that they have no competing interests.

Consent for publication
Yes.

Author details
[1]Health and Rehabilitation Research Institute, Auckland University of Technology, 90 Akoranga Drive, Northcote, Auckland 0627, New Zealand. [2]Waitemata Pain Service, Department of Anaesthesiology and Perioperative Medicine, North Shore Hospital, Waitemata DHB, 124 Shakespeare Road, Westlake, Takapuna, Auckland 0622, New Zealand.

References
1. Zhang Y, Niu J, Kelly-Hayes M, Chaisson CE, Aliabadi P, Felson DT. Prevalence of symptomatic hand osteoarthritis and its impact on functional status among the elderly: the Framingham Study. Am J Epidemiol. 2002;156(11):1021–7.
2. Kloppenburg M. Hand osteoarthritis-nonpharmacological and pharmacological treatments. Nat Rev Rheumatol. 2014;10(4):242–51.
3. da Costa BR, Nüesch E, Kasteler R, Husni E, Welch V, Rutjes AWS, Jüni P. Oral or transdermal opioids for osteoarthritis of the knee or hip. Cochrane Database Syst Rev. 2014;9:1–95.
4. Kjeken I, Smedslund G, Moe RH, Slatkowsky-Christensen B, Uhlig T, Hagen KB. Systematic review of design and effects of splints and exercise programs in hand osteoarthritis. Arthritis Care Res. 2011;63(6):834–48.
5. Ye L, Kalichman L, Spittle A, Dobson F, Bennell K. Effects of rehabilitative interventions on pain, function and physical impairments in people with hand osteoarthritis: a systematic review. Arthritis Res Ther. 2011;13(1):R28.

6. Oppong R, Jowett S, Nicholls E, Whitehurst DGT, Hill S, Hammond A, Hay EM, Dziedzic K. Joint protection and hand exercises for hand osteoarthritis: an economic evaluation comparing methods for the analysis of factorial trials. Rheumatology. 2015;54(5):876–83.

7. Nguyen C, Lefèvre-Colau M-M, Poiraudeau S, Rannou F. Rehabilitation (exercise and strength training) and osteoarthritis: a critical narrative review. Ann Phys Rehabil Med. 2016;59(3):190–5.

8. McDonough CM, Jette AM. The contribution of osteoarthritis to functional limitations and disability. Clin Geriatr Med. 2010;26(3):387–99.

9. Li Y, Su Y, Chen S, Zhang Y, Zhang Z, Liu C, Lu M, Liu F, Li S, He Z, et al. The effects of resistance exercise in patients with knee osteoarthritis: a systematic review and meta-analysis. Clin Rehabil. 2015;30(10):947–59.

10. van Baar ME, Assendelft WJ, Dekker J, Oostendorp RA, Bijlsma JW. Effectiveness of exercise therapy in patients with osteoarthritis of the hip or knee: a systematic review of randomized clinical trials. Arthritis Rheum. 1999;42(7):1361–9.

11. Hochberg MC, Altman RD, April KT, Benkhalti M, Guyatt G, McGowan J, Towheed T, Welch V, Wells G, Tugwell P. American College of Rheumatology 2012 recommendations for the use of nonpharmacologic and pharmacologic therapies in osteoarthritis of the hand, hip and knee. Arthritis Care Res. 2012; 41(1):465–74.

12. Zhang W, Doherty M, Leeb BF, Alekseeva L, Arden NK, Bijlsma JW, Dinçer F, Dziedzic K, Häuselmann HJ, Herrero-Beaumont G, et al. EULAR evidence based recommendations for the management of hand osteoarthritis: report of a task force of the EULAR Standing Committee for International Clinical Studies Including Therapeutics (ESCISIT). Ann Rheum Dis. 2007;66(3):377–88.

13. Bagis S, Sahin G, Yapici Y, Cimen OB, Erdogan C. The effect of hand osteoarthritis on grip and pinch strength and hand function in postmenopausal women. Clin Rheumatol. 2003;22(6):420–4.

14. Kjeken I, Dagfinrud H, Slatkowsky-Christensen B, Mowinckel P, Uhlig T, Kvien TK, Finset A. Activity limitations and participation restrictions in women with hand osteoarthritis: patients' descriptions and associations between dimensions of functioning. Ann Rheum Dis. 2005;64(11):1633–8.

15. Kalichman L, Hernández-Molina G. Hand osteoarthritis: an epidemiological perspective. Semin Arthritis Rheum. 2010;39(6):465–76.

16. Nunes MP, de Oliveira D, Aruin AS, Dos Santos JM. Relationship between hand function and grip force control in women with hand osteoarthritis. J Rehabil Res Dev. 2012;49(6):855–65.

17. Valdes K, von der Heyde R. An exercise program for carpometacarpal osteoarthritis based on biomechanical principles. J Hand Ther. 2012;25(3): 251–63.

18. Bertozzi L, Valdes K, Vanti C, Negrini S, Pillastrini P, Villafañe JH. Investigation of the effect of conservative interventions in thumb carpometacarpal osteoarthritis: systematic review and meta-analysis. Disabil Rehabil. 2015; 37(22):2025–43.

19. Mahendira D, Towheed TE. Systematic review of non-surgical therapies for osteoarthritis of the hand: an update. Osteoarthr Cartilage. 2009;17(10):1263–8.

20. Liberati A, Altman DG, Tetzlaff J, Mulrow C, Gotzsche PC, Ioannidis JP, Clarke M, Devereaux PJ, Kleijnen J, Moher D. The PRISMA statement for reporting systematic reviews and meta-analyses of studies that evaluate healthcare interventions: explanation and elaboration. BMJ. 2009;339:b2700.

21. Higgins JPT, Altman DG, Gøtzsche PC, Jüni P, Moher D, Oxman AD, Savović J, Schulz KF, Weeks L, Sterne JAC. The Cochrane Collaboration's tool for assessing risk of bias in randomised trials. BMJ. 2011;343:d5928.

22. Grade Working Group. Grading quality of evidence and strength of recommendations. BMJ. 2004;328(7454):1490.

23. Schünemann H, Brozek J, Guyatt G, Oxman A. GRADE handbook. 2009. http://www.gradeworkinggroup.org/. Accessed 30 Aug 2016.

24. Lipsey MW, Wilson DB. Practical meta-analysis. Thousand Oaks, CA: Sage Publications; 2001.

25. Guyatt GH, Thorlund K, Oxman AD, Walter SD, Patrick D, Furukawa TA, Johnston BC, Karanicolas P, Akl EA, Vist G, et al. GRADE guidelines: 13. Preparing Summary of Findings tables and evidence profiles—continuous outcomes. J Clin Epidemiol. 2012;66(2):173–83.

26. Borenstein M, Higgins JPT, Hedges LV, Rothstein HR. Basics of meta-analysis: I^2 is not an absolute measure of heterogeneity. Res Synth Methods. 2017;8(1):5–18. doi:10.1002/jrsm.1230.

27. Dziedzic K, Nicholls E, Hill S, Hammond A, Handy J, Thomas E, Hay E. Self-management approaches for osteoarthritis in the hand: a 2x2 factorial randomised trial. Ann Rheum Dis. 2015;74(1):108–18.

28. Lefler C, Armstrong WJ. Exercise in the treatment of osteoarthritis in the hands of the elderly. Clin Kinesiol. 2004;58(2):13–7.

29. Østerås N, Hagen KB, Grotle M, Sand-Svartrud AL, Mowinckel P, Kjeken I. Limited effects of exercises in people with hand osteoarthritis: results from a randomized controlled trial. Osteoarthr Cartilage. 2014;22(9):1224–33.

30. Rogers MW, Wilder FV. Exercise and hand osteoarthritis symptomatology: a controlled crossover trial. J Hand Ther. 2009;22(1):10–8.

31. Hennig T, Hæhre L, Hornburg VT, Mowinckel P, Norli ES, Kjeken I. Effect of home-based hand exercises in women with hand osteoarthritis: a randomised controlled trial. Ann Rheum Dis. 2015;74(8):1501–8.

32. Østerås N, Kjeken I, Smedslund G, Moe RH, Slatkowsky-Christensen B, Uhlig T, Hagen KB. Exercise for hand osteoarthritis. Cochrane Database Syst Rev. 2017;1:Cd010388.

33. Pelland L, Brosseau L, Wells G, MacLeay L, Lambert J, Lamothe C, Robinson V, Tugwell P. Efficacy of strengthening exercises for osteoarthritis (Part I): a meta-analysis. Phys Ther Rev. 2004;9(2):77–108.

34. Wilson G. Strength and power in sport. In: Bloomfield J, Ackland TR, Elliott B, editors. Applied anatomy and biomechanics in sport. London, England: Blackwell Scientific Publications; 1994. p. 110–224.

35. Garber CE, Blissmer B, Deschenes MR, Franklin BA, Lamonte MJ, Lee IM, Nieman DC, Swain DP. American College of Sports Medicine position stand. Quantity and quality of exercise for developing and maintaining cardiorespiratory, musculoskeletal, and neuromotor fitness in apparently healthy adults: guidance for prescribing exercise. Med Sci Sports Exerc. 2011;43(7):1334–59.

36. Bryk FF, Dos Reis AC, Fingerhut D, Araujo T, Schutzer M, Cury Rde P, Duarte Jr A, Fukuda TY. Exercises with partial vascular occlusion in patients with knee osteoarthritis: a randomized clinical trial. Knee Surg Sports Traumatol Arthrosc. 2016;24(5):1580–6.

37. Jorge RT, Souza MC, Chiari A, Jones A, Fernandes Ada R, Lombardi Junior I, Natour J. Progressive resistance exercise in women with osteoarthritis of the knee: a randomized controlled trial. Clin Rehabil. 2015;29(3):234–43.

38. Kjeken I, Grotle M, Hagen KB, Østerås N. Development of an evidence-based exercise programme for people with hand osteoarthritis. Scand J Occup Ther. 2015;22(2):103–16.

39. Farrar JT, Young Jr JP, LaMoreaux L, Werth JL, Poole RM. Clinical importance of changes in chronic pain intensity measured on an 11-point numerical pain rating scale. Pain. 2001;94(2):149–58.

40. Runhaar J, Luijsterburg P, Dekker J, Bierma-Zeinstra SMA. Identifying potential working mechanisms behind the positive effects of exercise therapy on pain and function in osteoarthritis: a systematic review. Osteoarthr Cartilage. 2015; 23(7):1071–82.

41. Daenen L, Varkey E, Kellmann M, Nijs J. Exercise, not to exercise, or how to exercise in patients with chronic pain? Applying science to practice. Clin J Pain. 2015;31(2):108–14.

42. Nijs J, Kosek E, Van Oosterwijck J, Meeus M. Dysfunctional endogenous analgesia during exercise in patients with chronic pain: to exercise or not to exercise? Pain Physician. 2012;15 Suppl 3:205–13.

43. Galdino G, Romero T, Silva JF, Aguiar D, Paula AM, Cruz J, Parrella C, Piscitelli F, Duarte I, Di Marzo V, et al. Acute resistance exercise induces antinociception by activation of the endocannabinoid system in rats. Anesth Analg. 2014;119(3): 702–15.

44. Lundberg IE, Nader GA. Molecular effects of exercise in patients with inflammatory rheumatic disease. Nat Clin Pract Rheumatol. 2008;4(11): 597–604.

45. Hoeksma HL, Dekker J, Ronday HK, Heering A, van der Lubbe N, Vel C, Breedveld FC, van den Ende CH. Comparison of manual therapy and exercise therapy in osteoarthritis of the hip: a randomized clinical trial. Arthritis Rheum. 2004;51(5):722–9.

46. Slade SC, Dionne CE, Underwood M, Buchbinder R, Beck B, Bennell K, Brosseau L, Costa L, Cramp F, Cup E, et al. Consensus on Exercise Reporting Template (CERT): Modified Delphi Study. Phys Ther. 2016;96(10):1514–24.

47. Kim JK, Park MG, Shin SJ. What is the minimum clinically important difference in grip strength? Clin Orthop Relat Res. 2014;472(8):2536–41.

CX3CL1 promotes MMP-3 production via the CX3CR1, c-Raf, MEK, ERK, and NF-κB signaling pathway in osteoarthritis synovial fibroblasts

Sheng-Mou Hou[1], Chun-Han Hou[2] and Ju-Fang Liu[3]* (iD)

Abstract

Background: Osteoarthritis (OA) is a degenerative joint disease that affects the cartilage, synovium, and subchondral bone and is the leading cause of disability in older populations. Specific diagnostic biomarkers are lacking; hence, treatment options for OA are limited. Synovial inflammation is very common in OA joints and has been associated with both OA's symptoms and pathogenesis. Confirming the role of the synovium in OA pathogenesis is a promising strategy for mitigating the symptoms and progression of OA. CX3CL1 is the only member of the CX3C class of chemokines that combines the properties of chemoattractants and adhesion molecules. CX3CL1 levels in the synovium and serum were both discovered to be positively associated with OA pathogenesis. CX3CL1 and its receptor CX3CR1 belong to a family of G protein-coupled receptors. Matrix metalloproteinases (MMPs), which are responsible for matrix degradation, play a crucial role in OA progression. The relationship between CX3CL1 and MMPs in the pathophysiology of OA is still unclear.

Methods: CX3CL1-induced MMP-3 production was assessed with quantitative real-time PCR and ELISA. The mechanisms of action of CX3CL1 in different signaling pathways were studied using western blot analysis, quantitative real-time PCR and ELISA. Neutralization antibodies of integrin were achieved to block the CX3CR1 signaling pathway. Luciferase assays were used to study NF-κB promoter activity.

Results: We investigated the signaling pathway involved in CX3CL1-induced MMP-3 production in osteoarthritis synovial fibroblasts (OASFs). CX3CL1 was found to induce MMP-3 production in a concentration-dependent and time-dependent manner. Using pharmacological inhibitors and CX3CR1 small interfering RNA to block CX3CR1 revealed that the CX3CR1 receptor was involved in the CX3CL1-mediated upregulation of MMP-3. CX3CL1-mediated MMP-3 production was attenuated by c-Raf inhibitors (GW5074) and MEK/ERK inhibitors (PD98059 and U0126). The OASFs were stimulated using CX3CL1-activated p65 phosphorylation.

Conclusions: Our results demonstrate that CX3CL1 activates c-Raf, MEK, ERK, and NF-κB on the MMP-3 promoter through CX3CR1, thus contributing to cartilage destruction during OA.

Keywords: CX3CL1, CX3CR1, Osteoarthritis, Matrix metalloproteinase 3

* Correspondence: anti0822@hotmail.com; T010615@ms.skh.org.tw
[3]Central Laboratory, Shin-Kong Wu Ho-Su Memorial Hospital, No. 95, Wenchang Road, Shilin, Taipei 111, Taiwan
Full list of author information is available at the end of the article

CX3CL1 promotes MMP-3 production via the CX3CR1, c-Raf, MEK, ERK, and NF-κB signaling pathway...

81

Background

Osteoarthritis (OA), a common progressive degenerative disease, is the most frequent cause of physical disability, which affects more than 12.4 million individuals aged 65 years and older. The prevalence of OA in the United States is estimated to increase by approximately 9 million from 1995 to 2020 [1]. The etiology of OA is currently unclear. Its main pathological characteristics are cartilage loss, change in the subchondral bone, and thickening of the synovium [2]. The goals of OA therapy are joint pain reduction and joint function improvement. The available strategies for preventing or treating OA are limited. The normal synovial membrane comprises an intimal lining one or two cell layers thick. A typical feature of OA is synovial lining hyperplasia, which increases the number of synovial fibroblasts (SFs) [3]. These OASFs are a source of proinflammatory cytokines and proteolytic enzymes, including matrix-degrading enzymes (matrix metalloproteinases (MMPs) and aggrecanases), which contribute to articular matrix degradation [4–8]. Therefore, elucidating the molecular mechanisms of OA can facilitate the development of novel anti-OA strategies.

Human chemokines are divided into four families (C, CC, CXC, and CX3C) depending on the conserved cysteine motif. Chemokines are chemoattractant proteins that regulate leukocyte trafficking, inflammation, and immune responses. Numerous studies have established a correlation between chemokine expression and inflammatory diseases including arthritis, atherosclerosis, asthma, and metabolic syndrome. CX3CL1 is expressed in many cell types, including neurons, intestinal epithelium, and activated vascular endothelium, and is structurally distinct from other chemokines. Several studies have indicated that CX3CL1 plays a central role in inflammatory diseases. In 2002, Cockwell et al. [9] discovered that CX3CL1 expression was increased in acute human renal inflammation. In 2003, Ollivier et al. [10] reported that CX3CL1 triggered not only monocyte adhesion but also chemotactic function and was involved in the pathogenesis of atherosclerosis. CX3CR1 is a seven-transmembrane domain G protein-coupled receptor and the specific receptor for CX3CL1. CX3CR1 mediates several intracellular signaling pathways, such as the p38MAPK signaling pathway [11] and the Akt pathway [12]. Several pieces of evidence have suggested that CX3CL1–CX3CR1 interactions contribute to the development of inflammatory diseases such as rheumatoid arthritis (RA) [13, 14]. CX3CL1 is overexpressed in the serum, synovium, synovial fluid, and cartilage of patients with RA [14, 15].

CX3CL1 may also promote MMP-2 production in SFs [16]. This confirms the role of CX3CL1 in the pathogenesis of OA; however, the molecular connections between CX3CL1 and OA remain largely elusive. Therefore, we explored the signaling pathways involved in CX3CL1-induced MMP-3 production in human OASFs in addition to the role of CX3CL1 in the pathogenesis of OA to determine whether CX3CL1 is an appropriate target for drug intervention in OA in the future.

Methods

Cell culture

Written informed consent was obtained from all patients recruited into this study, and the study was approved by the Institutional Review Board of Shin Kong Wu Ho-Su Memorial Hospital. Synovial tissue was obtained from patients with OA, and SFs were isolated. Human SFs were isolated by collagenase treatment of synovial tissue samples obtained from 10 patients with OA during knee-replacement surgeries and eight samples of nonarthritic synovial tissues obtained at arthroscopy after trauma/joint derangement. Fresh synovial tissues were finely minced and digested in Dulbecco's modified Eagle's medium (DMEM) containing 2 mg/ml type II collagenase (Sigma-Aldrich, St. Louis, MO, USA) for 4 h at 37 °C and under 5% CO_2. The isolated cells were placed in DMEM containing 10% fetal bovine serum (FBS), 100 units/ml penicillin, 100 μg/ml streptomycin, and 2 mM L-glutamine at 37 °C with 5% CO_2. Passages 4–6 of the obtained OASFs were used in this study. Results of four independent experiments are presented [4, 17].

Materials

DMEM, Lipofectamine3000, and Trizol were purchased from Invitrogen (Carlsbad, CA, USA). Cell culture dishes, FBS, six-well plates, and 12-well plates were purchased from Corning (Corning, NY, USA). Polyvinyldifluoride (PVDF) membranes and an Immobilon Western Chemiluminescent HRP Substrate detection system were purchased from Millipore (Billerica, MA, USA). Polyclonal antibodies specific for MMP3, CX3CL1, CX3CR1 and IKKα/β were purchased from Santa Cruz Biotechnology (Santa Cruz, CA, USA). Monoclonal antibodies specific for c-Raf, MEK, ERK, IκBα, p65, and β-Actin were purchased from Santa Cruz Biotechnology (Santa Cruz, CA, USA). Polyclonal rabbit antibodies specific for c-Raf phosphorylated at Ser338 and IKKα/β phosphorylated at ser176/180 were purchased from Cell Signaling and Neuroscience (Danvers, MA, USA). Monoclonal rabbit antibodies specific for MEK1/2 phosphorylated at Ser217/221, ERK1/2 phosphorylated at Thr202/204, IκBα phosphorylated at ser32/36, and p65 phosphorylated at ser536 were purchased from Cell Signaling and Neuroscience (Danvers, MA, USA).3-(3,5-Dibromo-4-hydroxybenzyliden)-5-iodo-1,3-dihydroindol-2-one (GW5074), 1,4-diamino-2,3-dicyano-1,4-

bis(o-aminophenylmercapto)butadiene monoethanolate (U0126), 2-(2-amino-3-methoxyphenyl)-4H-1-benzo-pyran-4-one (PD98059), pyrrolidine dithiocarbamate (PDTC), and L-1-tosylamido-2-phenylenylethyl chloro-methyl ketone (TPCK) were purchased from Sigma-Aldrich. Recombinant human CX3CL1 was purchased from PeproTech (Rocky Hill, NJ, USA). The small interfering RNA (siRNA) of the control and CX3CR1 siRNA were purchased from Santa Cruz Biotechnology. Nuclear factor kappa B (NF-κB) lucif-erase plasmid was purchased from Stratagene (La Jolla, CA, USA). A pSV-β-galactosidase vector and a luciferase assay kit were purchased from Promega (Madison, MA, USA). All other chemicals were pur-chased from Sigma-Aldrich.

RNA extraction and quantitative real-time polymerase chain reaction

Total RNA was extracted from cells using Trizol reagent (Invitrogen) following the manufacturer's protocol. In brief, cells were added to 0.5 ml Trizol, homogenized, and incubated at room temperature for 3 min. After ex-traction with chloroform (0.1 ml) and precipitation with isopropanol (0.4 ml), RNA was washed with 75% etha-nol, and finally the RNA pellet was dissolved in 10 μl of RNase-free water. The RNA yield and purity were deter-mined by measuring absorbance at 260 and 280 nm using a Nanodrop spectrophotometer (Thermo Fisher Scientific, Inc., Waltham, MA, USA). RNA was then used to synthesize complementary DNA (cDNA) using reverse transcriptase (Invitrogen) according to the man-ufacturer's instructions.

Real-time quantitative polymerase chain reaction (qPCR) was performed using SYBR Green (KAPA Biosystems, Woburn, MA, USA) according to the manufacturer's protocol, and reactions were performed using a StepOne-Plus machine (Applied Biosystems, Foster City, CA, USA). Human MMP-1, MMP-2, MMP-3, MMP-7, MMP-9, MMP-12, MMP-3, and glyceraldehyde 3-phosphate de-hydrogenase (GAPDH) purchased from Sigma-Aldrich were used as primers to amplify the target genes. The expression levels of the target genes were determined by normalizing them to the GAPDH levels. We calculated the results using the following equation:

$$\text{Ratio} = 2^{-\Delta\Delta Ct},$$
$$\text{where } \Delta\Delta Ct = \left(Ct_{target} - Ct_{GADPH}\right)_{Sample}$$
$$- \left(Ct_{target} - Ct_{GADPH}\right)_{Control}.$$

Each sample was assayed in triplicate, and the data represent three independent experiments.

Western blot analysis

Cellular lysates were prepared using the methods out-lined in previous studies. Proteins were resolved using sodium dodecyl sulfate polyacrylamide gel electrophor-esis and transferred to Immobilon PVDF membranes. The blots were blocked with 5% BSA for 1 h at room temperature and then probed using antihuman anti-bodies against MMP-3, CX3CL1, CX3CR1, c-Raf, MEK, ERK, IKKα/β, IκB, p65, and β-Actin (1:1000) for 1 h at room temperature. After three washes, the blots were in-cubated with secondary antibodies (1:10,000) for 1 h at room temperature. The blots were then visualized using a charge-coupled device camera-based detection system (UVP Inc., Upland, CA, USA). Quantitative data were obtained using ImageJ software (National Institute of Health, USA).

Determination of MMP-3 secretions using enzyme-linked immunosorbent assay

MMP-3 in the cell culture supernatants was then deter-mined using a Quantikine enzyme-linked immunosorb-ent assay (ELISA) kit (R&D Systems, Minneapolis, MN, USA) according to the manufacturer's protocol. In brief, OASFs were seeded in 100-mm culture dishes at a dens-ity of 5×10^6 cells per dish and then treated under differ-ent conditions. Following 24 h of incubation, the culture supernatant was collected and centrifuged at 10,000 rpm for 10 min and stored at −80 °C in fresh tubes.

Transfection and luciferase receptor activity

Transfection was performed using Lipofectamine 3000 transfection reagent (LF3000; Invitrogen) according to the manufacturer's instructions. Cells were transfected with control siRNA, CX3CR1 siRNA, vector, dominant negative MEK mutants, dominant negative ERK mutants, dominant negative IKKα mutants, dominant negative IKKβ mutants, and luciferase plasmid using Li-pofectamine 3000 in optiMEM medium. After 24 h of transfection, cells were incubated with the indicated agents. After 24 h of incubation, the luciferase activity in the transfected cells was measured using a Luciferase Reporter Assay System (Promega) according to the man-ufacturer's instructions. Transactivation was determined by monitoring the firefly luciferase levels in the pGL2 vector. The luciferase assay was performed by adding lysis buffer (100 μl) and harvesting the cells through centrifugation (13,000 rpm for 5 min). The supernatant was transferred to fresh tubes, and 20 μl of cell lysate was added to 80 μl of fresh luciferase assay buffer in an assay tube. The luciferase activity was measured using a microplate luminometer. Luciferase activity was normal-ized to transfection efficiency based on the cotransfected β-galactosidase expression vector.

Chromatin immunoprecipitation assay

Crosslinked chromatin was prepared from OASF cells, and a chromatin immunoprecipitation (ChIP) assay was performed using a Pierce Magnetic ChIP kit (Thermo Fisher Scientific, Inc.) according to the manufacturer's protocol. After immunoprecipitation with anti-p65 antibody or control IgG, protein A/G magnetic beads were added. DNA was purified and analyzed using PCR. The following MMP-3 primers were used: 5′-AATTCACATCACTGCCACCA-3′ (forward) and 5′-CTCTGTGGCAATAAGATCCC-3′ (reverse).

Statistics

Values are reported as mean ± standard error of the mean (SEM). A statistical comparison between two samples was performed using the Student t test. Statistical comparisons of more than two groups were performed using one-way analysis of variance with the Bonferroni post-hoc test. In all comparisons, $p < 0.05$ was considered significant.

Results

CX3CL1-induced MMP-3 production in human OASFs

CX3CL1 is known to participate in the pathogenesis of OA and RA pathogenesis [14, 18]. Therefore, we first compared the CX3CL1 levels in normal human SFs (normal SFs) and OASFs. The mRNA expression of CX3CL1 was higher in the OASFs than in the normal SFs (Fig. 1a). Because CX3CL1 stimulates MMP expression in chronic liver diseases [19], we hypothesized that any of these MMPs could be involved in CX3CL1-directed OA pathogenesis. We used qPCR to detect mRNA expression levels of MMPs in normal SFs and OASFs. The expression of MMP-3 was significantly higher than that of other MMPs in OASFs compared with the basal level expressed in normal SFs (Fig. 1b, c). To understand the relationship between CX3CL1 and MMP-3 in normal SFs and OASFs, we examined the level of MMP-3 after CX3CL1 treatment. The level of MMP-3 was significantly elevated in OASFs compared with normal SFs. CX3CL1 induced MMP-3 production in a concentration-dependent manner (Fig. 1d–f), and induction occurred in a time-dependent manner in OASFs (Fig. 1 g–i). These results indicated that CX3CL1 increased MMP-3 production in human OASFs.

CX3CL1–CX3CR1 interaction induced MMP-3 expression in OASFs

The CX3CL1–CX3CR1 axis plays a crucial role in the development of inflammatory diseases [10, 20]. Therefore, we hypothesized that CX3CR1 is involved in CX3CL1-induced MMP-3 production. We knocked down CX3CR1 expression by transfecting the OASFs with CX3CR1 siRNA and determined that CX3CR1 siRNA inhibited CX3CL1-induced MMP-3 production at the mRNA and protein expression levels (Fig. 2a, b). Furthermore, a CX3CL1 monoclonal antibody (mAb), but not the control IgG, effectively suppressed CX3CL1-induced MMP-3 mRNA and protein expression (Fig. 2c–e). These results suggest that CX3CR1 activation may be responsible for CX3CL1-induced MMP-3 expression.

CX3CL1-induced MMP-3 production through the c-Raf/MEK/ERK pathway

To examine the mechanism by which CX3CL1 induces MMP-3 production, we directly measured the c-Raf phosphorylation in response to CX3CL1. The results revealed that the stimulation of cells using CX3CL1 induced c-Raf phosphorylation in a time-dependent manner (Fig. 3a). Pretreatment of cells with the CX3CR1 antibody attenuated c-Raf phosphorylation, suggesting that CX3CR1 serves as the upstream regulator of c-Raf-mediated signaling (Fig. 3b). Furthermore, to examine whether CX3CL1 stimulates the production of MMP-3 through c-Raf signaling, we used pharmacological inhibitor (GW5704) and c-Raf shRNA. Pretreatment of cells with GW5074 was found to antagonize CX3CL1-induced MMP-3 production at the mRNA and protein levels (Fig. 3c–e). As shown in Fig. 3f, g, CX3CL1-induced MMP-3 production at the mRNA and protein levels was strongly reduced in shRNA against c-Raf.

Subsequently, we investigated whether CX3CL1 can activate MEK/ERK, which is a critical downstream target of c-Raf. Stimulation of cells with CX3CL1 was discovered to induce the time-dependent phosphorylation of MEK and ERK (Fig. 4a). However, this CX3CL1-induced phosphorylation of MEK/ERK was markedly decreased by inhibiting upstream signaling events using the c-Raf inhibitor (GW5704) (Fig. 4b). To further evaluate whether the MEK/ERK pathway can induce MMP-3 expression, we pretreated cells with PD98059 (10 μM) and U0126 (10 μM). CX3CL1 induced the mRNA and significantly reduced the protein levels of MMP-3 when cells were pretreated with PD98059 and U0126 (Fig. 4c–e). To further confirm this stimulation-specific mediation by MEK and ERK, we assessed the role of MEK and ERK using dominant negative mutations. Transfection of cells with dominant negative MEK and dominant negative ERK reduced MEK and ERK expression, respectively (Fig. 4f, upper panel). Transfection of cells with dominant negative MEK and dominant negative ERK effectively inhibited CX3CL1-induced MMP-3 mRNA and protein expression (Fig. 4e–g). These results indicate that CX3CL1 induces MMP-3 production through CX3CR1 activation, which consequently activates the c-Raf/MEK/ERK signaling pathways in OASFs.

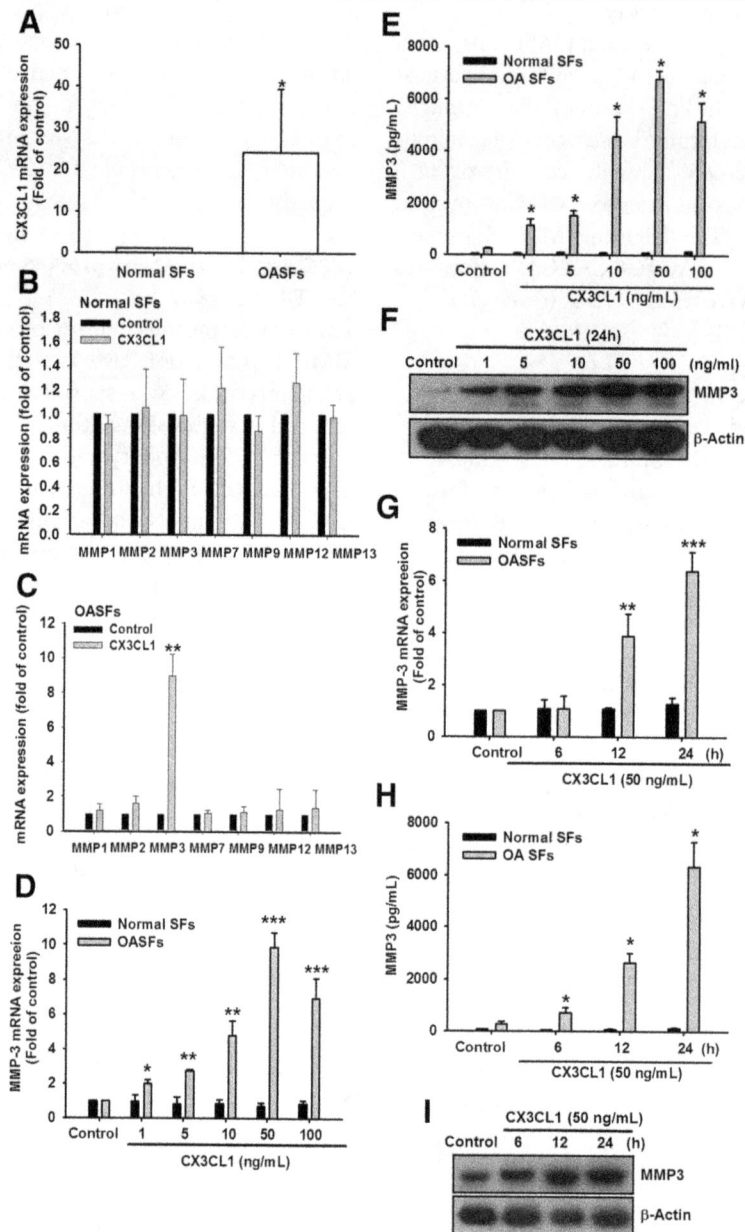

Fig. 1 Concentration-dependent and time-dependent increases in MMP-3 production by CX3CL1. **a** Human SFs were obtained from healthy patients ($n = 8$) or patients with OA ($n = 10$). CX3CL1 expression examined using qPCR. **b, c** OASFs and normal SFs were incubated with CX3CL1 (50 ng/ml) for 24 h. mRNA expression of MMPs examined using qPCR ($n = 4$). **d, g** OASFs and normal SFs were incubated with various concentrations of CX3CL1 for 24 h or with CX3CL1 (50 ng/ml) for 6, 12, or 24 h. mRNA expression of MMP-3 examined using qPCR ($n = 4$). **e, h** OASFs and normal SFs were incubated with various concentrations of CX3CL1 for 24 h or with CX3CL1 (50 ng/ml) for 6, 12, or 24 h; supernatants and cell lysates were then collected. MMP-3 level in culture media measured using a Quantikine ELISA kit ($n = 4$). **f, i** MMP-3 protein levels in cell lysates determined using western blot analysis. Both protein levels and enzymatic activity increased in a dose-dependent and time-dependent manner. Results expressed as mean ± SEM. * represents $P < 0.05$, ** represents $P < 0.01$, ***represents $P < 0.001$, as compared to respective control by using one-way ANOVA followed by Bonferroni's post-hoc test.. MMP matrix metalloproteinase, OASF osteoarthritis synovial fibroblast

Involvement of NF-κB in CX3CL1-induced MMP-3 production

The activation of NF-κB can induce MMP-3 production in the cells of patients with RA or OA [21]. NF-κB is a transcriptional activator that plays a vital role in OA pathogenesis [22]. To examine whether NF-κB is involved in the signal transduction pathway leading to CX3CL1-induced MMP-3 production, we used NF-κB inhibitors (PDTC) and IκB protease inhibitors (TPCK). Pretreatment of cells with PDTC and TPCK was discovered to inhibit CX3CL1-induced MMP-3 mRNA and protein expression (Fig. 5a–c). We further examined the

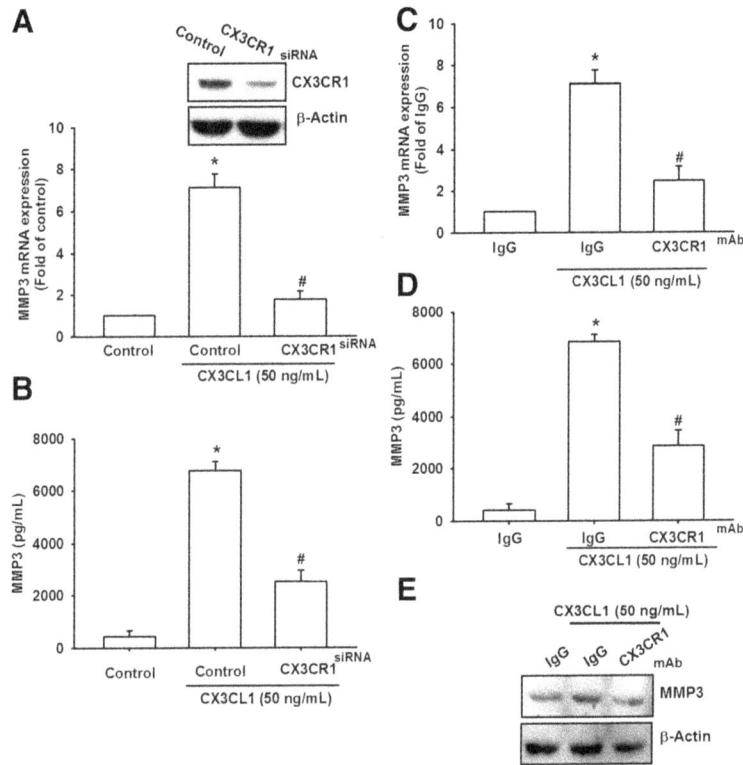

Fig. 2 CX3CR1 is involved in CX3CL1-mediated MMP-3 production in OASFs. **a, b** OSAFs were transfected for 24 h with CX3CR1 siRNA, followed by stimulation with CX3CL1 for 24 h. MMP-3 expression examined using qPCR and ELISA. **c–e** OASFs were pretreated for 30 min with CX3CR1 mAb followed by stimulation with CX3CL1 for 24 h. MMP-3 expression was examined using qPCR, ELISA and western blot. Results expressed as mean ± SEM ($n = 3$). *$p < 0.05$ compared with control; #$p < 0.05$ compared with CX3CL1-treated group. mAb monoclonal antibody, MMP matrix metalloproteinase, siRNA small interfering RNA

upstream molecules involved in CX3CL1-induced NF-κB activation. The stimulation of OASFs using CX3CL1 increased IKKα/β, IkBα, and p65 phosphorylation in a time-dependent manner (Fig. 5d). In addition, transfection of cells with IKKα and IKKβ mutants reduced CX3CL1-induced MMP-3 production and MMP-3 mRNA expression (Fig. 5e, f).

To confirm that NF-κB is involved in CX3CL1-induced MMP-3 expression, we performed transient transfection using NF-κB promoter–luciferase constructs. When OASFs were incubated with CX3CL1, the NF-κB promoter activity increased in a dose-dependent manner (Fig. 6a). The increase in NF-κB activity induced by CX3CL1 was antagonized by c-Raf inhibitor (GW5704), MEK inhibitors (PD98059 and U0126), and c-Raf shRNA, MEK, ERK, IKKα, and IKKβ mutants (Fig. 6b, c). Furthermore, GW5704, PD98059, and U0126 reduced CX3CL1-mediated p65 phosphorylation (Fig. 6d). In addition, these inhibitors (Gw5074, PD98059, and U0126) reduced the CX3CL1-induced binding of p65 to an NF-κB element (Fig. 6e). To further investigate CX3CL1-mediated MMP-3 expression in OASFs, we established CX3CL1-shRNA expression cells.

Western blot analyses were employed to compare the CX3CL1 expression levels in stable transfectants. CX3CL1 expression was drastically inhibited in OASF/CX3CL1-shRNA cells (Fig. 6f–h). In addition, CX3CL1 knockdown downregulated the expression of MMP-3 in OASFs (Fig. 6f–h). These data suggest that the CX3CR1, c-Raf, MEK, ERK, and NF-κB pathways must be activated if CX3CL1-induced MMP-3 production is to occur in human OASFs.

Discussion

The present study provided compelling data to support the novel role of CX3CL1 in the severity of OA through its induction of MMP-3 production via the NF-κB pathway. Accumulating evidence suggests that CX3CL1 plays a vital role in the pathogenesis and progression of OA [14, 23]. In the present study, the CX3CL1 levels in OASFs were significantly higher than those in normal SFs (Fig. 1). Previous studies have demonstrated that patients with knee OA had significantly higher levels of serum, synovial fluid, and synovial CX3CL1 than is found in normal synovial fluid [24–26], which is consistent with the present study's results. In addition, the role

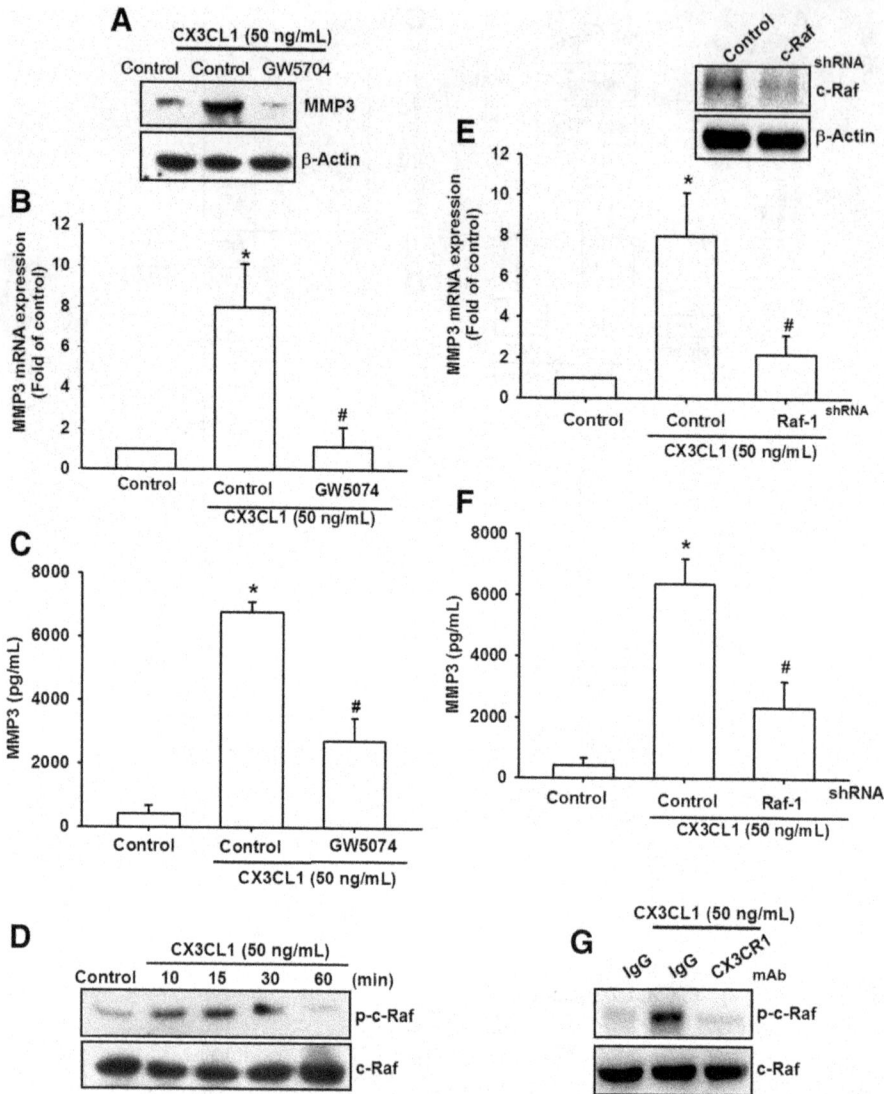

Fig. 3 c-Raf is involved in CX3CL1-mediated MMP-3 production in SFs. **a** OASFs were incubated with CX3CL1 for the indicated time intervals. c-Raf phosphorylation examined using western blot analysis. **b** OASFs were pretreated for 30 min with CX3CR1 mAb followed by stimulation with CX3CL1 for 15 min. c-Raf protein levels in the cell lysates determined using western blot analysis. **c–e** OASFs were pretreated for 30 min with c-Raf inhibitor (GW5074, 10 μM), followed by stimulation with CX3CL1 for 24 h. MMP-3 expression examined using qPCR, western blot analysis, and ELISA. **f, g** OASFs were transfected for 24 h with c-Raf shRNA followed by stimulation with CX3CL1 for 24 h. MMP-3 expression examined using qPCR and ELISA. Results expressed as mean ± SEM ($n = 3$). *$p < 0.05$ compared with control; #$p < 0.05$ compared with CX3CL1-treated group. MMP matrix metalloproteinase, shRNA small hairpin RNA

of CX3CL1 has been reported in inflammatory diseases [27]. CX3CL1 induces tumor necrosis factor alpha (TNF-α), interferon gamma, and interleukin 1 beta (IL-1β) production in chronic obstructive pulmonary disease, pulmonary hypertension, atherosclerosis, RA, HIV infection, and cancer [28–30]. In joint cartilage cells, the increase in CX3CL1 mRNA expression correlated with IL-1β [31]. Accumulating evidence suggests that CX3CL1 plays a more critical role in stimulating the inflammatory process in OA. The findings indicate that CX3CL1 may be considered a chemokine suitable for developing new therapeutic approaches for OA.

The MMP family comprises a group of zinc-ion-dependent endopeptidases that play an important role in normal and OA synovial tissue [32]. Unregulated MMP production results in excessive extracellular matrix degradation and leads to OA. MMP-3 (also known as stromelysin-1) is capable of degrading aggrecan and collagen types *I*, **II**, **III**, **IX**, **X and XI** in joints [33]. Accumulated evidence indicates that MMP-3 is not expressed in normal adult cartilage, but is highly expressed in the cartilage of patients with OA [34]. In addition, some studies have reported that CX3CL1 induces MMP production, including that of MMP-2 and

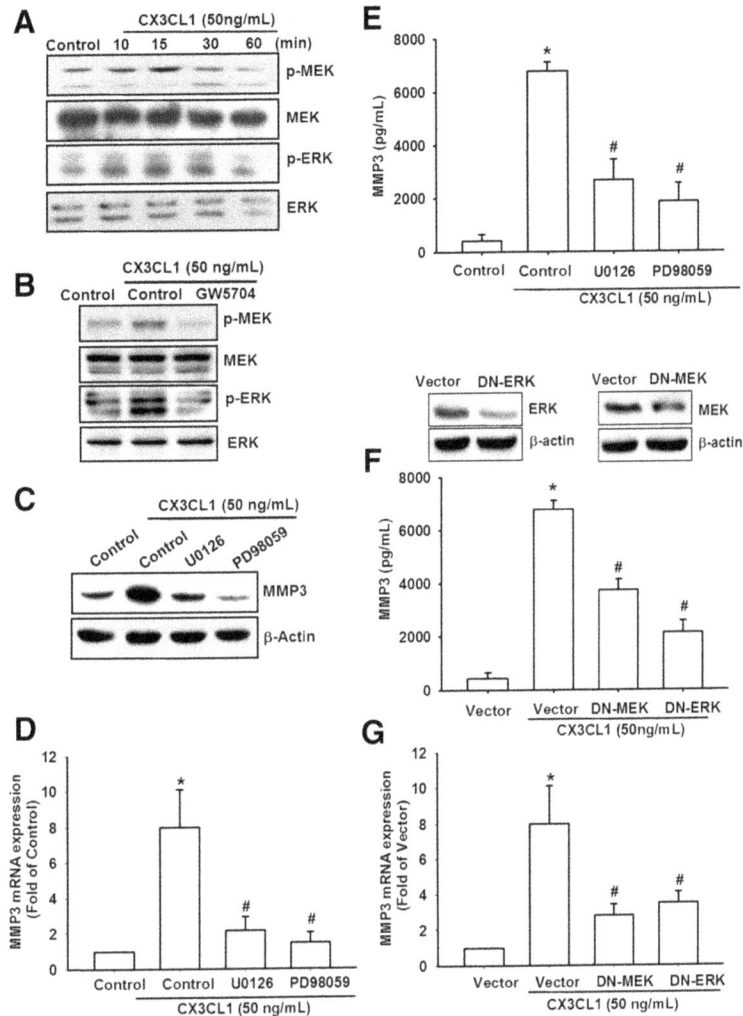

Fig. 4 MEK/ERK is involved in CX3CL1-mediated MMP-3 production in OASFs. **a** OASFs were incubated with CX3CL1 for the indicated time intervals. MEK/ERK phosphorylation examined using western blot analysis. **b** OASFs were pretreated for 30 min with c-Raf inhibitor (GW5074) followed by stimulation with CX3CL1 for 15 min. MEK/ERK protein levels in the cell lysates determined using western blot analysis. **c–e** OASFs were pretreated for 30 min with MEK/ERK inhibitors (U0126 and PD98059) followed by stimulation with CX3CL1 for 24 h. MMP-3 expression examined using qPCR, western blot analysis, and ELISA. **f, g** OASFs were transfected for 24 h with MEK and ERK mutants followed by stimulation with CX3CL1 for 24 h. MMP-3 expression examined using qPCR and ELISA. Results expressed as mean ± SEM ($n = 3$). *$p < 0.05$ compared with control; #$p < 0.05$ compared with CX3CL1-treated group. MMP matrix metalloproteinase

MMP-9 [16, 35]. We identified MMP-3 as the target protein of the CX3CL1 signaling pathway, which regulates cartilage breakdown. CX3CL1 was discovered to induce MMP-3 mRNA and protein expression in a dose-dependent and time-dependent manner in OASFs. These results suggest that CX3CL1 acts as an inducer of MMPs and enhances cartilage breakdown.

A previous study indicated that the activation of CX3CR1 signaling may be a causal factor of OA [31]. The high expression of CX3CR1 in the synovial membranes of patients with OA may be directly involved in the pathophysiology of OA [31]. The results of our study indicated that CX3CL1 protein levels were significantly higher in OASFs than in normal SFs. We also discovered

that CX3CR1 was required for CX3CL1-induced MMP-3 production. The incubation of cells with the CX3CR1 mAb inhibited CX3CL1-induced MMP-3 expression. In addition, CX3CR1 siRNA inhibited the increase in CX3CL1-induced MMP-3 production. These findings suggest that CX3CR1 is involved in CX3CL1-induced MMP-3 production in human OASFs.

In 2006, Lee et al. [36] demonstrated that the activation of CX3CL1 signaling in the c-Raf/MEK/ERK and PI3K/Akt/eNOS/NO signal pathways plays a vital role in molecular biological functions. However, the mechanisms for inducing MMP expression in different cell types may be regulated differently. The c-Raf/MEK/ERK signaling pathways that induce

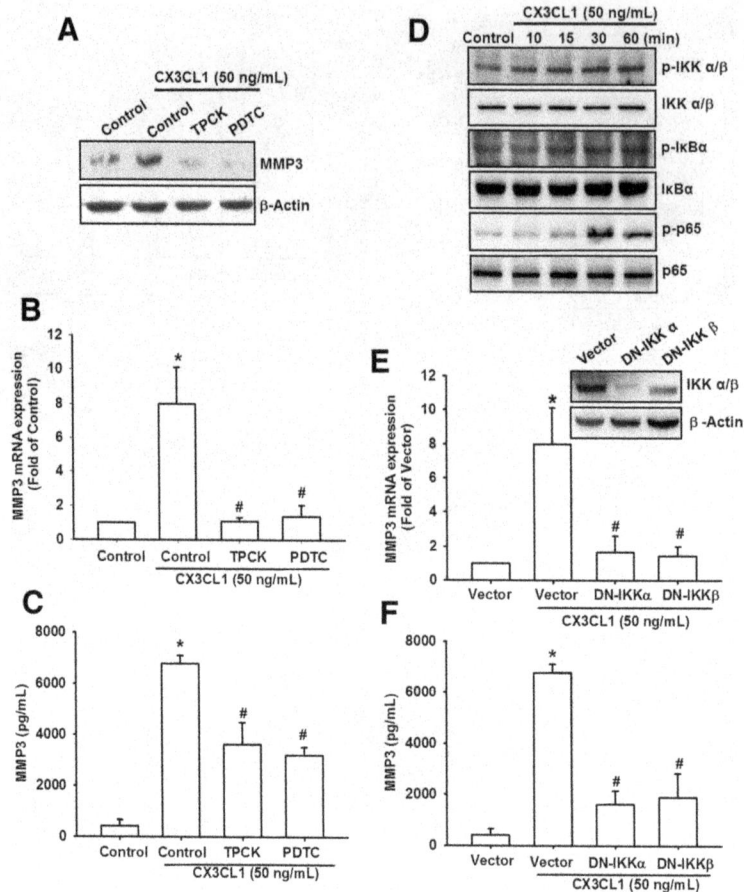

Fig. 5 NF-κB is involved in the potentiation of MMP-3 production by CX3CL1. **a–c** OASFs were pretreated for 30 min with PDTC (10 μM) and TPCK (10 μM) followed by stimulation with CX3CL1 for 24 h. MMP-3 expression examined using qPCR, western blot analysis, and ELISA. **d** OASFs were incubated with CX3CL1 for the indicated time intervals. p-IKKα/β, p-IκBα, and p-p65 expression determined using western blot analysis. **e, f** OASFs were transfected for 24 h with IKKα and IKKβ mutants followed by stimulation with CX3CL1 for 24 h. MMP-3 expression examined using qPCR and ELISA. Results expressed as mean ± SEM (*n* = 3). *$p < 0.05$ compared with control; #$p < 0.05$ compared with CX3CL1-treated group. MMP matrix metalloproteinase, PDTC pyrrolidine dithiocarbamate, TPCK L-1-tosylamido-2-phenylenylethyl chloromethyl ketone

MMP expression in OASFs have not been reported. In this study, we demonstrated that the ability of CX3CL1 to induce MMP-3 production is mediated by the interaction between CX3CL1 and CX3CR1 and the subsequent activation of the c-Raf/MEK/ERK pathway. Our results demonstrated that treatment of OASFs with c-Raf inhibitor or transfection of cells with c-Raf shRNA reduced the CX3CL1-induced MMP-3 expression. However, we also found that CX3CL1 treatment increased the level of c-Raf phosphorylation. Moreover, the CX3CR1 antibody inhibited CX3CL1-mediated c-Raf phosphorylation. These results suggest that CX3CL1 induced MMP-3 production through CX3CR1 and the c-Raf signaling pathway in SFs. The activation of the MAPK pathway by G-coupled protein receptors generally involves c-Raf [37, 38]. In our experiments, GW0574 completely inhibited CX3CL1-induced MEK and ERK activation and MMP-3 production, suggesting that these effects of CX3CL1 require c-Raf activation.

Accumulating evidence suggests that MMP production is regulated by activation of the ubiquitous transcription factor NF-κB. In addition, the critical role of NF-κB in the pathophysiology of OA has been reported [39, 40]. Under normal conditions, the p65 subunit of NF-κB is retained in the cytoplasm with the inhibitory protein IκB; however, when NF-κB is activated by stimuli such as IL-1β or TNF-α, the phosphorylated p65 subunit of NF-κB translocates to the nucleus to regulate the expression of inflammatory mediators and MMPs [41, 42]. In the present study, we used NF-κB inhibitors to explore these pathways. We demonstrated that NF-κB activation contributed to CX3CL1-induced MMP-3 expression in human SFs. The pretreatment of cells with NF-κB inhibitors TPCK and PDTC reduced the CX3CL1-induced MMP-3 expression. Therefore, the NF-κB binding site is important in CX3CL1-induced MMP-3 production. The NF-κB sequence binds to members of the p65 and p50 families of transcription factors, and the results of this study revealed

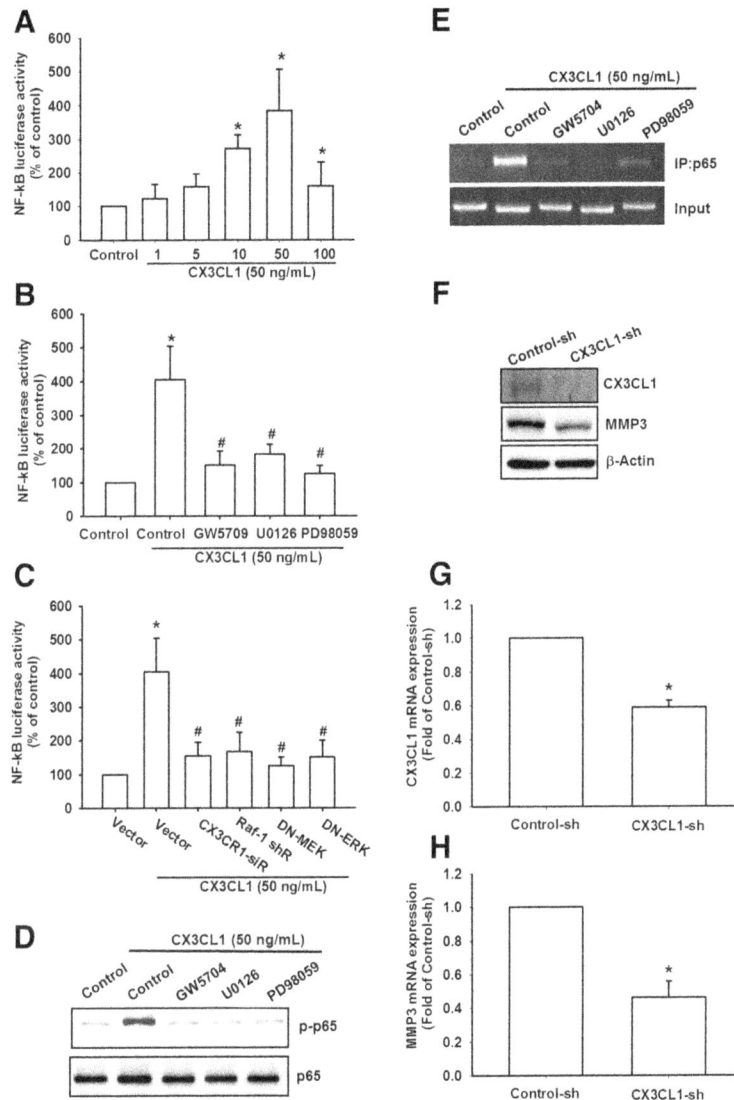

Fig. 6 CX3CL1 induced NF-κB activation through the CX3CR1/c-Raf/MEK/ERK pathway. **a–c** OASFs were incubated with various concentrations of CX3CL1 or pretreated with c-Raf inhibitors (GW5074) or MEK/ERK inhibitors (U0126 and PD98059) for 30 min or transfected with c-Raf shRNA, MEK, ERK, IKKα, and IKKβ mutants before exposure to CX3CL1. NF-κB luciferase activity measured, and results normalized to the β-galactosidase activity. **d** OASFs were pretreated with c-Raf inhibitors (GW5074) or MEK/ERK inhibitors (U0126 and PD98059) for 30 min followed by stimulation with CX3CL1 for 60 min. p-p65 expression examined using western blot analysis. **e** Cells were pretreated with 0.1% dimethyl sulfoxide as control, c-Raf inhibitors (GW5074), or MEK/ERK inhibitors (U0126 and PD98059) for 30 min, followed by CX3CL1 treatment for 120 min. ChIP performed using an antibody against p65. One percent of immunoprecipitated chromatin was assayed to verify equal loading (input). **f–h** Protein and mRNA levels of CX3CL1 and MMP-3 in control-shRNA and CX3CL1-shRNA OASFs examined using western blotting and qPCR. Results expressed as mean ± SEM ($n = 4$). *$p < 0.05$ compared with control; #$p < 0.05$ compared with CX3CL1-treated group. MMP matrix metalloproteinase, NF-κB nuclear factor kappa B, sh short hairpin

that CX3CL1 induced p65 phosphorylation and nuclear accumulation. Furthermore, the use of transient transfection with NF-κB-luciferase as an indicator of NF-κB activity revealed that CX3CL1 increased NF-κB activation. In addition, the c-Raf inhibitor (GW5074), MAPK inhibitors (U0126 and PD98059) or c-Raf shRNA or MEK, and the ERK mutant reduced CX3CL1-increased NF-κB promoter activity. These results indicate that CX3CL1 increases NF-κB activation through the CX3CR1/c-Raf/MAPK signaling pathway in human OASFs. The discovery of this CX3CL1 signaling pathway elucidates the mechanism underlying OA pathogenesis, which may lead to the development of effective therapies in the future.

Conclusion

We explored the signaling pathways involved in CX3CL1-induced MMP-3 production in human SFs. We determined that CX3CL1 increases MMP-3 production by binding to CX3CR1 and activating c-Rad, MEK, and ERK signaling, which enhances NF-κB transcription activity and results in the transactivation of MMP-3 production. Furthermore, the discovery of CX3CL1/CX3CR1-mediated signaling pathways increases the understanding of the mechanism of OA pathogenesis and could facilitate the development of effective therapies for OA in the future.

Abbreviations

cDNA: Complementary DNA; ChIP: Chromatin immunoprecipitation; DMEM: Dulbecco's modified Eagle's medium; ELISA: Enzyme-linked immunosorbent assay; FBS: Fetal bovine serum; GAPDH: Glyceraldehyde 3-phosphate dehydrogenase; mAb: Monoclonal antibody; MMP: Matrix metalloproteinase; NF-κB: Nuclear factor kappa B; OA: Osteoarthritis; OASF: Osteoarthritis synovial fibroblast; PVDF: Polyvinyldifluoride; qPCR: Real-time quantitative polymerase chain reaction; SEM: Standard error of the mean

Acknowledgements

The authors thank the staff of the Eighth Core Lab, Department of Medical Research, National Taiwan University Hospital for technical support during the study. This manuscript was edited by Wallace Academic Editing.

Funding

This study was supported by grants from the Ministry of Science and Technology, Taiwan, R.O.C. (MOST105-2314-B-341-001 and MOST105-2314-B-002-012), Shin-Kong Wu Ho-Su Memorial Hospital (SKH-8302-105-0301), and National Taiwan University Hospital (NTUH.106-S3464).

Authors' contributions

J-FL conceived and designed the experiments. C-HH and S-MH performed the experiments. S-MH and J-FL analyzed the data. C-HH and J-FL contributed reagents, materials, and analysis tools. C-HH and J-FL wrote the paper. All authors read and approved the final manuscript.

Consent for publication

Not applicable.

Competing interests

The authors declare that they have no competing interests.

Author details

[1]Department of Orthopedic Surgery, Shin Kong Wu Ho-Su Memorial Hospital, No. 95, Wen Chang Road, Taipei 111, Taiwan. [2]Department of Orthopedic Surgery, National Taiwan University Hospital, No. 1, Jen-Ai Road, Taipei 100, Taiwan. [3]Central Laboratory, Shin-Kong Wu Ho-Su Memorial Hospital, No. 95, Wenchang Road, Shilin, Taipei 111, Taiwan.

References

1. von Bernstorff M, Feierabend M, Jordan M, Glatzel C, Ipach I, Hofmann UK. Radiographic hip or knee osteoarthritis and the ability to drive. Orthopedics. 2017;40(1):e82–9.

2. Dziri C, Aloulou I, Loubiri I, Rekik M, Zohra Ben Salah F, Abdallah A. Assessment of disability in osteoarthritis of the knee. Ann Phys Rehabil Med. 2016;59S:e115.

3. Scanzello CR, Goldring SR. The role of synovitis in osteoarthritis pathogenesis. Bone. 2012;51(2):249–57.

4. Chen YT, Hou CH, Hou SM, Liu JF. The effects of amphiregulin induced MMP-13 production in human osteoarthritis synovial fibroblast. Mediators Inflamm. 2014;2014:759028.

5. Zeng GQ, Chen AB, Li W, Song JH, Gao CY. High MMP-1, MMP-2, and MMP-9 protein levels in osteoarthritis. Genet Mol Res. 2015;14(4):14811–22.

6. Jiang Q, Qiu YT, Chen MJ, Zhang ZY, Yang C. Synovial TGF-beta1 and MMP-3 levels and their correlation with the progression of temporomandibular joint osteoarthritis combined with disc displacement: a preliminary study. Biomed Rep. 2013;1(2):218–22.

7. Felson DT. Clinical practice. Osteoarthritis of the knee. N Engl J Med. 2006; 354(8):841–8.

8. Achari Y, Reno CR, Frank CB, Hart DA. Carrageenan-induced transient inflammation in a rabbit knee model: molecular changes consistent with an early osteoarthritis phenotype. Inflamm Res. 2012;61(8):907–14.

9. Cockwell P, Chakravorty SJ, Girdlestone J, Savage CO. Fractalkine expression in human renal inflammation. J Pathol. 2002;196(1):85–90.

10. Ollivier V, Faure S, Tarantino N, Chollet-Martin S, Deterre P, Combadiere C, de Prost D. Fractalkine/CX3CL1 production by human aortic smooth muscle cells impairs monocyte procoagulant and inflammatory responses. Cytokine. 2003;21(6):303–11.

11. Wu XM, Liu Y, Qian ZM, Luo QQ, Ke Y. CX3CL1/CX3CR1 axis plays a key role in ischemia-induced oligodendrocyte injury via p38MAPK signaling pathway. Mol Neurobiol. 2016;53(6):4010–8.

12. Li D, Chen H, Luo XH, Sun Y, Xia W, Xiong YC. CX3CR1-mediated Akt1 activation contributes to the paclitaxel-induced painful peripheral neuropathy in rats. Neurochem Res. 2016;41(6):1305–14.

13. Clark AK, Staniland AA, Malcangio M. Fractalkine/CX3CR1 signalling in chronic pain and inflammation. Curr Pharm Biotechnol. 2011;12(10):1707–14.

14. Nanki T, Imai T, Kawai S. Fractalkine/CX3CL1 in rheumatoid arthritis. Mod Rheumatol. 2017;27(3):392–7.

15. Odai T, Matsunawa M, Takahashi R, Wakabayashi K, Isozaki T, Yajima N, Miwa Y, Kasama T. Correlation of CX3CL1 and CX3CR1 levels with response to infliximab therapy in patients with rheumatoid arthritis. J Rheumatol. 2009; 36(6):1158–65.

16. Blaschke S, Koziolek M, Schwarz A, Benohr P, Middel P, Schwarz G, Hummel KM, Muller GA. Proinflammatory role of fractalkine (CX3CL1) in rheumatoid arthritis. J Rheumatol. 2003;30(9):1918–27.

17. Hou CH, Tang CH, Hsu CJ, Hou SM, Liu JF. CCN4 induces IL-6 production through alphavbeta5 receptor, PI3K, Akt, and NF-kappaB singling pathway in human synovial fibroblasts. Arthritis Res Ther. 2013;15(1):R19.

18. Zhao L, Wang Q, Zhang C, Huang C. Genome-wide DNA methylation analysis of articular chondrocytes identifies TRAF1, CTGF, and CX3CL1 genes as hypomethylated in osteoarthritis. Clin Rheumatol. 2017; 36(10)2335-42.

19. Bourd-Boittin K, Basset L, Bonnier D, L'Helgoualc'h A, Samson M, Theret N. CX3CL1/fractalkine shedding by human hepatic stellate cells: contribution to chronic inflammation in the liver. J Cell Mol Med. 2009; 13(8A):1526–35.

20. Ferretti E, Pistoia V, Corcione A. Role of fractalkine/CX3CL1 and its receptor in the pathogenesis of inflammatory and malignant diseases with emphasis on B cell malignancies. Mediators Inflamm. 2014;2014:480941.

21. Tzeng HE, Chen JC, Tsai CH, Kuo CC, Hsu HC, Hwang WL, Fong YC, Tang CH. CCN3 increases cell motility and MMP-13 expression in human chondrosarcoma through integrin-dependent pathway. J Cell Physiol. 2011; 226(12):3181–9.

22. Imagawa K, de Andres MC, Hashimoto K, Pitt D, Itoi E, Goldring MB, Roach HI, Oreffo RO. The epigenetic effect of glucosamine and a nuclear factor-kappa B (NF-kB) inhibitor on primary human chondrocytes—implications for osteoarthritis. Biochem Biophys Res Commun. 2011;405(3):362–7.

23. Huo LW, Ye YL, Wang GW, Ye YG. Fractalkine (CX3CL1): a biomarker reflecting symptomatic severity in patients with knee osteoarthritis. J Investig Med. 2015;63(4):626–31.

24. Yano R, Yamamura M, Sunahori K, Takasugi K, Yamana J, Kawashima M, Makino H. Recruitment of CD16+ monocytes into synovial tissues is mediated by fractalkine and CX3CR1 in rheumatoid arthritis patients. Acta Med Okayama. 2007;61(2):89–98.

25. Klosowska K, Volin MV, Huynh N, Chong KK, Halloran MM, Woods JM. Fractalkine functions as a chemoattractant for osteoarthritis synovial fibroblasts and stimulates phosphorylation of mitogen-activated protein kinases and Akt. Clin Exp Immunol. 2009;156(2):312–9.

26. Zou Y, Li Y, Lu L, Lin Y, Liang W, Su Z, Wang X, Yang H, Wang J, Yu C, et al. Correlation of fractalkine concentrations in serum and synovial fluid with the radiographic severity of knee osteoarthritis. Ann Clin Biochem. 2013;50(Pt 6):571–5.

27. Shimoda S, Harada K, Niiro H, Taketomi A, Maehara Y, Tsuneyama K, Kikuchi K, Nakanuma Y, Mackay IR, Gershwin ME, et al. CX3CL1 (fractalkine): a signpost for biliary inflammation in primary biliary cirrhosis. Hepatology. 2010;51(2):567–75.

28. Jones BA, Beamer M, Ahmed S. Fractalkine/CX3CL1: a potential new target for inflammatory diseases. Mol Interv. 2010;10(5):263–70.

29. Zhang J, Patel JM. Role of the CX3CL1-CX3CR1 axis in chronic inflammatory lung diseases. Int J Clin Exp Med. 2010;3(3):233–44.

30. Xiong Z, Leme AS, Ray P, Shapiro SD, Lee JS. CX3CR1+ lung mononuclear phagocytes spatially confined to the interstitium produce TNF-alpha and IL-6 and promote cigarette smoke-induced emphysema. J Immunol. 2011;186(5):3206–14.

31. Wojdasiewicz P, Poniatowski LA, Kotela A, Deszczynski J, Kotela I, Szukiewicz D. The chemokine CX3CL1 (fractalkine) and its receptor CX3CR1: occurrence and potential role in osteoarthritis. Arch Immunol Ther Exp (Warsz). 2014;62(5):395–403.

32. van den Bosch MH, Blom AB, van de Loo FA, Koenders MI, Lafeber FP, van den Berg WB, van der Kraan PM, van Lent PL. Brief Report: Induction of Matrix Metalloproteinase Expression by Synovial Wnt Signaling and Association With Disease Progression in Early Symptomatic Osteoarthritis. Arthritis Rheumatol. 2017; 69(10)1978-83.

33. Ma JD, Zhou JJ, Zheng DH, Chen LF, Mo YQ, Wei XN, Yang LJ, Dai L. Serum matrix metalloproteinase-3 as a noninvasive biomarker of histological synovitis for diagnosis of rheumatoid arthritis. Mediators Inflamm. 2014;2014:179284.

34. Tong Z, Liu Y, Chen B, Yan L, Hao D. Association between MMP3 and TIMP3 polymorphisms and risk of osteoarthritis. Oncotarget. 2017; 8(48)83563-9.

35. Ancuta P, Wang J, Gabuzda D. CD16+ monocytes produce IL-6, CCL2, and matrix metalloproteinase-9 upon interaction with CX3CL1-expressing endothelial cells. J Leukoc Biol. 2006;80(5):1156–64.

36. Lee SJ, Namkoong S, Kim YM, Kim CK, Lee H, Ha KS, Chung HT, Kwon YG, Kim YM: Fractalkine stimulates angiogenesis by activating the Raf-1/MEK/ERK- and PI3K/Akt/eNOS-dependent signal pathways. Am J Physiol Heart Circ Physiol 2006, 291(6):H2836-46.

37. Robinson JD, Pitcher JA. G protein-coupled receptor kinase 2 (GRK2) is a Rho-activated scaffold protein for the ERK MAP kinase cascade. Cell Signal. 2013;25(12):2831–9.

38. Filardo EJ, Quinn JA, Frackelton Jr AR, Bland KI. Estrogen action via the G protein-coupled receptor, GPR30: stimulation of adenylyl cyclase and cAMP-mediated attenuation of the epidermal growth factor receptor-to-MAPK signaling axis. Mol Endocrinol. 2002;16(1):70–84.

39. Shakibaei M, John T, Schulze-Tanzil G, Lehmann I, Mobasheri A. Suppression of NF-kappaB activation by curcumin leads to inhibition of expression of cyclo-oxygenase-2 and matrix metalloproteinase-9 in human articular chondrocytes: implications for the treatment of osteoarthritis. Biochem Pharmacol. 2007;73(9):1434–45.

40. Tong KM, Chen CP, Huang KC, Shieh DC, Cheng HC, Tzeng CY, Chen KH, Chiu YC, Tang CH. Adiponectin increases MMP-3 expression in human chondrocytes through AdipoR1 signaling pathway. J Cell Biochem. 2011; 112(5):1431–40.

41. Liu FL, Chen CH, Chu SJ, Chen JH, Lai JH, Sytwu HK, Chang DM. Interleukin (IL)-23 p19 expression induced by IL-1beta in human fibroblast-like synoviocytes with rheumatoid arthritis via active nuclear factor-kappaB and AP-1 dependent pathway. Rheumatology (Oxford). 2007;46(8):1266–73.

42. Montaseri A, Busch F, Mobasheri A, Buhrmann C, Aldinger C, Rad JS, Shakibaei M. IGF-1 and PDGF-bb suppress IL-1beta-induced cartilage degradation through down-regulation of NF-kappaB signaling: involvement of Src/PI-3 K/AKT pathway. PLoS One. 2011;6(12):e28663.

9

New insights on the MMP-13 regulatory network in the pathogenesis of early osteoarthritis

Heng Li[1], Dan Wang[1], Yongjian Yuan[1] and Jikang Min[1,2*]

Abstract

Osteoarthritis (OA) is the most common joint disorder and affects approximately half of the aged population. Current treatments for OA are largely palliative until the articular cartilage has been deeply damaged and irreversible morphological changes appear. Thus, effective methods are needed for diagnosing and monitoring the progression of OA during its early stages when therapeutic drugs or biological agents are most likely to be effective. Various proteinases involved in articular cartilage degeneration in pre-OA conditions, which may represent the earliest reversible measurable changes, are considered diagnostic and therapeutic targets for early OA. Of these proteinases, matrix metalloproteinase 13 (MMP-13) has received the most attention, because it is a central node in the cartilage degradation network. In this review, we highlight the main MMP-13-related changes in OA chondrocytes, including alterations in the activity and expression level of MMP-13 by upstream regulatory factors, DNA methylation, various non-coding RNAs (ncRNAs), and autophagy. Because MMP-13 and its regulatory networks are suitable targets for the development of effective early treatment strategies for OA, we discuss the specific targets of MMP-13, including upstream regulatory proteins, DNA methylation, non-coding RNAs, and autophagy-related proteins of MMP-13, and their therapeutic potential to inhibit the development of OA. Moreover, the various entities mentioned in this review might be useful as early biomarkers and for personalized approaches to disease prevention and treatment by improving the phenotyping of early OA patients.

Keywords: Matrix metalloproteinases, MMP-13, Osteoarthritis, Non-coding RNA, DNA methylation, Autophagy

Background

Osteoarthritis (OA) is the most common joint disorder, affecting approximately half of the aged population (>65 years) and is characterized by the progressive degeneration of articular cartilage. The major clinical manifestation includes symptoms of knee pain, knee swelling, ankylosis, and limited activity [1]. OA results in mobility problems and severe pain during the intermediate or advanced stages and represents a leading socioeconomic burden in the developed world [2].

Currently, clinical diagnosis and monitoring of OA mainly rely on symptomatic and radiographic assessments and certain traditional laboratory tests [3–5]. Although their sensitivity and accuracy are relatively high, these methods fail to distinctively identify the developmental stages of OA. Similarly, the current treatments for OA are largely palliative until the articular cartilage has been deeply damaged and irreversible morphological changes have occurred; during the progression of OA the joints become completely dysfunctional and prosthetic replacement becomes necessary [6]. Thus, effective methods for diagnosing OA during its early stages are imperative and OA-related changes can likely be reversed by effective therapeutic drugs.

However, the development of disease-modifying drugs and the verification of their effectiveness in clinical trials are difficult to achieve due to the lack of a biomarker for the identification of patients with early OA-related changes. Articular cartilage damage is one of the most significant hallmarks of the early stages of OA [7]. Recently, studies have focused on the identification of biomarkers involved in articular cartilage degeneration in very early OA, which may represent the earliest reversible measurable changes.

* Correspondence: mjk@medmail.com.cn
[1]The First Affiliated Hospital of Huzhou Teachers College, Zhejiang Province 313000, China
[2]Department of Orthopaedics, The First Affiliated Hospital of Huzhou Teachers College, The First People's Hospital of Huzhou, Zhejiang Province 313000, China

Biomarkers that are related to the onset of articular cartilage degeneration during the early phase of OA include a number of matrix-degrading enzymes, such as the matrix metalloproteinase (MMP) family, the a disintegrin and metalloproteinase with thrombospondin type-1 motifs (ADAMTS) family, aggrecanases, etc. [8]. Of these proteinases, attention has focused on MMP-13 because it is significantly over-expressed in the joints and articular cartilage in patients with OA and can hardly be detected in normal adult tissues. MMP-13 is known to function as an extracellular matrix (ECM)-degrading enzyme in OA joints [9, 10]. In an experimental mouse OA model using a microsurgical technique, MMP-13 levels correlate with the presence of pathological chondrocytes that undergo hypertrophic differentiation in the early stage of OA development [11] and its over-expression can induce the onset of OA through excessive ECM degradation [12]. In contrast, OA progression is inhibited in MMP-13 knockout mice through protecting cartilage from proteoglycan loss and structural damage in an experimental OA model derived using medial meniscal destabilization surgery [13]. In clinical samples, MMP-13 was abnormally expressed during different stages of the OA process and was found to up-regulated during the early stage and down-regulated during the late stage in human OA cartilage [14]. Therefore, because MMP-13 is a central node in the cartilage degradation network [15], an understanding of the contribution of MMP-13 to the initiation/onset of OA is necessary. The activity of MMP-13 can be regulated at multiple levels [16], including epigenetic modification [17–19], transcriptional regulation, post-transcriptional regulation by ncRNAs [20, 21], and the activation or inhibition of proenzymes [9, 22]. In this review, we focus on new insights on the role of the MMP-13 regulatory network in the pathogenesis of early OA, considering transcriptional regulation [20, 21], different epigenetic alterations (such as DNA methylation and deregulation of non-coding RNA [17–19]), and autophagy [23]. We also discuss whether MMP-13 and its regulatory network could be useful in the diagnosis of early OA.

Recent investigations into the role of MMP-13 in the onset of OA

The MMP family in humans comprises 24 different MMP genes and 23 different MMP proteins that are structurally related and characterized as zinc-dependent endopeptidases that degrade various components of the ECM and basement membrane [24]. Based on their domain organization, their sequence similarities, and the specificity of their substrates, the MMPs can be classified into the following four groups: gelatinases, matrilysins, archetypal, and furin-activated. The archetypal MMPs can be classified into the following three subgroups according to their substrate specificities: collagenases, stromelysins, and other archetypal MMPs [25]. MMP-13, also known as collagenases-3, is a member of the collagenase subgroup [25].

Recently, the mRNA and protein expression of MMP-13 were shown to be increased during the process of OA onset. In rat initial/onset OA models, the increased expression of MMP-13 was detected using both immunohistochemistry and qRT-PCR, suggesting that MMP-13 was a factor responsible for early-onset OA [26, 27]. A similar result was observed in anterior cruciate ligament transection (ACLT) or ACLT with partial medial meniscectomy (ACLT + MMx) rat OA models in which a significant increase in the mRNA levels of MMP-13 was observed as early as the first week post-surgery, and the increased expression remained elevated throughout the 10-week study [28].

In addition to MMP-13, its regulatory factors, including interacting protein of MMP-13, were involved in the process of OA onset. For example, low-density lipoprotein receptor-related protein 1 (LRP1) binds both pro- and activated MMP-13, and is a key modulator of the extracellular levels of MMP-13. LRP1 was associated with the function of MMP-13 in the physiological turnover of the ECM [17]. Thus, MMP-13 plays a key role in the initiation of the shift from normal chondrocytes to the pathological phase, at least partially, by driving the shedding of LRP1 in cartilage, which may help us develop a new approach for controlling the onset of OA. A similar function was observed in leptin-targeted gene therapy. Leptin, which is a 16-kDa non-glycosylated protein product of the obese (ob) gene, exhibits a detrimental effect on articular cartilage. Small interference RNA against leptin could directly deactivate MMP-13 in the OA chondrocyte and possibly has therapeutic potential for OA treatment [29]. Similarly, high temperature requirement A1 (HTRA1) is increased in both human OA cartilage and the articular cartilage in mouse models of OA [30]. Once HTRA1 activity disrupts the pericellular matrix, which may occur early before the overt symptoms of OA develop, chondrocyte receptors such as DDR2 may be activated by type II collagen in the fibrillar form, leading to the preferential up-regulation of MMP-13 and further degradation of the interterritorial matrix [31].

Another kind of protein that interacts with MMP-13 functions by activating the latent form of the MMP-13 protein. Activators of pro-MMP-13 are potential therapeutic targets for early OA since activation of the zymogen form of MMP-13 occurs relatively early in the OA course. Recently, Magarinos et al. [32] constructed an ex vivo mouse femoral head explant system and studied the effects of tryptase-β and MCP-6 on MMP-13 enzymatic activity. The results show that tetramer-forming tryptases initiated aggrecanolysis by proteolytically activating the latent proenzyme form of MMP-13. There is specificity as to which neutral proteinase zymogen of MMP-13 in the joint is susceptible to tryptase-dependent activation, although no evidence of direct interaction between tryptase-β and/or MCP-6 with latent pro-MMP-13 has so far been provided [32].

Furthermore, the function of MMP-13 in the onset/initiation of OA may be mediated by specific signaling pathways. Many transcription factors are involved during different stages of OA, such as LEF1, NF-κB, ELF3, HIF2α, and Runx2, and most transcription factors directly or indirectly impact MMP-13 transcription. For example, Yun et al. [33] found that LEF1, interacting with β-catenin, directly binds the 3′ region of the MMP13 gene and transactivates MMP13 promoter activity, possibly through a change of DNA conformation. SIRT1 represses MMP-13 in human OA chondrocytes, which appears to be mediated, at least in part, through repression of the transcription activity of LEF1. In the SIRT1 knockout (KO) mouse model, LEF1 and MMP-13 appeared elevated in the superficial zone of articular cartilage, which suggested the initiation of OA [34]. NF-κB activation results in the activation of ELF3 and HIF2α, which leads to activation of MMP-13 and facilitates the shift of normal articular chondrocytes to a hypertrophic-like differentiated state, subsequently initiating OA onset [35].

In addition, MMP inhibitors could be developed to control the onset of OA. For example, Wang et al. [36] and Julovi et al. [37] investigated the effects of high molecular weight hyaluronic acid (HMW-HA) on the gene expression of 16 OA-associated cytokines and enzymes. These authors found that HMW-HA has a structure-modifying effect on early OA by effectively inhibiting the production of MMP-1, MMP-3, and MMP-13 in human articular cartilage.

Mechanical stress also plays a key role in the pathogenesis of OA cartilage destruction and MMP-13 has been proven to be involved in the early stage in a series of in vivo and in vitro experiments. For example, Kamekura et al. [11] created a mechanical stress-induced OA mouse model and found MMP-13 was markedly induced and colocalized in the early stage OA cartilage in vivo. Subsequently, studies have demonstrated that mechanical stress upregulated MMP-13 expression rapidly in chondrocytes in vitro: cyclic tensile stress (CTS) induced MMP-13 expression in rat cultured normal chondrocytes. The upregulation of MMP-13 was observed within 3 h, which was earlier than that of IL-1β [38]; a static load exceeding 40 psi initiated extracellular matrix degradation through an increase of catabolic MMP-13 encoding gene expression within 24 h [39]. In addition, MMP-13 genes were also significantly enhanced when chondrocytes were co-cultured with excessively mechanically stressed osteoblasts [40]. These results demonstrate that alterations in cartilage metabolism can be induced by stressed chondrocytes and osteoblasts through a MMP-13-dependent pathway, indicating a possible explanation for the onset and progression of OA.

Although CTS is known to upregulate MMP-13 expression via the Runx-2/Cbfa1 [41] and NF-κB [42] pathways, the detailed regulatory mechanisms of mechanical stress on MMP-13 remain unknown. It has long been known that the integrin signal pathway serves as a mechanotransducer in chondrocytes by "integrating" the extracellular matrix with cytoskeletal structures and signals in response to mechanical forces. Its effect on MMP-13 could partially account for the regulatory mechanisms of mechanical stress on MMP-13 [43]. For instance, the matrix protein fibronectin fragment (FN-f), which is generated by the action of MMP-13, stimulates chondrocytes to produce MMP-13 through binding with α3β1, α4β1, α5β1, and αVβ1 integrins [43]. Similarly, angiopoietin-like 4 (ANGPTL4) promotes ECM degradation through induction of MMP-13 by binding integrins β1 and β5 and modulating integrin-mediated signaling [44]. Thus, MMP-13 is a well-known key player in the pathology of early OA due to its capacity to directly or indirectly initiate the degradation of a wide range of downstream matrix and collagen components via its regulatory factors through specific signaling pathways (Fig. 1). A few of its regulatory factors and inhibitors could be explored as potential targets for therapeutic interventions in early OA.

Role of ncRNA-mediated MMP-13 regulation in early OA

The human transcriptome includes many transcripts without protein-coding potential, namely ncRNAs. The deregulation of ncRNAs is closely associated with diverse diseases, including OA [45]. MicroRNAs (miRNAs) are single-stranded ncRNA molecules that are typically 19 to 25 nucleotides long. Recently, alterations in the expression levels of miRNAs have been linked to a variety of disease processes and provide a new horizon in OA [12]. In fact, several differentially expressed miRNA profiles were identified in normal articular cartilage and mild to severe OA auricular cartilage [46]. Certain miRNAs were considered suppressors or promoters of the early steps in the chondrogenic program [47]. Due to the significant role of MMP-13 in promoting the initiation of OA, an understanding of the miRNA-mediated regulatory network of MMP-13 is necessary for the identification of valid alternative therapeutic approaches for the early disease process.

Jones et al. [48] compared the miRNA expression profiles in human cartilage and bone between late-stage OA patients and normal donors. In this study, 17 miRNAs in the cartilage and 30 miRNAs in the bone showed differential expression greater than fourfold in the diseased tissue compared to that in the normal tissue [48]. Among the miRNAs, miR-9 was subsequently shown to directly target MMP-13. miR-9 was up-regulated in late-stage OA cartilage and bone samples compared with normal specimens. The over-expression of miR-9 in isolated chondrocytes decreased the secretion of MMP-13, while the inhibition of

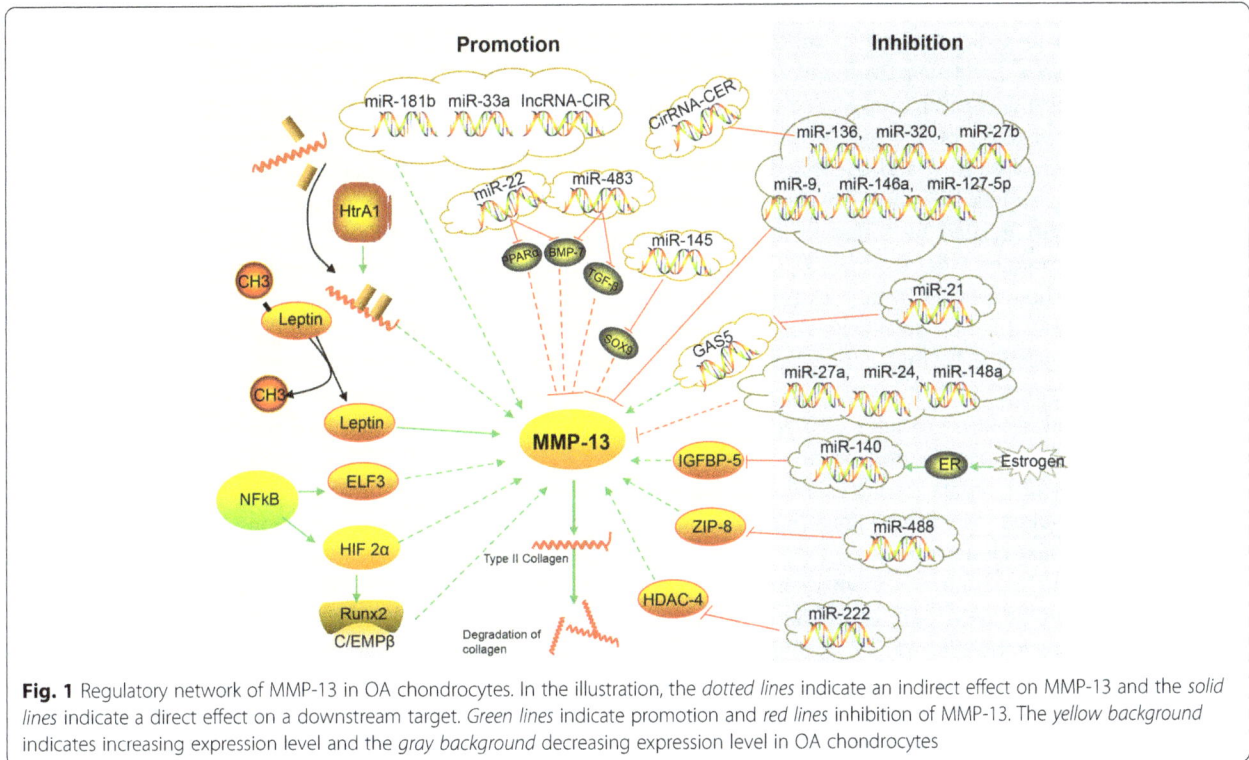

Fig. 1 Regulatory network of MMP-13 in OA chondrocytes. In the illustration, the *dotted lines* indicate an indirect effect on MMP-13 and the *solid lines* indicate a direct effect on a downstream target. *Green lines* indicate promotion and *red lines* inhibition of MMP-13. The *yellow background* indicates increasing expression level and the *gray background* decreasing expression level in OA chondrocytes

miR-9 increased the levels of this metalloproteinase. Consistently, MMP-13 has been shown to be down-regulated in late-stage human OA cartilage, which was based on an experiment in which MMP-13 showed a higher gene expression level in the intact region of the OA cartilage than in the damaged region of the OA cartilage [14]. Furthermore, miR-9 was found to inhibit the secretion of collagen type II in isolated human chondrocytes, which was based on the mechanism of targeting MMP-13 [48]. Due to a shortage of early OA samples, however, the variations in the expression of miR-9 and MMP-13 during OA onset could not be explored.

In addition to miR-9, four other miRNAs, miR-146a, miR-127-5p, miR-27b, and miR-320, target MMP-13 in chondrocytes. Okuhara et al. [49] investigated the relative expression levels of miR-146a in peripheral blood mononuclear cells derived from OA patients with different K-L grades (Kellgren and Lawrence grading scale). The expression level of miR-146a at grade 0 was significantly lower than those at K-L grades 2, 3, and 4. However, the expression level of miR-146a decreased as the K-L classification grade increased. Therefore, the expression of miR-146a was significantly higher during the early stages of OA than during the later stages [49]. Similar results were observed in cartilage samples derived from patients with different grades according to a modified Mankin scale [50]. Yamasaki et al. [50] found that miR-146a was significantly higher in cartilage in patients with grade I OA and lower in cartilage in patients with grade II and III OA. Furthermore, the

variation in the expression of miR-146a in cartilage in patients with grade II OA was inversely related to the expression level of MMP-13. Specifically, the expression of MMP-13 was significantly increased in grade II OA [50] but subsequently decreased in the grade III OA cartilage, which is consistent with the level of miR-146a. Further studies have demonstrated that miR-146a suppressed the expression of aggrecan, Col2, MMP-13, and ADAMTS-5 in human chondrocytes [51] and functions as a suppressor of autoimmunity and myeloproliferation and particularly as a negative feedback regulator of MMP-13 [52]. Notably, during certain stages of OA, such as in grade I and III patients, the expression of MMP-13 was not entirely reversed by miR-146a. This discrepancy can be explained by two aspects: First, the clinical samples differ from OA cell models. The expression levels of MMP-13 and miR-146a in various clinical samples were affected not only in the chondrocytes but also in synovial cells and their microenvironments, which cannot be anticipated as a perfect one-to-one correspondence. Second, Yamasaki et al. assayed the mRNA expression of MMP-13 using only RT-PCR [50]. However, miRNAs can regulate their targets at the post-transcription level, such as by inhibiting the translation process. Therefore, further assays should be performed to detect MMP-13 protein levels.

Park et al. [20] found a significant reduction in miR-127-5p expression in OA cartilage compared with normal cartilage. The up-regulation of MMP-13 expression by IL-1β was correlated with the down-regulation of miR-127-

5p expression in human chondrocytes. MMP-13 has been shown to function as a direct target of miR-127-5p [20] and miR-27b is also a direct negative regulator of MMP-13, as shown by several research groups. Akhtar et al. [53] investigated the expression of 352 human miRs in chondrocytes stimulated with IL-1 and identified 44 significantly differentially expressed miRs. Among these miRs, miR-27b was down-regulated by threefold in the IL-1β-stimulated OA chondrocytes compared with in the unstimulated OA chondrocytes. In the OA cell model, the expression of MMP-13 was inversely correlated with miRNA-27b expression [53]. miR-27b targets MMP-13 mRNA and is suppressed by mitogen-activated protein kinase (MAPK) and NF-kB signaling [53]. Recently, Meng et al. [54] reported that over-expression of miR-320 suppressed the activity of a reporter construct containing the 3′ UTR and inhibited MMP-13 expression in IL-1β-treated primary mouse chondrocytes.

Several other miRNAs that are down-regulated in OA also indirectly inhibit MMP-13 expression, including miR-27a, miR-140, miR-488, miR-24, miR-148a, and miR-222, and these miRNAs were decreased in OA chondrocytes. miR-27a may indirectly regulate the levels of MMP-13 and proanabolic insulin-like growth factor binding protein (IGFBP)-5 by targeting the upstream effectors of both genes [55]. Similarly to miR-27a, miR-140 is reduced in OA tissue and its functions include the indirect regulation (through post-transcriptional inhibition) of IGFBP-5 and MMP-13 [55]. 17-β-Estradiol (E2) has been recently shown to suppress the expression of MMP-13 in human articular chondrocytes, which was accompanied by an up-regulation of the expression of miR-140. Furthermore, the estrogen receptor (ER) directly binds the miR-140 promoter, and estrogen acts via the ER and miR-140 pathway to inhibit the expression of MMP-13. Therefore, the ER/miR-140/IGFBP/MMP-13 signaling pathway may be a potential target for therapeutic interventions for OA patients. In addition, more potential targets have been reported. For example, a decrease in the expression of miR-488 was observed in OA chondrocytes and miR-488 inhibits MMP-13 activity by targeting ZIP-8 [56]. Philipot et al. [15] reported that the down-regulation of miR-24 was consistent with the increased production of MMP-13 in human OA chondrocytes. Chondrocytes from OA patients also showed a decrease in the expression of miRNA-148a, while its over-expression inhibited the presence of MMP-13. Consequently, different approaches that increase miRNA-148a have been suggested to inhibit chondrocyte hypertrophy [57]. miR-222 was significantly down-regulated in OA chondrocytes [58] and its over-expression was accompanied by the down-regulation of HDAC-4 and MMP-13 levels. HDAC-4 has been shown to be a direct target of miR-222; the treatment of chondrocytes with the HDAC inhibitor trichostatin A (TSA)

suppressed the MMP-13 protein level, whereas the over-expression of HDAC-4 displayed the opposite effects. The introduction of miR-222 into the cartilage of medial meniscus-destabilized mice significantly reduced the cartilage destruction and MMP-13 level. Altogether, miR-222 may be involved in cartilage destruction by targeting HDAC-4 and regulating the MMP-13 level [58].

However, several miRNAs are up-regulated in OA and indirectly increase MMP-13 expression, including miR-22, miR-33a, miR-181b, miR-145, and miR-483. Iliopoulos et al. [59] measured the expression of 365 miRNAs in articular cartilage obtained from OA patients and normal individuals. These authors identified nine up-regulated miRNAs and seven down-regulated miRNAs in the OA cartilage. Of these miRNAs, the inhibition of endogenous miR-22 blocks MMP-13 activity by up-regulating bone morphogenetic protein (BMP)-7 and peroxisome proliferator activated receptor alpha (PPARα) expression [59]. miR-181b was significantly up-regulated in OA chondrocytes and the use of an inhibitor to attenuate miR-181b can reduce MMP-13 expression [60]. Similarly to miR-181b, the expression of miR-33a is increased in OA chondrocytes and exogenous miR-33a significantly elevated MMP-13 expression levels [61]. miR-145 is also increased in OA chondrocytes and its over-expression increased MMP-13 expression. The effect of miR-145 on MMP-13 may be mediated by Sox9, i.e., miR-145 negatively regulates endogenous Sox9 by directly targeting Sox9 in human articular chondrocytes, while MMP-13 was down-regulated in Sox9-over-expressing hypertrophic chondrocytes [62]. The expression of miR-483 was significantly up-regulated in an operative murine model of OA, particularly one week after surgery, suggesting that miR-483 may play critical roles in the early pathogenesis of OA. The expression of miR-483 was negatively correlated with the mRNA expression of BMP-7 and TGF-β and positively correlated with MMP-13 according to a Pearson correlation analysis [63].

Although studies investigating miRNAs have dominated the field of RNA biology in recent years, multiple studies have indicated that long non-coding RNAs (lncRNAs) are involved in a variety of biologic processes. The lncRNAs have been defined as ncRNAs of < 200 nucleotides in length and are characterized by the complexity and diversity of their sequences and mechanisms of action [64, 65]. The deregulation of lncRNA is closely associated with the OA process [45]. Regarding the differential expression profiles of lncRNAs in the process of OA, up to 152 lncRNAs have been found to be differentially expressed (more than eightfold) between OA and normal cartilage. lncRNA-CIR was particularly over-expressed in OA cartilage compared with in normal cartilage. The expression of lncRNA-CIR is increased in OA tissues, which is consistent with the up--regulation of MMP-13. Furthermore, the silencing of lncRNA-CIR reduced the expression of MMP-13 and vice versa, suggesting a co-regulation of lncRNA-CIR and MMP-13 in articular cartilage [66]. GAS5 is another lncRNA that was up-regulated in OA chondrocytes compared with non-OA and normal chondrocytes [67]. Furthermore, GAS5 was identified as a direct target of miR-21 and the over-expression of GAS5 was subsequently found to promote OA pathogenesis by increasing MMP-13 expression levels [67].

In addition, circular RNAs (circRNAs) are a newly reported family of ncRNAs that function as miRNA "sponges" that naturally sequester and competitively suppress miRNA activity. Liu et al. identified 71 circRNAs that were differentially expressed between OA and normal cartilage using an Arraystar Human circRNA Array. CircRNA-CER was confirmed to be over-expressed in OA, which is consistent with the up-regulation of MMP-13. It was also shown to act as a decoy for MMP13 by functioning as a competing sponge of miR-136. The sequence of the circRNA-CER 3′ UTR matches miR-136, and MMP-13 is the direct target of miR-136 [68].

In summary, considering the critical role of MMP-13 in the onset of cartilage degradation, clarifying the regulatory network of ncRNA-mediated MMP-13 is critical for an understanding of the pathogenesis of OA and exploring new potential diagnostic and therapeutic targets (Fig. 1).

Role of DNA methylation in MMP-13 gene expression in OA

DNA methylation, which is one of the most well-clarified epigenetic changes, targets DNA sequences by adding a methyl (CH3) group to the carbon 5 (C5) position of cytosine and results in the phenotype of gene silencing [69–71]. These modified sites are high-density CpG regions, namely CpG islands, which are typically located in the gene promoter regions [72, 73]. More importantly, while DNA methylation is heritable at the cellular level, it is potentially reversible. Therefore, the DNA methylation status could be a new molecular target for OA progression, particularly during the early stages of the disease [74].

Several genome-wide DNA methylation studies involving OA patients found many differentially methylated CpG sites in promoters of genes associated with OA development [75–77], which suggested that DNA methylation modifications play an important role in the development of OA [29, 77, 78]. In these studies, promoter hypomethylation events were associated with the increased expression of several MMPs involved in cartilage degradation [74, 79]. For example, Roach et al. [79] first compared the DNA methylation status of four degradative enzymes (i.e., MMP-3, MMP-9, MMP-13, and ADAMTS-4) between OA and non-OA samples. Of the MMPs, MMP-13 was the most heavily methylated in the non-OA samples (95.8%), and its methylation rate decreased to 79.8% in OA samples. The authors identified that both the −134 and −110 sites in the MMP-13 promoter became demethylated during the OA process, even at the early stage. Subsequently, the −104 CpG site in the MMP-13 promoter was also shown to be consistently demethylated and correlated with increased MMP-13 expression. cAMP response binding element (CREB) was identified as a regulating factor that is able to bind the MMP-13 promoter only when the CpG −104 is demethylated [80]. Subsequently, the demethylation of specific CpG sites at −110 bp in the MMP-13 promoter was observed in chondrocytes derived from human OA cartilage, which strongly correlated with higher levels of MMP-13 expression. The methylation status resides within a HIF consensus motif, which results in the most marked suppression of MMP-13 activities. In chromatin immuno-precipitation assays, the methylation of the −110 CpG site in the MMP-13 promoter inhibited its HIF-2α-driven transactivation and decreased HIF-2α binding to the MMP-13 proximal promoter, which may attenuate the process of OA [81]. Recently, Moazedi-Fuerst and colleagues [82] performed a genome-wide methylation screening to identify potential differences between paired mild and severe OA human cartilage. However, the authors could not confirm the presence of differential methylation of MMP-13 in OA, which may be because their "target probe set" did not cover the MMP-13 promoter. Therefore, the CpG sites −104, −110, and −134 are demethylated in OA cartilage and are correlated with elevated MMP-13 expression and cartilage destruction. The highly novel link between the epigenetic status of MMP-13 and OA development may help develop a new strategy to treat early OA [71].

DNA methylation is involved in the MMP-13-driven OA process not only through directly targeting the MMP-13 promoter, but also by targeting the promoters of genes encoding MMP-13-mediated proteins. For example, RunX2 cooperates with the CCAAT/enhancer binding protein β to drive MMP-13 transactivation, because the protein complex of Runx2 and C/EBPβ is located between −144 and −89 bp of the MMP-13 promoter (which contains a C/EBPβ-binding motif at residues −103 to − 97 and a RunX2 binding motif at −138 to −132). HIF-2α is a transcriptional inducer of C/EBPβ in chondrocytes and is located between −103 and −46 bp of the C/EBPβ promoter [83]. Therefore, HIF-2α regulated MMP-13 expression not only by directly binding the MMP-13 promoter but also by binding the upstream protein promoter of MMP-13. Jeffries et al. [76] performed a genome-wide DNA methylation study to identify the DNA methylation changes in OA cartilage tissue and identified that RUNX2 was hypomethylated, which may result in high expression of its protein product and further promote the transcriptional activity of MMP-13 in OA. In addition, the Ingenuity Pathways Analysis (IPA) system (Ingenuity Systems) identified miR-27a to be enriched among the differentially methylated genes, which linked to MMP-13 in vitro [55]. DNA methylation was also involved in the regulation of leptin expression in OA, which affects its downstream target, MMP-13 [29].

Altogether, MMP-13 expression was directly or indirectly regulated by epigenetic mechanisms during early OA (Fig. 2), suggesting that DNA methylation could be a new target for the treatment and diagnosis of early OA.

Relationship between MMP-13 and autophagy

The wide range of MMP-13 proteolytic capacities suggests that it is a powerful, potentially destructive proteinase; thus, it was believed for a long time that MMP-13 is not produced in most adult human tissues in the steady state. However, recent studies have revealed that human chondrocytes isolated from healthy adults constitutively express and secrete MMP-13, but MMP-13 is rapidly endocytosed and degraded by chondrocytes, which is suggestive of the key role of autophagy in the regulation of the MMP-13 protein [17]. Autophagy is a cellular self-protection mechanism that removes damaged organelles and intracellular unfolded proteins [84]. During this process, the expression levels of several autophagy regulators, including autophagy-related genes (Atgs), Beclin-1, and the LC3-II/LC3-I ratio, are increased. Recently, a few studies have suggested that autophagy protects against cartilage degradation under MMP-13-mediated OA conditions [5–87].

Firstly, in some OA models, researchers found that the patterns of variation of autophagy levels and MMP-13 expression levels were reversed. For instance, during the insulin-induced OA pathological process, the increased MMP-13 expression was consistent with the reduced LC3 II expression as well as the decreased autophagy [88, 89]. In a computational model of aging OA established by Hui et al., an increase in the MMP-13 levels was accompanied by a gradual decline in lysosome activity and Bcl-2 levels, which was similar to the experimental data [90]. Furthermore, the process of age-associated spontaneous OA can be accelerated by the loss of the von Hippel-Lindau (VHL) gene in adult articular cartilage, which was illustrated by an earlier study on MMP-13 over-expression and compromised chondrocyte autophagy [91]. The over-expression of GAS5 in articular chondrocytes was another novel method of establishing an OA model, which consistently showed increasing MMP-13 levels and suppressed autophagy responses during OA pathogenesis [67].

Secondly, MMP-13 expression levels were changed when autophagy activities were inhibited or stimulated in chondrocytes. For example, sucrose treatment and Torin 1 (a chemical autophagy inducer) treatment can induce autophagy and significantly inhibited the mRNA expression of MMP-13 in human OA chondrocytes [92–94]. In contrast, 3-methyladenine (a chemical autophagy inhibitor) treatment induced the loss of autophagy, which is linked to increased MMP-13 mRNA expression and the development of OA [93, 94]. In addition, Bouderlique et al. [95] generated mice which lack the Atg5 gene in their chondrocytes (Atg5cKO). Development of OA was observed in Atg5cKO mice, associated with an increase in MMP-13 levels in the articular cartilage.

In conclusion, current studies report opposite variation tendencies between autophagy and MMP-13 levels in OA models as well as in autophagy-regulated models, which implies that autophagy may play a protective role in the pathogenesis of OA by inhibiting MMP-13 production. However, closer links between autophagy and MMP-13 levels in OA progression need far more supporting evidence. For example, whether or how will autophagy change when MMP-13 activities are inhibited or stimulated in chondrocytes? Thus, the detailed molecular mechanism and effect of MMP-13 on autophagy should be further explored.

Discussion

Because abnormal MMP expression levels have been linked to OA progression, the MMPs are attractive targets for the development of specific inhibitors that

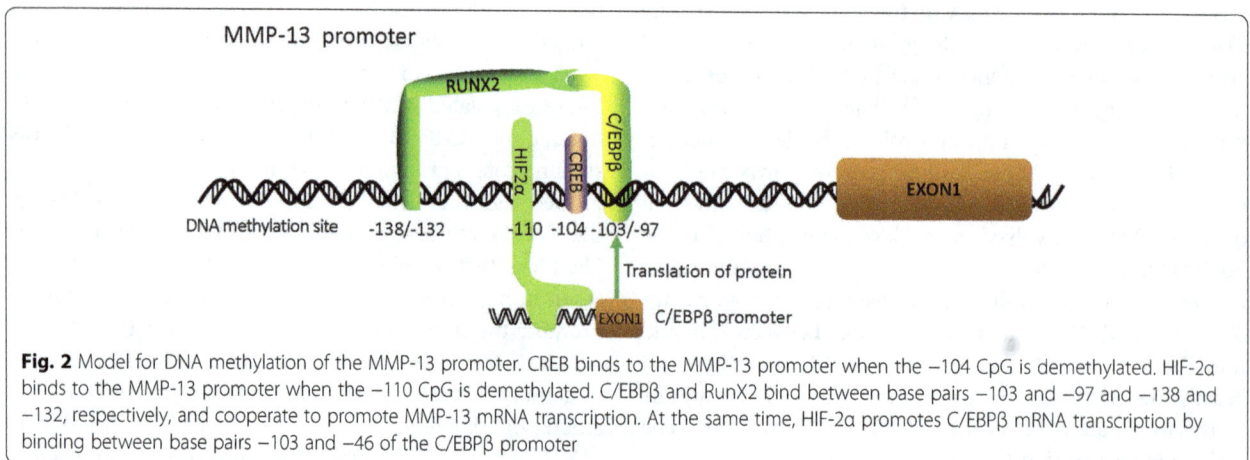

Fig. 2 Model for DNA methylation of the MMP-13 promoter. CREB binds to the MMP-13 promoter when the −104 CpG is demethylated. HIF-2α binds to the MMP-13 promoter when the −110 CpG is demethylated. C/EBPβ and RunX2 bind between base pairs −103 and −97 and −138 and −132, respectively, and cooperate to promote MMP-13 mRNA transcription. At the same time, HIF-2α promotes C/EBPβ mRNA transcription by binding between base pairs −103 and −46 of the C/EBPβ promoter

Table 1 Functional and pathological implications of MMP regulation in OA

Regulatory factor	Direct/indirect target of MMP-13	Effect on MMP-13	Function in OA onset/progression
LRP1 [17]	Directly binds to MMP-13	Endocytosed and degraded MMP-13	Inhibits OA onset
leptin [29]	Direct	Activate MMP-13	Promotes OA onset
HTRA1 [30]	Indirect/DDR2	Upregulate MMP-13	Promotes OA onset
LEF1/ELF3/HIF2α/Runx2/CEBPβ [34, 35]	Directly binds to promoter	Upregulate MMP-13	Promotes OA onset
HMW-HA [36, 37]	Indirect	Inhibits production of MMP-13	Inhibits OA onset
miR-9 [41]	Targets MMP-13	Inhibits production of MMP-13	Promotes progression of late-stage OA
miR-146a [42–45]	Targets MMP-13	Inhibits production of MMP-13	Promotes OA onset
miR-127-5p [20]	Targets MMP-13	Inhibits production of MMP-13	Inhibits OA progression
miR-27b [46]	Targets MMP-13	Inhibits production of MMP-13	Inhibits OA progression
miR-320 [47]	Targets MMP-13	Inhibits production of MMP-13	Inhibits OA progression
miR-136 [61]	Targets MMP-13	Inhibits production of MMP-13	Inhibits OA progression
miR-27a [48]	Indirect	Inhibits production of MMP-13	A slight decrease in OA
miR-140 [48]	Indirect/IGFBP-5	Inhibits production of MMP-13	Inhibits OA progression
	Indirect/ER binding miR-140 promoter	Inhibits production of MMP-13	Inhibits OA progression
miR-488 [49]	Indirect/ZIP-8	Inhibits MMP-13 activity	Inhibits OA progression
miR-24 [15]	Indirect	Inhibits production of MMP-13	Inhibits OA progression
miRNA-148a [50]	Indirect	Inhibits production of MMP-13	Inhibits chondrocyte hypertrophy
miR-222 [51]	Indirect/HDAC-4	Inhibits production of MMP-13	Inhibits OA onset
miR-22 [52]	Indirect/BMP-7, PPARα	Activates MMP-13	Promotes OA progression
miR-181b [53]	Indirect	Increases production of MMP-13	Promotes OA progression
miR-33a [54]	Indirect	Increases production of MMP-13	Promotes OA progression
miR-145 [55]	Indirect/Sox9	Increases production of MMP-13	Promotes OA progression
miR-483 [56]	Indirect/BMP-7, TGF-β	Increases production of MMP-13	Promotes OA onset
LncRNA-CIR [59]	Indirect	Increases production of MMP-13	Promotes OA onset and progression
GAS5 [60]	Indirect/miR-21	Increases production of MMP-13	Promotes OA progression
circRNA-CER [61]	Competes with miR-136 as a 'sponge'	Up-regulation of MMP-13	Promotes OA progression

may have clinical applications. In a model of explanted human OA cartilage, an MMP inhibitor targeting MMP-13 could block the ECM degradation in OA cartilage [96]. Therefore, certain synthetic MMP-13 inhibitors have been developed as promising agents to treat OA [97]. To the best of our knowledge, however, few MMP-13 inhibitors have been successfully utilized as therapeutic agents thus far. Although many factors may have contributed to this failure of MMP inhibitors in the clinic, we identified two possible reasons in this review.

First, as we mentioned in another review [25], MMP-13 shares generally similar active site structures with other members of the MMP family, has overlapping specificities, and plays numerous key roles in important biological processes other than OA development; therefore, designing MMP inhibitors that are highly selective and have low side effect profiles is challenging.

Therefore, to improve the selectivity of therapeutic agents for OA therapy, new therapeutic agents targeting MMP-13 should be able to inhibit MMP-13 expression indirectly by targeting key central nodes in its interaction network rather than targeting the MMP-13 protein. Therefore, DNA methylation sites and ncRNA-mediated MMP-13 expression are potential promising targets for selectively inhibiting MMP-13 expression, without interfering with the structural similarities of the MMP catalytic domains. Moreover, epigenetic regulators can target multiple molecules, frequently in the context of a network, which makes them extremely efficient at regulating distinct biological processes that are relevant to the OA process [25].

Second, all clinical trials conducted to date involved patients with stage III–IV OA, and several overlapping pathways may contribute to the irreversible and uncontrolled cartilage degradation. Therefore, targeting MMP-13 and its regulators for early detection and intervention in OA could be feasible because the process of cartilage degradation is irreversible and the onset mechanism of OA is relatively controllable.

It should be noted that current knowledge on MMP13 expression regulation is still limited and the specific roles of MMP-13 during different stages of joint degeneration also should be further explored, although they have been focused on for more than 20 years. For example, a close correlation between MMP-13 expression and osteophyte development was noted by several studies [28, 98, 99]. However, how to explain the observation that MMP-13-deficient mice are not resistant to osteophyte development [13]? We try to explain it based on the speculation that MMP-13 may play a key role in the early OA process, mainly degrading ECM and cartilage, while osteophytes develop in the late stage when MMP-13 has less function in joints. During the late stage, although MMP-13 is still expressed in the majority of osteophyte tissues, its function can be substituted for by other factors in its regulatory network. Anyway, the speculation should be proved or revised by more evidence; therefore, more detailed research on MMP-13 function should be done during different OA stages and in more types of joint tissues, including not only chondrocytes or articular cartilage but also synovial fibroblasts, synovial mast cells, subchondral bone, and osteophytes.

Conclusions

In this review, we discuss how MMP-13-mediated regulation may improve or inhibit the onset of OA through the functions of interacting factors, the autophagy process, and epigenetic modification (Table 1). Multiple regulatory pathways are involved in MMP-13-mediated regulation, and many of these pathways remain unknown. Based on the growing relevance of the autophagy process and epigenetic modification in the regulation of the OA process, it is likely that further work in this field will reveal additional interacting factors that can modulate MMP-13, thus contributing to their functional regulation in the different physiological and pathological contexts. A thorough understanding of MMP-13-mediated regulatory mechanisms governing OA onset and development should provide new insights into the diagnosis and treatment of early OA.

Abbreviations

ACLT: Anterior cruciate ligament transaction; ADAMTS: A disintegrin and metalloproteinase with thrombospondin type-1 motifs; ANGPTL4: Angiopoietin-like 4; BMP: Bone morphogenetic protein; circRNA: Circular RNA; CTS: Cyclic tensile stress; ECM: Extracellular matrix; ER: Estrogen receptor; FN-f: fibronectin fragment; HIF: Hypoxia-inducible factor; HMW-HA: High molecular weight hyaluronic acid; HTRA1: High temperature requirement A1; IGFBP: Proanabolic insulin-like growth factor binding protein; K-L grade: Kellgrane and Lawrence grading scale; KO: Knockout; LEF1: Lymphoid enhancer factor-1; lncRNA: Long non-coding RNA; LRP1: Low-density lipoproteinreceptor-related protein 1; MAPK: Mitogen-activated protein kinase; MMP: Matrix metalloproteinase; ncRNA: Non-coding RNA; OA: Osteoarthritis; PPARα: Peroxisome proliferator activated receptor alpha; SIRT1: Silent mating type information regulation 2 homolog 1 (sirtuin-1)

Acknowledgements

Not applicable.

Funding

This work was supported by Zhejiang Provincial Natural Science Foundation of China (grant number LY14H060001); Science and Technology Project of Huzhou City (grant number 2016GY26); Zhejiang Provincial Technological Research Project for Public Welfare (grant number 2017C33227).

Authors' contributions

Dr. HL described the role of MMP-13 and non-coding RNA-mediated MMP-13 regulation in the early OA; Dr. YY described the relationship between MMP-13 and autophagy; Dr. DW described the role of DNA methylation on MMP-13 gene expression in OA. Dr. JM organized and revised this manuscript. All authors read and approved the final manuscript.

Authors' information

All authors read and approved this manuscript.

Consent for publication

Not applicable.

Competing interests

The authors declare that they have no competing interests.

References

1. Brooks P. Impact of osteoarthritis on individuals and society: how much disability? Social consequences and health economic implications. Curr Opin Rheumatol. 2002;14:573–7.
2. Bijlsma J, Berenbaum F, Lafeber F. Osteoarthritis: an update with relevance for clinical practice. Lancet (London, England). 2011;377:2115–26.
3. Sinusas K. Osteoarthritis: diagnosis and treatment. Am Fam Physician. 2012;85:49–56.
4. McCormack PL. Celecoxib: a review of its use for symptomatic relief in the treatment of osteoarthritis, rheumatoid arthritis and ankylosing spondylitis. Drugs. 2011;71:2457–89.
5. Abhishek A, Doherty M. Diagnosis and clinical presentation of osteoarthritis. Rheum Dis Clin N Am. 2013;39:45–66.
6. Arabelovic S, McAlindon TE. Considerations in the treatment of early osteoarthritis. Curr Rheumatol Rep. 2005;7:29–35.
7. Goldring MB, Marcu KB. Epigenomic and microRNA-mediated regulation in cartilage development, homeostasis, and osteoarthritis. Trends Mol Med. 2012;18:109–18.
8. Matyas J, Atley L, Ionescu M, Eyre D, Poole A. Analysis of cartilage biomarkers in the early phases of canine experimental osteoarthritis. Arthritis Rheum. 2004;50:543–52.
9. Knäuper V, López-Otín C, Smith B, Knight G, Murphy G. Biochemical characterization of human collagenase-3. J Biol Chem. 1996;271:1544–50.
10. Knauper V, Cowell S, Smith B, Lopez-Otin C, O'Shea M, Morris H. The role of the C-terminal domain of human collagenase-3 (MMP-13) in the activation of procollagenase-3, substrate specificity, and tissue inhibitor of metalloproteinase interaction. J Biol Chem. 1997;272:7608–16.
11. Kamekura S, Hoshi K, Shimoaka T, Chung U, Chikuda H, Yamada T, et al. Osteoarthritis development in novel experimental mouse models induced by knee joint instability. Osteoarthr Cartil. 2005;13:632–41.
12. Nugent M. MicroRNAs: exploring new horizons in osteoarthritis. Osteoarthr Cartil. 2016;24:573–80.
13. Little CB, Barai A, Burkhardt D, Smith SM, Fosang AJ, Werb Z, et al. Matrix metalloproteinase 13-deficient mice are resistant to osteoarthritic cartilage erosion but not chondrocyte hypertrophy or osteophyte development. Arthritis Rheum. 2009;60:3723–33.
14. Sato T, Konomi K, Yamasaki S, Aratani S, Tsuchimochi K, Yokouchi M. Comparative analysis of gene expression profiles in intact and damaged regions of human osteoarthritic cartilage. Arthritis Rheum. 2006;54:808e–17e.
15. Philipot D, Guerit D, Platano D, Chuchana P, Olivotto E, Espinoza F, et al. p16INK4a and its regulator miR-24 link senescence and chondrocyte terminal differentiation-associated matrix remodeling in osteoarthritis. Arthritis Res Ther. 2014;16:R58.
16. Barter MJ, Bui C, Young DA. Epigenetic mechanisms in cartilage and osteoarthritis: DNA methylation, histone modifications and microRNAs. Osteoarthr Cartil. 2012;20:339–49.
17. Yamamoto K, Okano H, Miyagawa W, Visse R, Shitomi Y, Santamaria S, et al. MMP-13 is constitutively produced in human chondrocytes and co-endocytosed with ADAMTS-5 and TIMP-3 by the endocytic receptor LRP1. Matrix Biol. 2016;56:57–73.
18. Pendas AM, Balbin M, Llano E, Jimenez MG, López-Otín C. Structural analysis and promoter characterization of the human collagenase-3 gene (MMP13). Genomics. 1997;140:222–33.
19. Rydziel S, Delany AM, Canalis E. AU-rich elements in the collagenase 3 mRNA mediate stabilization of the transcript by cortisol in osteoblasts. J Biol Chem. 2004;279:5397–404.
20. Park S, Cheon E, Lee M, Kim H. MicroRNA-127-5p regulates matrix metalloproteinase 13 expression and interleukin-1beta-induced catabolic effects in human chondrocyte. Arthritis Rheum. 2013;65:3141–52.
21. Xu N, Lingyun Z, Florian M, Harada M, Heilborn J, Homey B, et al. MicroRNA-125b down-regulates matrix metallopeptidase 13 and inhibits cutaneous squamous cell carcinoma cell proliferation, migration, and invasion. J Biol Chem. 2012;287:29899–908.
22. Knäuper V, Will H, López-Otín C, Smith B, Atkinson SJ, Stanton H, et al. Cellular mechanisms for human procollagenase-3 (MMP-13) activation. Evidence that MT1-MMP (MMP-14) and gelatinase a (MMP-2) are able to generate active enzyme. J Biol Chem. 1996;271:17124–31.
23. Li YS, Zhang FJ, Zeng C, Luo W, Xiao WF, Gao SG, et al. Autophagy in osteoarthritis. Joint Bone Spine. 2016;83:148–8.
24. Chowdhury TT, Schulz RM, Rai SS, Thuemmler CB, Wuestneck N, Bader A, et al. Biomechanical modulation of collagen fragment-induced anabolic and catabolic activities in chondrocyte/agarose constructs. Arthritis Res Ther. 2010;12:R82.
25. Li LQ, Li H. Role of microRNA-mediated MMP regulation in the treatment and diagnosis of malignant tumors. Cancer Biol Ther. 2013;14:796–805.
26. Bo N, Peng W, Xinghong P, Ma R. Early cartilage degeneration in a rat experimental model of developmental dysplasia of the hip. Connect Tissue Res. 2012;53:513–20.
27. Xu L, Polur I, Lim C, Servais JM, Dobeck J, Li Y, et al. Early-onset osteoarthritis of mouse temporomandibular joint induced by partial discectomy. Osteoarthr Cartil. 2009;17:917–22.
28. Pickarski M, Hayami T, Zhuo Y, Duong LT. Molecular changes in articular cartilage and subchondral bone in the rat anterior cruciate ligament transection and meniscectomized models of osteoarthritis. BMC Musculoskelet Disord. 2011;12:197.
29. Iliopoulos D, Malizos KN, Tsezou A. Epigenetic regulation of leptin affects MMP-13 expression in osteoarthritic chondrocytes: possible molecular target for osteoarthritis therapeutic intervention. Ann Rheum Dis. 2007;66:1616–21.
30. Polur N, Lee PL, Servais JM, Xu L. Role of HTRA1, a serine protease, in the progression of articular cartilage degeneration. Histol Histopathol. 2010;25:599–608.
31. Xu L, Servais J, Polur I, Kim D, Lee P, Chung K, et al. Attenuation of osteoarthritis progression by reduction of discoidin domain receptor 2 in mice. Arthritis Rheum. 2010;62:2736–44.
32. Magarinos NJ, Bryant KJ, Fosang AJ, Adachi R, Stevens RL, Patrick MNH. Mast cell-restricted, tetramer-forming tryptases induce aggrecanolysis in articular cartilage by activating matrix metalloproteinase-3 and -13 zymogens. J Immunol. 2013;191:1404–12.
33. Yun K, Im SH. Transcriptional regulation of MMP13 by Lef1 in chondrocytes. Biochem Biophys Res Commun. 2007;364:1009–14.
34. Elayyan J, Lee EJ, Gabay O, Smith CA, Qiq O, Reich E, et al. LEF1-mediated MMP13 gene expression is repressed by SIRT1 in human chondrocytes. 2017. doi: 10.1096/fj.201601253R.
35. Goldring MB, Otero M, Plumb DA, Dragomir C, Favero M, El HK, et al. Roles of inflammatory and anabolic cytokines in cartilage metabolism: signals and multiple effectors converge upon MMP-13 regulation in osteoarthritis. Eur Cell Mater. 2011;21:202–20.
36. Wang CT, Lin YT, Chiang BL, Lin YH, Hou SM. High molecular weight hyaluronic acid down-regulates the gene expression of osteoarthritis-associated cytokines and enzymes in fibroblast-like synoviocytes from patients with early osteoarthritis. Osteo Arthritis Cartilage. 2006;14:1237–47.
37. Julovi SM, Yasuda T, Shimizu M, Hiramitsu T, Nakamura T. Inhibition of interleukin-1beta-stimulated production of matrix metalloproteinases by CD44 in human articular cartilage. Arthritis Rheum. 2004;50:516–25.
38. Doi H, Nishida K, Yorimitsu M, Komiyama T, Kadota Y, Tetsunaga T, et al. Interleukin-4 downregulates the cyclic tensile stress-induced matrix metalloproteinases-13 and cathepsin B expression by rat normal chondrocytes. Acta Med Okayama. 2008;62:119–26.
39. Lin YY, Tanaka N, Ohkuma S, Iwabuchi Y, Tanne Y, Kamiya T, et al. Applying an excessive mechanical stress alters the effect of subchondral osteoblasts on chondrocytes in a co-culture system. Eur J Oral Sci. 2010;118:151–58.
40. Young IC, Chuang ST, Gefen A, Kuo WT, Yang CT, Hsu CH, et al. A novel compressive stress-based osteoarthritis-like chondrocyte system. Exp Biol Med (Maywood). 2017;242:1062–71.
41. Tetsunaga T, Nishida K, Furumatsu T, Naruse K, Hirohata S, Yoshida A, et al. Regulation of mechanical stress-induced MMP-13 and ADAMTS-5 expression by RUNX-2 transcriptional factor in SW1353 chondrocyte-like cells. Osteoarthr Cartil. 2011;19:222–32.

42. Saito T, Nishida K, Furumatsu T, Yoshida A, Ozawa M, Ozaki T. Histone deacetylase inhibitors suppress mechanical stress-induced expression of RUNX-2 and ADAMTS-5 through the inhibition of the MAPK signaling pathway in cultured human chondrocytes. Osteoarthr Cartil. 2013;21:165–74.

43. Loeser RF. Integrins and chondrocyte-matrix interactions in articular cartilage. Matrix Biol. 2014;39:11–6.

44. Mathieu M, Iampietro M, Chuchana P, Guerit D, Djouad F, Noel D, et al. Involvement of angiopoietin-like 4 in matrix remodeling during chondrogenic differentiation of mesenchymal stem cells. J Biol Chem. 2014;289:8402–12.

45. Marques-Rocha JL, Samblas M, Milagro FI, Bressan J, Martinez JA, Marti A. Noncoding RNAs, cytokines, and inflammation-related diseases. Faseb J. 2015;29:3595–611.

46. Portal-Nunez S, Esbrit P, Alcaraz MJ, Largo R. Oxidative stress, autophagy, epigenetic changes and regulation by miRNAs as potential therapeutic targets in osteoarthritis. Biochem Pharmacol. 2016;108:1–10.

47. Lin E, Li K, Bai X, Luan Y, Liu C. miR-199a*, a bone morphogenic protein 2-responsive microRNA, regulates chondrogenesis via direct targeting to Smad1. J Biol Chem. 2009;284:11326–35.

48. Jones SW, Watkins G, Le Good N, Roberts S, Murphy CL, Brockbank SM, et al. The identification of differentially expressed microRNA in osteoarthritic tissue that modulate the production of TNF-alpha and MMP13. Osteoarthr Cartil. 2009;17:464–72.

49. Okuhara A, Nakasa T, Shibuya H, Niimoto T, Adachi N, Deie M, et al. Changes in microRNA expression in peripheral mononuclear cells according to the progression of osteoarthritis. Mod Rheumatol. 2012;22:446–57.

50. Yamasaki K, Nakasa T, Miyaki S, Ishikawa M, Deie M, Adachi N, et al. Expression of microRNA-146a in osteoarthritis cartilage. Arthritis Rheum. 2009;60:1035–41.

51. Li X, Gibson G, Kim JS, Kroin J, Xu S, van Wijnen AJ, et al. MicroRNA-146a is linked to pain-related pathophysiology of osteoarthritis. Gene. 2011;480:34–41.

52. Boldin MP, Taganov KD, Rao DS, Yang L, Zhao JL, Kalwani M, et al. miR-146a is a significant brake on autoimmunity, myeloproliferation, and cancer in mice. J Exp Med. 2011;208:1189–201.

53. Akhtar N, Rasheed Z, Ramamurthy S, Anbazhagan AN, Voss FR, Haqqi TM. MicroRNA-27b regulates the expression of matrix metalloproteinase 13 in human osteoarthritis chondrocytes. Arthritis Rheum. 2010;62:1361–71.

54. Meng F, Zhang Z, Chen W, Huang G, He A, Hou C, et al. MicroRNA-320 regulates matrix metalloproteinase-13 expression in chondrogenesis and interleukin-1beta-induced chondrocyte responses. Osteoarthr Cartil. 2016;24:932–41.

55. Tardif G, Hum D, Pelletier JP, Duval N, Martel-Pelletier J. Regulation of the IGFBP-5 and MMP-13 genes by the microRNAs miR-140 and miR-27a in human osteoarthritic chondrocytes. BMC Musculoskelet Disord. 2009;10:148.

56. Song J, Kim D, Lee CH, Lee MS, Chun CH, Jin EJ. MicroRNA-488 regulates zinc transporter SLC39A8/ZIP8 during pathogenesis of osteoarthritis. J Biomed Sci. 2013;20:31.

57. Vonk L, Kragten A, Dhert W, Saris D, Creemers L. Overexpression of hsa-miR-148a promotes cartilage production and inhibits cartilage degradation by osteoarthritic chondrocytes. Osteoarthr Cartilage. 2014;22:145–53.

58. Song J, Jin EH, Kim D, Kim KY, Chun CH, Jin EJ. MicroRNA-222 regulates MMP-13 via targeting HDAC-4 during osteoarthritis pathogenesis. BBA Clin. 2015;3:79–89.

59. Iliopoulos D, MalizosK N, Oikonomou P, Tsezou A. Integrative microRNA and proteomic approaches identify novel osteoarthritis genes and their collaborative metabolic and inflammatory networks. PLoS One. 2008;3:e3740.

60. Song J, Lee M, Kim D, Han J, Chun C, Jin E. MicroRNA-181b regulates articular chondrocytes differentiation and cartilage integrity. Biochem Biophys Res Commun. 2013;431:210–4.

61. Kostopoulou F, Malizos K, Papathanasiou I, Tsezou A. MicroRNA-33a regulates cholesterol synthesis and cholesterol efflux-related genes in osteoarthritic chondrocytes. Arthritis Res Ther. 2015;17:42.

62. Martinez-Sanchez A, Dudek KA, Murphy CL. Regulation of human chondrocyte function through direct inhibition of cartilage master regulator SOX9 by microRNA-145 (miRNA-145). J Biol Chem. 2012;287:916–24.

63. Qi Y, Ma N, Yan F, Yu Z, Wu G, Qiao Y, et al. The expression of intronic miRNAs, miR-483 and miR-483*, and their host gene, Igf2, in murine osteoarthritis cartilage. Int J Biol Macromol. 2013;61:43–9.

64. Wang Z, Jin Y, Ren H, Ma X, Wang B, Wang Y. Downregulation of the long non-coding RNA TUSC7 promotes NSCLC cell proliferation and correlates with poor prognosis. Am J Transl Res. 2016;8:680–7.

65. Wu Y, Yu DD, Hu Y, Yan D, Chen X, Cao HX, et al. Genome-wide profiling of long non-coding RNA expression patterns in the EGFR-TKI resistance of lung adenocarcinoma by microarray. Oncol Rep. 2016;35:3371–86.

66. Liu Q, Zhang X, Dai L, Hu X, Zhu J, Li L, et al. Long noncoding RNA related to cartilage injury promotes chondrocyte extracellular matrix degradation in osteoarthritis. Arthritis Rheumatol. 2014;66:969–78.

67. Song J, Ahn C, Chun CH, Jin EJ. A long non-coding RNA, GAS5, plays a critical role in the regulation of miR-21 during osteoarthritis. J Orthop Res. 2014;32:1628–35.

68. Liu Q, Zhang X, Hu X, Dai L, Fu X, Zhang J, et al. Circular RNA related to the chondrocyte ECM regulates MMP13 expression by functioning as a miR-136 'Sponge' in human cartilage degradation. Sci Rep. 2016;6:22572.

69. Ooi SK, Bestor TH. The colorful history of active DNA demethylation. Cell. 2008;133:1145–8.

70. Han L, Liu Y, Duan S, Perry B, Li W, He Y. DNA methylation and hypertension: emerging evidence and challenges. Brief Funct Genomics. 2016;15:3–14.

71. Xiao JL, Meng JH, Gan YH, Li YL, Zhou CY, Ma XC. DNA methylation profiling in different phases of temporomandibular joint osteoarthritis in rats. Arch Oral Biol. 2016;68:105–15.

72. Schubeler D. Function and information content of DNA methylation. Nature. 2015;517:321–6.

73. Bergman Y, Cedar H. DNA methylation dynamics in health and disease. Nat Struct Mol Biol. 2013;20:274–81.

74. Roach H, Aigner T. DNA methylation in osteoarthritic chondrocytes: a new molecular target. Osteoarthr Cartil. 2007;15:128–37.

75. Fernandez-Tajes J, Soto-Hermida A, Vazquez-Mosquera ME. Genome-wide DNA methylation analysis of articular chondrocytes reveals a cluster of osteoarthritic patients. Ann Rheum Dis. 2014;73:668–77.

76. Takahashi A, de Andres MC, Hashimoto K, Itoi E, Otero M, Goldring MB, et al. DNA methylation of the RUNX2 P1 promoter mediates MMP13 transcription in chondrocytes. Sci Rep. 2017;7:7771.

77. Rushton MD, Reynard LN, Barter MJ. Characterization of the cartilage DNA methylome in knee and hip osteoarthritis. Arthritis Rheum. 2014;66:2450–60.

78. Jeffries MA, Donica M, Baker LW, Stevenson ME, Annan AC, Humphrey MB, et al. Genome-wide DNA methylation study identifies significant epigenomic changes in osteoarthritic cartilage. Arthritis Rheum. 2014;66:2804–15.

79. Roach HI, Yamada N, Cheung KS, Tilley S, Clarke NM, Oreffo RO, et al. Association between the abnormal expression of matrix-degrading enzymes by human osteoarthritic chondrocytes and demethylation of specific CpG sites in the promoter regions. Arthritis Rheum. 2005;52:3110–24.

80. Bui C, Barter MJ, Scott JL, Xu Y, Galler M, Reynard LN, et al. cAMP response element-binding (CREB) recruitment following a specific CpG demethylation leads to the elevated expression of the matrix metalloproteinase 13 in human articular chondrocytes and osteoarthritis. Faseb J. 2012;26:3000–11.

81. Hashimoto K, Otero M, Imagawa K, Carmen De Andrés M, Coico JM, Roach HI, et al. Regulated transcription of human matrix metalloproteinase 13 (MMP13) and interleukin-1 beta (IL1B) genes in chondrocytes depends on methylation of specific proximal promoter CpG sites. J Biol Chem. 2013;288:10061–72.

82. Florentine C, Moazedi-Fuerst MHGG, Daniela Peischler BLMG. Epigenetic differences in human cartilage between mild and severe OA. J Orthop Res. 2014;32:1636–45.

83. Hirata M, Kugimiya F, Fukai A, Saito T, Yano F, Ikeda T, et al. C/EBPbeta and RUNX2 cooperate to degrade cartilage with MMP-13 as the target and HIF-2alpha as the inducer in chondrocytes. Hum Mol Genet. 2012;21:1111–23.

84. Mizushima N. Physiological functions of autophagy. Curr Top Microbiol Immunol. 2009;335:71–84.

85. Caramés B, Taniguchi N, Otsuki S, Blanco FJ, Lotz M. Autophagy is a protective mechanism in normal cartilage, and its aging-related loss is linked with cell death and osteoarthritis. Arthritis Rheumatism. 2010;62:791–801.

86. Sasaki H, Takayama K, Matsushita T, Ishida K, Kubo S, Matsumoto T, et al. Autophagy modulates osteoarthritis-related gene expression in human chondrocytes. Arthritis Rheum. 2012;64:1920–8.

87. Zhang M, Zhang J, Lu L, Qiu Z, Zhang X, Yu S, et al. Enhancement of chondrocyte autophagy is an early response in the degenerative cartilage of the temporomandibular joint to biomechanical dental stimulation. Apoptosis. 2013;18:423–34.

88. Ribeiro M, Lopez DFP, Blanco FJ, Mendes AF, Carames B. Insulin decreases autophagy and leads to cartilage degradation. Osteoarthr Cartil. 2016;24:731–9.

89. Ribeiro M, Lopez DFP, Nogueira-Recalde U, Centeno A, Mendes AF, Blanco FJ, et al. Diabetes-accelerated experimental osteoarthritis is prevented by autophagy activation. Osteoarthr Cartil. 2016;24:2116–25.

90. Hui W, Young DA, Rowan AD, Xu X, Cawston TE, Proctor CJ. Oxidative changes and signalling pathways are pivotal in initiating age-related changes in articular cartilage. Ann Rheum Dis. 2016;75:449–58.

91. Weng T, Xie Y, Yi L, Huang J, Luo F, Du X, et al. Loss of Vhl in cartilage accelerated the progression of age-associated and surgically induced murine osteoarthritis. Osteoarthr Cartil. 2014;22:1197–205.

92. Khan NM, Ansari MY, Haqqi TM. Sucrose, but not glucose, blocks IL1-beta-induced inflammatory response in human chondrocytes by inducing autophagy via AKT/mTOR pathway. J Cell Biochem. 2017;118:629–39.

93. Cheng NT, Guo A, Cui YP. Intra-articular injection of Torin 1 reduces degeneration of articular cartilage in a rabbit osteoarthritis model. Bone Joint Res. 2016;5:218–24.

94. Cheng NT, Guo A, Meng H. The protective role of autophagy in experimental osteoarthritis, and the therapeutic effects of Torin 1 on osteoarthritis by activating autophagy. BMC Musculoskelet Disord. 2016;17:150.

95. Bouderlique T, Vuppalapati KK, Newton PT, Li L, Barenius B, Chagin AS. Targeted deletion of Atg5 in chondrocytes promotes age-related osteoarthritis. Ann Rheum Dis. 2016;75:627–31.

96. Billinghurst RC, Dahlberg L, Ionescu M, Reiner A, Bourne R, Rorabeck C, et al. Enhanced cleavage of type II collagen by collagenases in osteoarthritic articular cartilage. J Clin Invest. 1997;99:1534–45.

97. Murphy G, Nagase H. Reappraising metalloproteinases in rheumatoid arthritis and osteoarthritis: destruction or repair? Nat Clin Pract Rheumatol. 2008;4:128–35.

98. Li P, Raitcheva D, Hawes M, Moran N, Yu X, Wang F, et al. Hylan G-F 20 maintains cartilage integrity and decreases osteophyte formation in osteoarthritis through both anabolic and anti-catabolic mechanisms. Osteoarthr Cartil. 2012;11:1336–46.

99. Latourte A, Cherifi C, Maillet J, Ea HK, Bouaziz W, Funck-Brentano T, et al. Systemic inhibition of IL-6/Stat3 signalling protects against experimental osteoarthritis. Ann Rheum Dis. 2017;76:748–55.

10

Are estrogen-related drugs new alternatives for the management of osteoarthritis?

Ya-Ping Xiao[1], Fa-Ming Tian[2], Mu-Wei Dai[3], Wen-Ya Wang[4], Li-Tao Shao[1] and Liu Zhang[1*]

Abstract

Osteoarthritis (OA) is a chronic degenerative disease involving multiple physiopathological mechanisms. The increased prevalence of OA after menopause and the presence of estrogen receptors in joint tissues suggest that estrogen could help prevent development of OA. This review summarizes OA research with a focus on the effects of estrogen and selective estrogen receptor modulators (SERMs). Preclinical studies and clinical trials of estrogen therapy have reported inconsistent results. However, almost all studies assessing SERM treatment have obtained more consistent and favorable effects in OA with a relatively safety and tolerability profiles. At present, some SERMs including raloxifene and bazedoxifene have been approved for the treatment of osteoporosis. In summary, estrogen-related agents may exert both a direct effect on subchondral bone and direct and/or indirect effects upon the surrounding tissues, including the articular cartilage, synovium, and muscle, to name a few. Estrogen and SERMs may be particularly favorable for postmenopausal patients with early-stage OA or osteoporotic OA, a phenotype defined by reduced bone mineral density related to high remodeling in subchondral bone. At present, no single drug exists that can prevent OA progression. Although estrogen-related drugs provide insight into the continued work in the field of OA drug administration, further research is required before SERMs can become therapeutic alternatives for OA treatment.

Keywords: Osteoarthritis, Estrogen, Selective estrogen receptor modulators, Joint, Bazedoxifene

Background

Osteoarthritis (OA) is a chronic, progressive disease that affects the entire joint organ and eventually leads to joint organ dysfunction [1]. An OA subset of high remodeling and/or low subchondral bone mineral density (BMD) may benefit from management with anti-resorptive agents to inhibit OA progression [2–5]. OA is the main cause of disability in the older population and is a socioeconomic burden worldwide.

Observational studies indicate that the prevalence of OA is increased immensely in postmenopausal women [6]. Further research has identified the presence of estrogen receptors (ERs) in joint tissues [7]. Moreover, the aromatase gene involved in estrogen secretion and ER gene mutation are associated with OA severity of the lower limb large joint [8]. Similarly, polymorphisms in the ERα gene might also be

associated with a higher OA risk [9, 10]. Taken together, evidence strongly suggests that estrogen may be involved in the development of OA.

Selective estrogen receptor modulators (SERMs) are synthetic nonsteroidal agents with different chemical structures that elicit diverse estrogen agonist and antagonist activities within different tissues [11]. However, SERMs have shown consistent agonist activities in joint tissues. An ideal SERM would exert favorable tissue-selective estrogenic agonist activities in the bone, cardiovascular system, brain, urogenital system, vagina, and skin, with ER neutral or anti-estrogenic activities in the endometrium, breast, and pelvic floor [12, 13]. Importantly, SERM treatment has not resulted in any long-term estrogen treatment-related adverse events to date.

Recent studies have supported that estrogen or SERMs may have beneficial effects on joint tissues (Table 1). In this review, relevant English-language articles concerning the effects of estrogen or SERMs in OA progression or on joint tissues were identified using the PubMed database. The aim of this literature review was to

* Correspondence: zhliu130@sohu.com
[1]Department of Orthopedic Surgery, The Affiliated Hospital of North China University of Science and Technology, No. 73 Jianshe South Road, Tangshan, Hebei Province, China
Full list of author information is available at the end of the article

Table 1 Effects of estrogen-related drugs on joint tissues

Tissue	Main effects
Articular cartilage	Reduction of articular cartilage turnover and destruction, regulation of cartilage metabolism, improvement of mechanical properties
Subchondral bone	Regulation of bone growth and remodeling, promotion of matrix production and mineralization, regulation of osteoblast and osteoclast development and function
Synovial membrane	Decrease of the proliferation of rheumatoid arthritis-like synovial cells, decrease of proinflammatory cytokine production, reversion of experimental arthritis
Muscle	Promotion of myoblast proliferation and differentiation, reduction of muscle cell apoptosis, reversion of muscle atrophy and contractile dysfunction

identify evidence suggesting that early-stage OA patients, particularly osteoporotic OA patients, may benefit from treatment with estrogen or SERMs. The findings highlight that, at present, no single drug can prevent OA progression, while estrogen-related drugs analyzed together provide insight into the ongoing work on OA administration.

Estrogen therapy: inconclusive results

Direct binding of estrogen to ERs acts on joint tissues, protecting their biomechanical structure and function, thus maintaining overall joint health (Table 2). However, the exact effect of estrogen on OA remains controversial and in some cases inconsistent, likely owing to the methodological drawbacks or the varying OA phenotypes as detailed in the research.

Preclinical studies

A systematic review comprising controlled studies found estrogen to have confounding effects on articular cartilage in ovariectomized (OVX) animals [14]. Interestingly, only 11 out of 22 animal studies report beneficial actions of estrogen on OA, suggesting that the estrogenic effect is inconclusive, which is consistent with the majority of recently published literature [15]. In fact, intraarticular injection of estrogen was reported to actually damage the knee articular cartilage in OVX rabbits [16, 17], with long-term estrogen treatment being beneficial for articular cartilage in other animal models [18, 19]. Early studies of estrogen administration may therefore overestimate the positive effect of estrogen on articular cartilage [20].

In-vivo estrogen treatment has shown inconclusive results in OA. Gao et al. [21] found that serum-free estradiol levels and total serum estradiol levels were significantly lower in postmenopausal compared with premenopausal OA women. Afzal and Khanam [22] found that estrogen deficiency may lead to increased serum IL-6 in postmenopausal patients with OA, which

has been found to promote OA progression. In a murine model of knee OA, exogenous estrogen suppressed tibia and patella subchondral cortical bone thinning and prevented patellar cartilage damage, supporting an etiological role for altered estrogen signaling in OA [23]. Similarly, in an osteopenic mouse, estrogen treatment recovered bone mass of the subchondral bone, but although it reduced the expression of cartilage ADAMTS-4 and ADAMTS-5, cartilage damage was not significantly prevented [19]. However, estrogen has been shown to improve the histological integrity of articular cartilage and reduced cartilage and bone turnover in a murine OA model [18]. Furthermore, in an OA OVX rat model, 17β-estradiol treatment significantly reduced the density of substance P and calcitonin gene-related peptide immunoreactive nerve fibers in the synovial membrane, suggesting that estrogen partly regulates intraarticular neurogenic inflammation in OA joints by modulating the expression of neuropeptides in the synovial membrane [24]. However, in an iodoacetate-induced temporomandibular joint OA rat model, estrogen administration promoted cartilage degeneration, subchondral bone erosion, and expression of apoptosis genes [25]. Intraarticular injection of estrogen was also reported to actually damage the knee articular cartilage in rabbits OA models [16, 17].

Estrogen appears to have a potential protective effect on chondrocytes in vitro. In rabbit articular chondrocytes, 17β-estradiol has been shown to upregulate collagen type II expression by Sp1/3, Sox-9, and ERα [26]. In another study, 17β-estradiol treatment prevented injury-related cell death and glycosaminoglycan release in mature articular cartilage explants, suggesting that 17β-estradiol may be useful for treating either cartilage-related sports injuries or OA [27]. Kumagai et al. [28] also found that 17β-estradiol suppressed doxorubicin-induced apoptosis by blocking volume-sensitive Cl⁻ current in rabbit articular chondrocytes. In cultured chondrocytes from a rat OA model, 17β-estradiol promoted chondrocyte proliferation via the PI3K/Akt pathway [29].

Clinical studies

Consistent with these preclinical studies, comprehensive analysis of a multitude of clinical studies has shown that the effects of estrogen on hand OA or other joint OA failed to reach clear conclusions [15, 30].

On the one hand, estrogen appears to have a potential protective effect on OA in many clinical studies. A cross-sectional study found that postmenopausal women who received long-term estrogen treatment had a significantly reduced risk of any radiographic hip OA, indicating that postmenopausal estrogen management may ameliorate hip OA [31]. In the Women's Health Initiative study [32], women receiving conjugated equine

Table 2 Effects of estrogen on joint tissues

Drug name	Type of study	Effects on joint tissues	Reference
Estradiol	In-vivo OVX + OA rabbits	Cartilage degeneration	[16]
β-estradiol	In-vivo OVX rabbits	Loss of glycosaminoglycans and collagen	[17]
17β-estradiol	In-vivo OVX rats	Decrease of CTX-II; prevention of cartilage lesions	[20]
17β-estradiol	In-vivo postmenopausal OA women	Decrease of 17β-estradiol after menopause	[21]
Estrogen	In-vivo postmenopausal OA women	Estrogen deficiency may lead to increase of serum IL-6	[22]
17β-estradiol	In-vivo murine with knee OA	Inhibition of tibial and patellar subchondral cortical thinning and tibial cartilage damage	[23]
17β-estradiol	In-vivo OVX + OA mice	Inhibition of bone resorption; decreased ADAMTS-4 and ADAMTS-5 expression	[19]
β-estradiol	In-vivo OA + OVX murine	Reduction of cartilage and bone turnover	[18]
β-estradiol	In-vivo OVX + ACLT murine	Regulation of intraarticular neurogenic inflammation	[24]
17β-estradiol	In-vivo OA + OVX murine	Potentiation of cartilage degradation and subchondral bone erosion and mRNA expression of Fas, FasL, caspase 3, and caspase 8	[25]
17β-estradiol	In-vitro rabbit chondrocytes	Upregulation of type II collagen gene	[26]
17β-estradiol	In-vitro cow mature joint cartilage	Prevention injury-related cell death and GAG release	[27]
17β-estradiol	In-vitro rabbit chondrocytes	Inhibition of doxorubicin-induced apoptosis	[28]
17β-estradiol	In-vitro rat OA chondrocytes	Promotion of chondrocyte proliferation	[29]
Oral estrogen	CSS osteoporotic white women	Reduction of risk of any hip OA	[31]
HRT	CSS women around menopause	Inverse association of current HRT use and radiological OA of the knee	[35]
Oral estrogen	CSS women with OA	No positive association of estrogen use with radiographic knee OA	[36]
ERT	CSS older women	Protection moderately against worsening of radiographic knee OA, but not statistically significant	[37]
ERT	CSS women	Nonsignificant protective effect for incident knee osteophytes	[38]
CEE	RCT community-dwelling women	Lower rates of any arthroplasty	[32]
Estrogen	CSS women	Lower subchondral bone attrition and bone marrow edema-like abnormalities	[33]
Estrogen	CSS, older women	No significant correlation with knee replacement of OA	[39]
HT	Prospective study, women around menopause	Correlation highly with the hip or knee replacement rates of OA	[40]
17β-estradiol	RCT postmenopausal OP women	Decrease of levels of COMP	[34]

OA osteoarthritis, *OP* osteoporosis, *OVX* ovariectomy, *CTX-II* C-terminal cross-linked telopeptide type II collagen, *HRT* hormone replacement therapy, *ERT* estrogen replacement therapy, *COMP* cartilage oligomeric matrix protein, *ACLT* anterior cruciate ligament transaction, *CEE* conjugated equine estrogens, *HT* hormonal therapies, *CSS* cross-sectional study, *RCT* randomized controlled trial

estrogens had significantly lower rates of arthroplasty, particularly hip replacement rates. In a cross-sectional study, knee MRI scans identified that women receiving estrogen had significantly less subchondral bone attrition and bone marrow edema-like abnormalities in the knee compared with nontreated women [33]. Likewise, a case–control study found that estrogen treatment significantly reduced the serum level of cartilage oligomeric matrix protein, a marker associated with cartilage degeneration, suggesting that estrogen treatment may be a novel treatment modality to prevent OA joint degeneration [34].

Conversely, estrogen seems to have no protective or even damaging effect on OA in some other clinical studies. Two of the largest observational studies, the Britain Chingford Study and the US Framingham Osteoarthritis Study, and subsequent follow-up of these two studies found that estrogen treatment did not significantly reduce the radiographic severity of knee OA or hand OA [35–38]. In a recent longitudinal observational study, estrogen therapy had no significant correlation with OA knee replacement [39]. Furthermore, estrogen treatment is reported to increase the joint replacement rate of OA, which conflicts with its suggested protective effect [15]. A prospective study showed that postmenopausal estrogen treatment increased the risk of hip or knee replacement of OA [40].

In summary, although considerable studies have found that estrogen may have potential protective effects on OA joints, the exact effect of estrogen on OA remains controversial. The inconclusive results of estrogen in OA may be due to the following reasons. First, estrogen may have different effects on the initiation and progression of OA. Increasing numbers of experimental and human studies have demonstrated the existence of remodeling abnormalities in the subchondral bone, with increased bone turnover and subsequent bone loss in early stages of OA [41, 42]. These changes are followed by reduced bone turnover and further subchondral sclerosis in the late stages of OA [41–43]. Consequently, estrogen could decrease bone turnover and may have potential beneficial effects for early-stage OA. Conversely, the prevention of bone loss may result in effects that are not beneficial or are even harmful for late-stage OA, with some studies showing an association between high bone density and radiographic OA changes [36, 38]. Second, estrogen may have a beneficial effect on only certain subtypes of OA. Depending on the ratio between formation and resorption, subchondral bone remodeling can culminate in either a sclerotic or an osteoporotic phenotype. Patients with osteoporotic OA may thus achieve clinical and structural benefit from estrogen intervention [2, 3, 5].

Finally, outcome measurements in these studies vary widely. Although some studies have reported moderate but nonsignificant protective effects [36–38], those detecting serologic or radiographic changes have shown an overall protective effect [31, 33–35]. Conversely, inconsistent results are apparent in studies using joint replacement patients [32, 40]. In addition to differences in trial design, the association between estrogen replacement therapy and the incidence of joint replacement may be affected by nonbiological factors. For example, women who take estrogen replacement therapy may have easier access to health services and, as such, may be more likely to have a joint replacement for existing OA. Furthermore, it is reported that women that have undergone knee replacement are in higher socioeconomic groups and are more likely to have other operations, such as hysterectomy [40].

Taken together, although estrogen treatment elicits a potential protective effect on OA, the identification of OA patient phenotypes and specific OA stages should be considered alongside therapeutic interventions in future studies, which may lead to clearer conclusions regarding estrogen therapy on OA progression.

SERM treatment: consistent evidence

SERMs are a specific type of ER-binding estrogen that have selective effects on target tissues. Present studies support that SERMs have a more consistent beneficial effect on bone tissue, and therefore some have been approved for treatment of osteoporosis, such as lasofoxifene and bazedoxifene in Europe and the USA [44]. Subsequent studies have found that SERMs also have a beneficial role in other joint tissues, thus maintaining joint health as a whole. Compared with the controversial effects of estrogen administration on OA, SERMs have more stable and favorable effects on OA.

Preclinical studies

Basic research has shown that SERMs inhibit destruction of articular cartilage and subchondral bone, delaying OA progression. Meanwhile, SERMs have an anti-inflammatory effect and prevent OA-like joint degeneration as a whole (Table 3).

Intraarticular administration of tamoxifen was shown to reduce cartilage damage and antagonize chondrodestructive effects of high-dose estradiol in different rabbit OA models [45–48]. Tamoxifen played a protective effect on articular cartilage in intact male rabbits, suggesting that its therapeutic effect might not only be associated with its anti-estrogenic role [47]. Furthermore, both levormeloxifene and cis-3,4-7-hydroxy-3-phenyl-4-(4-(2pyrrolidinoethoxy)-phenyl)chromane suppressed OVX-induced acceleration of bone and cartilage turnover and ameliorated destruction of cartilage in female rats [49, 50]. Andersson et al. [51] found recently that the anti-osteoporotic drugs lasofoxifene and bazedoxifene ameliorated cartilage and bone lesions and the histologic grade of synovitis, indicating that they are potent inhibitors of joint inflammation and destruction of cartilage and bone in experimental arthritis. Similarly, Saito et al. [52] found that bazedoxifene inhibited OVX-induced deterioration of structural properties of vertebral cancellous bone in monkeys and improved bone strength.

The consistent effect of SERMs in vivo indicates a protective effect on chondrocytes. Kavas et al. [53] reported that 1 µM of raloxifene reduced expression of OA-related genes, apoptosis, and extracellular matrix-degrading enzymes, and increased extracellular matrix deposition and improved mechanical properties in rat articular chondrocytes with OA-like degeneration. However, these effects were reversed with increased dose, demonstrating that low-dose raloxifene has the potential to cease or decrease cartilage degeneration in OA. In cultured human chondrocytes, when raloxifene and IL-1β were coincubated in the culture medium, proteoglycans were significantly and dose-dependently augmented, and matrix metalloproteinase-3 and nitric oxide (NO) levels were significantly decreased, demonstrating that raloxifene antagonized IL-1β-induced OA-like chondrocyte changes [54]. In another study, the natural SERM genistein antagonized lipopolysaccharide-induced OA-like chondrocyte changes with a significant decrease of COX-2 protein and NO level in the supernatant of cultured human chondrocytes, indicating that genistein may maintain joint health through an anti-inflammatory effect [55].

Clinical studies

SERMs appear to have protective effects on joint tissues. SERMs regulate metabolism of articular cartilage and subchondral bone, maintain their normal biomechanical structure and performance, and possibly delay disease progression of OA. In addition, SERMs may have a

Table 3 Effects of selective estrogen receptor modulators on joint tissues

Drug name	Type of study	Effects on joint tissues	Reference
Tamoxifen	In-vivo rabbit with OVX + MMX-OA	Reduction of cartilage damage	[48]
	In-vivo rabbit with MMX-OA	Reduction of cartilage damage	[46]
	In-vivo intact male rabbit with OA	Reduction of cartilage damage	[47]
	In-vivo rabbit with OVX + MMX-OA	Antagonism of chondrodestructive effects of high-dose estradiol intraarticular administration	[45]
CHPPPC	In-vivo Sprague–Dawley rats with OVX	Inhibition of the OVX-induced acceleration of bone and cartilage turnover, and suppression of cartilage damage	[49]
Levormeloxifene	In-vivo Sprague–Dawley rats with OVX	Prevention of the OVX-induced cartilage and bone changes	[50]
	RCT postmenopausal women	Decrease of CTX-I I by approximately 50 %	[50]
Lasofoxifene	In-vivo DBA/1 mice with OVX + arthritis	Reduction of the grade of histologic synovitis and erosions on cartilage and bone	[51]
Bazedoxifene	In-vivo DBA/1 mice with OVX + arthritis	Reduction of the grade of histologic synovitis and erosions on cartilage and bone	[51]
	In-vivo cynomolgus monkeys with OVX	Inhibition of OVX-induced vertebral deterioration of structural properties	[52]
	Prospective study in postmenopausal women with type 2 diabetes	Improvement of bone resorption markers	[57]
	RCT in postmenopausal women with OP	Lowered significantly the cumulative incidences of new vertebral fractures and maintained total hip bone mineral density	[58]
	Exploratory analysis women with increased fracture risk	Geometry-related improvements in bone strength	[59]
	RCT in women with menopausal symptoms	Improvement of lumbar spine and total hip BMD	[60]
	RCT in postmenopausal women with OP	Reduction of the incidences of vertebral and nonvertebral fractures	[61]
Raloxifene	In-vitro rat OA-like chondrocytes	Ceases or reduces the matrix degeneration in OA	[53]
	In-vitro human OA-like chondrocytes	Augmented in proteoglycans and a significant decrease of MMP-3 and NO levels	[54]
	Cross-sectional study in older women with knee OA	Less subchondral bone attrition and bone marrow edema-like abnormalities	[33]
	RCT in postmenopausal women with back or knee pain	Amelioration of bone and joint pain	[62]
Genistein	In-vitro human OA-like chondrocytes	Decrease of NO and IL-1β level in supernatant	[55]

OA osteoarthritis, *OVX* ovariectomy, *OP* osteoporosis, *MMX-OA* medial meniscectomy-induced OA, *CHPPPC* cis-3,4-7-hydroxy-3-phenyl-4-(4-(2-pyrrolidinoethox) phenyl)chromane, *RCT* randomized controlled trial, *CTX-II* C-terminal cross-linked telopeptide type II collagen, *BMD* bone mineral density, *MMP* matrix metalloproteinase, *NO* nitric oxide

potential analgesic effect in OA. Moreover, SERMs may play protective roles on the synovium and other joint tissues, maintaining joint health as a whole.

In the Health, Aging and Body Composition Study cohort, raloxifene significantly reduced subchondral bone attrition, bone marrow edema-like abnormalities, and knee pain according to Western Ontario and McMaster Universities Arthritis Index scores when compared with the control group [33]. A further study found that SERMs have a positive effect on cartilage metabolism. In this placebo-controlled trial, levormeloxifene reduced the urinary excretion of C-terminal cross-linked telopeptide type II collagen (CTX-II) by approximately 50 % and restored CTX-II levels to the premenopausal range compared with the control group, indicating that levormeloxifene inhibits degeneration of articular cartilage [50]. In another study, raloxifene not only reduced the

CTX-II level, but also decreased the level of the bone resorptive marker CTX-I in postmenopausal women [56]. Interestingly, when women ceased levormeloxifene treatment, CTX-II levels returned to baseline level, while CTX-I was still strongly suppressed. This suggests that SERMs may play a short-lived role on cartilage and a long-term role on bone [56]. In recent studies, bazedoxifene not only prevented bone loss and maintained BMD by reducing bone turnover in postmenopausal women, but also improved the microstructure of bone. Consequently, bazedoxifene enhanced bone strength and reduced the risk of vertebral and nonvertebral fractures in postmenopausal women [57–61]. Remarkably, Fujita et al. [62] reported that combined raloxifene and alfacalcidol treatment appeared to be more effective on bone and joint pain than alfacalcidol alone in postmenopausal women with either back or knee pain alone, or both, according to electroalgometry and visual rating scale measurements.

In summary, postmenopausal women with osteoporotic OA might benefit from treatment with SERMs. The mechanisms of action of SERMs within joint tissues are being gradually elucidated [53, 54, 63]. In addition to the role of SERMs on ERs and their interaction with coregulator proteins to produce transcriptional complexes, some clinical effects of SERMs may involve rapid actions mediated by G protein-coupled estrogen receptor 1 (GPER1), with subsequent activation of the PI3K/Akt and/or PKC/MAPK pathways. Consequently, tamoxifen and raloxifene have been identified as GPER1 agonists [53].

Estrogen-related drug mechanisms of action in OA

Recent research has confirmed that significant changes in the subchondral bone occur during OA progression [64]. Key changes in the subchondral bone include high bone turnover with decreased BMD and bone biomechanical structural damage in the early stages of OA, which either coincide with or precede cartilage degeneration [64]. Subchondral bone degeneration may be the trigger for changes in the cartilage biomechanical and biochemical microenvironment, thus promoting cartilage erosion and ultimately OA progression [65]. Consequently, subchondral bone is a potential therapeutic target, and drugs acting on subchondral bone represent potential disease-modifying OA drugs [2–4]. Similarly, the main pathological change in OA is degeneration of the articular cartilage that promotes subchondral bone lesions during progression of OA, particularly in late OA stages when cartilage erosion is extensive [4, 43]. Therefore, subchondral bone and cartilage are strongly dependent on each other during the progression of OA. In short, OA disease-modifying drugs must be able to act on both of these joint tissues to prevent the development and progression of OA.

Estrogen-related drugs that act on both subchondral bone and cartilage are good candidates for early-stage OA treatment, especially osteoporotic OA. These drugs are potent in antagonizing bone resorption, which can effectively decrease bone remodeling and prevent subchondral bone loss and the deterioration of microarchitecture and biomechanical properties [18, 19, 23]. Thus, the protective effect of these drugs on articular cartilage may be an indirect effect through protection of the subchondral bone. Additionally, these drugs directly target cartilage tissue, preventing cartilage damage and maintaining healthy cartilage [26, 66]. In addition to the direct or indirect protective role of these drugs on articular cartilage, subchondral bone, and the surrounding joint tissues, including the synovium and muscle, the joint tissues themselves interact with each other, thus

maintaining joint organ homeostasis as a whole and finally delaying joint degeneration [56].

Moreover, the beneficial effect of estrogen-related drugs on OA may be, at least in part, associated with amelioration of the abnormal mechanical stress via or by regulating ER. Mechanical stress has an important role in the pathogenesis of OA [67], whereby abnormal mechanical stress is reported to promote deterioration of the subchondral bone and articular cartilage during OA progression [68]. A recent study has reported that estrogen reduces mechanical injury-related cell death and proteoglycan degradation in an ER-mediated pathway in mature articular cartilage. This suggests that estrogen agents ameliorate abnormal mechanical stress to protect cartilage-related sports injuries or OA [27].

On the contrary, downregulation of ER expression is evident during cartilage degeneration [69, 70], which may be associated with abnormal mechanical stress [27]. More recently, lower serum estrogen has been shown to downregulate ER expression, with estrogen therapy upregulating ER expression [70, 71], a finding that may relate to the beneficial effects of estrogen agents on OA. In fact, these changes are similar to ER changes in disc degeneration and its estrogen therapy [69, 72].

In summary, abnormal mechanical stress changes the articular microenvironment to decrease expression of ERs, which is associated with subsequent joint degeneration. We therefore hypothesize that the upregulated expression of ER by estrogen may correlate with amelioration of abnormal mechanical stress, a hypothesis that warrants further investigation.

Efficacy of estrogen-related drugs on joint tissues

Current observational studies suggest that estrogen may be involved in the progression of OA and have potential protective effects on joint tissues. However, some studies suggest that the role of estrogen is controversial and warrants further study. In contrast, preclinical and clinical studies indicate that SERMs not only have consistently positive effects on OA [33, 36, 38, 39, 53, 54], but also significantly reduce estrogen treatment-related adverse events. However, the positive estrogen-like effects of SERMs on bone tissue are weaker than those of estrogen [44], and therefore need to be strengthened. A number of reasons may account for this interesting phenomenon. First, estrogen has an extensive effect in vivo, regulating many metabolic pathways within various tissues [73, 74]. However, the interaction of these metabolic pathways may weaken the effect of estrogen on articular tissues in vivo. Conversely, SERMs exhibit tissue-specific ER antagonist or agonist activity, with selective effects on specific tissues [11–13]. Consequently, the impact of other metabolic pathways on the effect of SERMs in articular tissues is weaker than that of estrogen. SERMs could thus produce greater estrogen-like effects in vivo [50]. New estrogen-like drugs are continuously reported. For example, tissue-selective estrogen complexes (TSECs) are a combination of an estrogen and one SERM, and demonstrate many features of ideal SERMs [14]. Theoretically, estrogen could reinforce the positive role of SERMs on bone tissue, making the effects of TESCs on bone tissue more effective than SERMs, which has been verified in a clinical trial [75]. Conversely, the many adverse reactions of estrogen could be antagonized by SERMs. We speculate that the effects of TESCs on joint tissues may be greater than those of SERMs, with a generally desirable safety and tolerability profile. In short, TESCs may become candidates for OA drugs in the future.

Safety and tolerability of estrogen-related drugs

Research has revealed that SERMs are suited for the treatment of OA with relatively favorable safety and tolerability profiles.

Long-term estrogen therapy stimulates breast and endometrial hyperplasia with significantly increased risk of breast and endometrial cancer [73]. Moreover, this drug increases the risk of cardiovascular events and stroke, especially thromboembolic diseases [74]. These adverse effects severely limit the clinical application of estrogen.

SERMs selectively act on ERs in target tissues and the adverse events of SERMs are significantly reduced compared with estrogen [11]. Almost all SERMs have anti-estrogenic action in the breast and do not increase the risk of breast cancer. Moreover, some SERMs such as tamoxifen, toremifene, and raloxifene can be used for the treatment or prevention of estrogen-sensitive breast cancer [44]. SERMs have relatively varied effects on the uterus. Furthermore, very few SERMs, such as tamoxifen, stimulate endometrial proliferation with the increased risk of endometrial cancer. In fact, the majority of SERMs have neutral or anti-estrogenic effects on the endometrium and do not increase the risk of endometrial cancer [13]. In addition, most SERMs do not increase the risk of cardiovascular events [11]. Although some SERMs are reported to slightly increase the incidence of hot flashes or vulvar vaginal atrophy, the symptoms are mild and do not affect the clinical application of SERMs. Currently, the primary limit of clinical application of most SERMs is the increased risk of venous thrombosis embolism [44].

Conclusion

At present, the roles of estrogen in joint tissues or OA are controversial. However, SERMs have consistently protective effects on joint tissues or in OA with relatively favorable safety and tolerability profiles. SERMs

and estrogen may represent therapeutic options to treat joint diseases in the future. In particular, SERMs and estrogen may be beneficial for postmenopausal women with osteoporotic OA or early-stage OA [2, 3, 5]. Although, there is a wide range of SERMs, their chemical structure and biological function are quite complex. Therefore, it is difficult to identify the optimal types of SERMs to treat OA. Further research is needed to identify the most suitable types of SERMs to treat OA and to clearly identify their action mechanisms on joint tissues. A new group of estrogen-related drugs, TSECs are reported to have a beneficial effect on bone tissue [75, 76]. Furthermore, TSECs may have the potential to protect other joint tissues, suggesting they may become favorable therapeutic alternatives for treatment of OA. These findings warrant further clarification in future preclinical and clinical studies.

Abbreviations
ADAMTS, a disintegrin and metalloproteinase with thrombospondin motifs; Akt, protein kinase B; BMD, bone mineral density; COX-2, cycloxygenase-2; CTX-I, C-terminal cross-linked telopeptide type I collagen; CTX-II, C-terminal cross-linked telopeptide type II collagen; ER, estrogen receptor; GPER, G protein-coupled estrogen receptor 1; IL, interleukin; MAPK, mitogen-activated protein kinase; NO, nitric oxide; OA, osteoarthritis; OVX, ovariectomized; PI3K, phosphatidyl inositol 3-kinase; PKC, protein kinase C; SERM, selective estrogen receptor modulator; Sox-9, Sry related HMG box-9; TSEC, tissue selective estrogen complex

Funding
This work was supported by grants from National Natural Science Foundation of China (Grant No. 31171136) and Hebei Province Nature Science Foundation (Grant No. H2013209257).

Authors' contributions
Y-P X and L Z conceived the study. Y-P X and L-T S performed the searches. Y-P X, W-Y W, and M-W D performed the analyses. Y-P X wrote the manuscript. F-M T, M-W D, W-Y W, and L Z shared expertise of review, and helped with interpretation of and critically revised the manuscript. All authors read and approved the final submitted manuscript.

Competing interests
The authors declare that they have no competing interests.

Author details
[1]Department of Orthopedic Surgery, The Affiliated Hospital of North China University of Science and Technology, No. 73 Jianshe South Road, Tangshan, Hebei Province, China. [2]Medical Research Center, North China University of Science and Technology, Tangshan, China. [3]Department of Orthopedic Surgery, Hebei Medical University, Shijiazhuang, China. [4]Department of Pathology, School of Basic Medical Sciences, North China University of Science and Technology, Tangshan, China.

References
1. Malfait AM. Osteoarthritis year in review 2015: biology. Osteoarthritis Cartilage. 2016;24:21–6.
2. Roman-Blas JA, Herrero-Beaumont G. Targeting subchondral bone in osteoporotic osteoarthritis. Arthritis Res Ther. 2014;16:494.
3. Roman-Blas JA, Castaneda S, Largo R, Lems WF, Herrero-Beaumont G. An OA phenotype may obtain major benefit from bone-acting agents. Semin Arthritis Rheum. 2014;43:421–8.
4. Karsdal MA, Bay-Jensen AC, Lories RJ, Abramson S, Spector T, Pastoureau P, et al. The coupling of bone and cartilage turnover in osteoarthritis: opportunities for bone antiresorptives and anabolics as potential treatments? Ann Rheum Dis. 2014;73:336–48.

5. Herrero-Beaumont G, Roman-Blas JA. Osteoarthritis: Osteoporotic OA: a reasonable target for bone-acting agents. Nat Rev Rheumatol. 2013;9:448–50.

6. Srikanth VK, Fryer JL, Zhai G, Winzenberg TM, Hosmer D, Jones G. A meta-analysis of sex differences prevalence, incidence and severity of osteoarthritis. Osteoarthritis Cartilage. 2005;13:769–81.

7. Roman-Blas JA, Castaneda S, Largo R, Herrero-Beaumont G. Osteoarthritis associated with estrogen deficiency. Arthritis Res Ther. 2009;11:241.

8. Riancho JA, Garcia-Ibarbia C, Gravani A, Raine EV, Rodriguez-Fontenla C, Soto-Hermida A, et al. Common variations in estrogen-related genes are associated with severe large-joint osteoarthritis: a multicenter genetic and functional study. Osteoarthritis Cartilage. 2010;18:927–33.

9. Yin YW, Sun QQ, Hu AM, Wang Q, Liu HL. Association of rs9340799 polymorphism in estrogen receptor alpha gene with the risk of osteoarthritis: evidence based on 8,792 subjects. Mol Genet Genomics. 2015;290:513–20.

10. Wang Q, Yan XB, Sun QQ, Hu AM, Liu HL, Yin YW. Genetic polymorphism of the estrogen receptor alpha gene and susceptibility to osteoarthritis: evidence based on 15,022 subjects. Curr Med Res Opin. 2015;31:1047–55.

11. Pinkerton JV, Thomas S. Use of SERMs for treatment in postmenopausal women. J Steroid Biochem Mol Biol. 2014;142:142–54.

12. Taylor HS. Designing the ideal selective estrogen receptor modulator—an achievable goal? Menopause. 2009;16:609–15.

13. Maximov PY, Lee TM, Jordan VC. The discovery and development of selective estrogen receptor modulators (SERMs) for clinical practice. Curr Clin Pharmacol. 2013;8:135–55.

14. Sniekers YH, Weinans H, Bierma-Zeinstra SM, van Leeuwen JP, van Osch GJ. Animal models for osteoarthritis: the effect of ovariectomy and estrogen treatment—a systematic approach. Osteoarthritis Cartilage. 2008;16:533–41.

15. de Klerk BM, Schiphof D, Groeneveld FP, Koes BW, van Osch GJ, van Meurs JB, et al. Limited evidence for a protective effect of unopposed oestrogen therapy for osteoarthritis of the hip: a systematic review. Rheumatology (Oxford). 2009;48:104–12.

16. Tsai CL, Liu TK. Estradiol-induced knee osteoarthrosis in ovariectomized rabbits. Clin Orthop Relat Res. 1993;291:295–302.

17. Hashem G, Zhang Q, Hayami T, Chen J, Wang W, Kapila S. Relaxin and β-estradiol modulate targeted matrix degradation in specific synovial joint fibrocartilages: progesterone prevents matrix loss. Arthritis Res Ther. 2006;8:R98.

18. Yang JH, Kim JH, Lim DS, Oh KJ. Effect of combined sex hormone replacement on bone/cartilage turnover in a murine model of osteoarthritis. Clin Orthop Surg. 2012;4:234–41.

19. Funck-Brentano T, Lin H, Hay E, Ah Kioon MD, Schiltz C, Hannouche D, et al. Targeting bone alleviates osteoarthritis in osteopenic mice and modulates cartilage catabolism. PLoS One. 2012;7:e33543.

20. Oestergaard S, Sondergaard BC, Hoegh-Andersen P, Henriksen K, Qvist P, Christiansen C, et al. Effects of ovariectomy and estrogen therapy on type II collagen degradation and structural integrity of articular cartilage in rats: implications of the time of initiation. Arthritis Rheum. 2006;54:2441–51.

21. Gao WL, Wu LS, Zi JH, Wu B, Li YZ, Song YC, et al. Measurement of serum estrogen and estrogen metabolites in pre- and postmenopausal women with osteoarthritis using high-performance liquid chromatography-electrospray ionization-tandem mass spectrometry. Braz J Med Biol Res. 2015;48:146–53.

22. Afzal S, Khanam A. Serum estrogen and interleukin-6 levels in postmenopausal female osteoarthritis patients. Pak J Pharm Sci. 2011;24:217–9.

23. Sniekers YH, Weinans H, van Osch GJ, van Leeuwen JP. Oestrogen is important for maintenance of cartilage and subchondral bone in a murine model of knee osteoarthritis. Arthritis Res Ther. 2010;12:R182.

24. Yoshida A, Morihara T, Matsuda K, Sakamoto H, Arai Y, Kida Y, et al. Immunohistochemical analysis of the effects of estrogen on intraarticular neurogenic inflammation in a rat anterior cruciate ligament transection model of osteoarthritis. Connect Tissue Res. 2012;53:197–206.

25. Wang XD, Kou XX, Meng Z, Bi RY, Liu Y, Zhang JN, et al. Estrogen aggravates iodoacetate-induced temporomandibular joint osteoarthritis. J Dent Res. 2013;92:918–24.

26. Maneix L, Servent A, Poree B, Ollitrault D, Branly T, Bigot N, et al. Up-regulation of type II collagen gene by 17β-estradiol in articular chondrocytes involves Sp1/3, Sox-9, and estrogen receptor alpha. J Mol Med (Berl). 2014;92:1179–200.

27. Imgenberg J, Rolauffs B, Grodzinsky AJ, Schunke M, Kurz B. Estrogen reduces mechanical injury-related cell death and proteoglycan degradation in mature articular cartilage independent of the presence of the superficial zone tissue. Osteoarthritis Cartilage. 2013;21:1738–45.

28. Kumagai K, Imai S, Toyoda F, Okumura N, Isoya E, Matsuura H, et al. 17β-Oestradiol inhibits doxorubicin-induced apoptosis via block of the volume-sensitive Cl(−) current in rabbit articular chondrocytes. Br J Pharmacol. 2012;166:702–20.

29. Huang JG, Xia C, Zheng XP, Yi TT, Wang XY, Song G, et al. 17β-Estradiol promotes cell proliferation in rat osteoarthritis model chondrocytes via PI3K/Akt pathway. Cell Mol Biol Lett. 2011;16:564–75.

30. Watt FE. Hand osteoarthritis, menopause and menopausal hormone therapy. Maturitas. 2016;83:13–8.

31. Nevitt MC, Cummings SR, Lane NE, Hochberg MC, Scott JC, Pressman AR, et al. Association of estrogen replacement therapy with the risk of osteoarthritis of the hip in elderly white women. Study of Osteoporotic Fractures Research Group. Arch Intern Med. 1996;156:2073–80.

32. Cirillo DJ, Wallace RB, Wu L, Yood RA. Effect of hormone therapy on risk of hip and knee joint replacement in the Women's Health Initiative. Arthritis Rheum. 2006;54:3194–204.

33. Carbone LD, Nevitt MC, Wildy K, Barrow KD, Harris F, Felson D, et al. The relationship of antiresorptive drug use to structural findings and symptoms of knee osteoarthritis. Arthritis Rheum. 2004;50:3516–25.

34. Seo SK, Yang HI, Lim KJ, Jeon YE, Choi YS, Cho S, et al. Changes in serum levels of cartilage oligomeric matrix protein after estrogen and alendronate therapy in postmenopausal women. Gynecol Obstet Invest. 2012;74:143–50.

35. Spector TD, Nandra D, Hart DJ, Doyle DV. Is hormone replacement therapy protective for hand and knee osteoarthritis in women?: The Chingford Study. Ann Rheum Dis. 1997;56:432–4.

36. Hannan MT, Felson DT, Anderson JJ, Naimark A, Kannel WB. Estrogen use and radiographic osteoarthritis of the knee in women. The Framingham Osteoarthritis Study. Arthritis Rheum. 1990;33:525–32.

37. Zhang Y, McAlindon TE, Hannan MT, Chaisson CE, Klein R, Wilson PW, et al. Estrogen replacement therapy and worsening of radiographic knee osteoarthritis: the Framingham Study. Arthritis Rheum. 1998;41:1867–73.

38. Hart DJ, Doyle DV, Spector TD. Incidence and risk factors for radiographic knee osteoarthritis in middle-aged women: the Chingford Study. Arthritis Rheum. 1999;42:17–24.

39. Wise BL, Niu J, Zhang Y, Felson DT, Bradley LA, Segal N, et al. The association of parity with osteoarthritis and knee replacement in the multicenter osteoarthritis study. Osteoarthritis Cartilage. 2013;21:1849–54.

40. Liu B, Balkwill A, Cooper C, Roddam A, Brown A, Beral V, et al. Reproductive history, hormonal factors and the incidence of hip and knee replacement for osteoarthritis in middle-aged women. Ann Rheum Dis. 2009;68:1165–70.

41. Burr DB, Gallant MA. Bone remodelling in osteoarthritis. Nat Rev Rheumatol. 2012;8:665–73.

42. Pastoureau PC, Chomel AC, Bonnet J. Evidence of early subchondral bone changes in the meniscectomized guinea pig. A densitometric study using dual-energy X-ray absorptiometry subregional analysis. Osteoarthritis Cartilage. 1999;7:466–73.

43. Herrero-Beaumont G, Roman-Blas JA, Largo R, Berenbaum F, Castaneda S. Bone mineral density and joint cartilage: four clinical settings of a complex relationship in osteoarthritis. Ann Rheum Dis. 2011;70:1523–5.

44. Komm BS, Mirkin S. An overview of current and emerging SERMs. J Steroid Biochem Mol Biol. 2014;143:207–22.

45. Tsai CL, Liu TK. Inhibition of estradiol-induced early osteoarthritic changes by tamoxifen. Life Sci. 1992;50:1943–51.

46. Rosner IA, Boja BA, Goldberg VM, Moskowitz RW. Tamoxifen therapy in experimental osteoarthritis. Curr Ther Res. 1983;34:409–14.

47. Colombo C, Butler M, Hickman L, Selwyn M, Chart J, Steinetz B. A new model of osteoarthritis in rabbits. II. Evaluation of anti-osteoarthritic effects of selected antirheumatic drugs administered systemically. Arthritis Rheum. 1983;26:1132–9.

48. Rosner IA, Malemud CJ, Goldberg VM, Papay RS, Getzy L, Moskowitz RW. Pathologic and metabolic responses of experimental osteoarthritis to estradiol and an estradiol antagonist. Clin Orthop Relat Res. 1982;171:280–6.

49. Hoegh-Andersen P, Tanko LB, Andersen TL, Lundberg CV, Mo JA, Heegaard AM, et al. Ovariectomized rats as a model of postmenopausal osteoarthritis: validation and application. Arthritis Res Ther. 2004;6:R169–80.

50. Christgau S, Tanko LB, Cloos PA, Mouritzen U, Christiansen C, Delaisse JM, et al. Suppression of elevated cartilage turnover in postmenopausal women and in ovariectomized rats by estrogen and a selective estrogen-receptor modulator (SERM). Menopause. 2004;11:508–18.

51. Andersson A, Bernardi AI, Stubelius A, Nurkkala-Karlsson M, Ohlsson C, Carlsten H, et al. Selective oestrogen receptor modulators lasofoxifene and bazedoxifene inhibit joint inflammation and osteoporosis in ovariectomised mice with collagen-induced arthritis. Rheumatology. 2015; kev355.

52. Saito M, Kida Y, Nishizawa T, Arakawa S, Okabe H, Seki A, et al. Effects of 18-month treatment with bazedoxifene on enzymatic immature and mature cross-links and non-enzymatic advanced glycation end products, mineralization, and trabecular microarchitecture of vertebra in ovariectomized monkeys. Bone. 2015;81:573–80.

53. Kavas A, Cagatay ST, Banerjee S, Keskin D, Tezcaner A. Potential of Raloxifene in reversing osteoarthritis-like alterations in rat chondrocytes: an in vitro model study. J Biosci. 2013;38:135–47.

54. Tinti L, Niccolini S, Lamboglia A, Pascarelli NA, Cervone R, Fioravanti A. Raloxifene protects cultured human chondrocytes from IL-1β induced damage: a biochemical and morphological study. Eur J Pharmacol. 2011;670:67–73.

55. Hooshmand S, do Soung Y, Lucas EA, Madihally SV, Levenson CW, Arjmandi BH. Genistein reduces the production of proinflammatory molecules in human chondrocytes. J Nutr Biochem. 2007;18:609–14.

56. Karsdal MA, Bay-Jensen AC, Henriksen K, Christiansen C. The pathogenesis of osteoarthritis involves bone, cartilage and synovial inflammation: may estrogen be a magic bullet? Menopause Int. 2012;18:139–46.

57. Yoshii T, Yamada M, Minami T, Tsunoda T, Sasaki M, Kondo Y, et al. The effects of bazedoxifene on bone, glucose, and lipid metabolism in postmenopausal women with type 2 diabetes: an exploratory pilot study. J Clin Med Res. 2015;7:762–9.

58. Palacios S, Silverman SL, de Villiers TJ, Levine AB, Goemaere S, Brown JP, et al. A 7-year randomized, placebo-controlled trial assessing the long-term efficacy and safety of bazedoxifene in postmenopausal women with osteoporosis: effects on bone density and fracture. Menopause. 2015;22:806–13.

59. Beck TJ, Fuerst T, Gaither KW, Sutradhar S, Levine AB, Hines T, et al. The effects of bazedoxifene on bone structural strength evaluated by hip structure analysis. Bone. 2015;77:115–9.

60. Pinkerton JV, Harvey JA, Lindsay R, Pan K, Chines AA, Mirkin S, et al. Effects of bazedoxifene/conjugated estrogens on the endometrium and bone: a randomized trial. J Clin Endocrinol Metab. 2014;99:E189–98.

61. Kim K, Svedbom A, Luo X, Sutradhar S, Kanis JA. Comparative cost-effectiveness of bazedoxifene and raloxifene in the treatment of postmenopausal osteoporosis in Europe, using the FRAX algorithm. Osteoporos Int. 2014;25:325–37.

62. Fujita T, Fujii Y, Munezane H, Ohue M, Takagi Y. Analgesic effect of raloxifene on back and knee pain in postmenopausal women with osteoporosis and/or osteoarthritis. J Bone Miner Metab. 2010;28:477–84.

63. Hattori Y, Kojima T, Kato D, Matsubara H, Takigawa M, Ishiguro N. A selective estrogen receptor modulator inhibits tumor necrosis factor-alpha-induced apoptosis through the ERK1/2 signaling pathway in human chondrocytes. Biochem Biophys Res Commun. 2012;421:418–24.

64. Funck-Brentano T, Cohen-Solal M. Subchondral bone and osteoarthritis. Curr Opin Rheumatol. 2015;27:420–6.

65. Bellido M, Lugo L, Roman-Blas JA, Castaneda S, Caeiro JR, Dapia S, et al. Subchondral bone microstructural damage by increased remodelling aggravates experimental osteoarthritis preceded by osteoporosis. Arthritis Res Ther. 2010;12:R152.

66. Liang Y, Duan L, Xiong J, Zhu W, Liu Q, Wang D, et al. E2 regulates MMP-13 via targeting miR-140 in IL-1β-induced extracellular matrix degradation in human chondrocytes. Arthritis Res Ther. 2016;18:105.

67. Varady NH, Grodzinsky AJ. Osteoarthritis year in review 2015: mechanics. Osteoarthr Cartil. 2016;24:27–35.

68. Levillain A, Boulocher C, Kaderli S, Viguier E, Hannouche D, Hoc T, et al. Meniscal biomechanical alterations in an ACLT rabbit model of early osteoarthritis. Osteoarthritis Cartilage. 2015;23:1186–93.

69. Kato M, Takaishi H, Yoda M, Tohmonda T, Takito J, Fujita N, et al. GRIP1 enhances estrogen receptor alpha-dependent extracellular matrix gene expression in chondrogenic cells. Osteoarthritis Cartilage. 2010;18:934–41.

70. Dai G, Li J, Liu X, Liu Q, Liu C. The relationship of the expression of estrogen receptor in cartilage cell and osteoarthritis induced by bilateral ovariectomy in guinea pig. J Huazhong Univ Sci Technolog Med Sci. 2005;25:683–6.

71. Li ZX, Chen CJ. The effect of lowered serum levels of estrogen on the expression of ERα, ERβ, OPG and RANKL in rat mandibular condylar cartilage. Shanghai Kou Qiang Yi Xue. 2015;24:437–41.

72. Song XX, Yu YJ, Li XF, Liu ZD, Yu BW, Guo Z. Estrogen receptor expression in lumbar intervertebral disc of the elderly: gender- and degeneration degree-related variations. Joint Bone Spine. 2014;81:250–3.

73. Komm BS, Mirkin S. The tissue selective estrogen complex: a promising new menopausal therapy. Pharmaceuticals (Basel). 2012;5:899–924.

74. Komm BS, Morgenstern D, Yamamoto AL, Jenkins SN. The safety and tolerability profile of therapies for the prevention and treatment of osteoporosis in postmenopausal women. Expert Rev Clin Pharmacol. 2015;8:769–84.

75. Lindsay R, Gallagher JC, Kagan R, Pickar JH, Constantine G. Efficacy of tissue-selective estrogen complex of bazedoxifene/conjugated estrogens for osteoporosis prevention in at-risk postmenopausal women. Fertil Steril. 2009;92:1045–52.

76. Komm BS, Vlasseros F, Samadfam R, Chouinard L, Smith SY. Skeletal effects of bazedoxifene paired with conjugated estrogens in ovariectomized rats. Bone. 2011;49:376–86.

Is the relationship between increased knee muscle strength and improved physical function following exercise dependent on baseline physical function status?

Michelle Hall[1], Rana S. Hinman[1], Martin van der Esch[2], Marike van der Leeden[2], Jessica Kasza[3], Tim V. Wrigley[1], Ben R. Metcalf[1], Fiona Dobson[4] and Kim L. Bennell[1*]

Abstract

Background: Clinical guidelines recommend knee muscle strengthening exercises to improve physical function. However, the amount of knee muscle strength increase needed for clinically relevant improvements in physical function is unclear. Understanding how much increase in knee muscle strength is associated with improved physical function could assist clinicians in providing appropriate strength gain targets for their patients in order to optimise outcomes from exercise. The aim of this study was to investigate whether an increase in knee muscle strength is associated with improved self-reported physical function following exercise; and whether the relationship differs according to physical function status at baseline.

Methods: Data from 100 participants with medial knee osteoarthritis enrolled in a 12-week randomised controlled trial comparing neuromuscular exercise to quadriceps strengthening exercise were pooled. Participants were categorised as having mild, moderate or severe physical dysfunction at baseline using the Western Ontario and McMaster Universities Osteoarthritis Index (WOMAC). Associations between 12-week changes in physical function (dependent variable) and peak isometric knee extensor and flexor strength (independent variables) were evaluated with and without accounting for baseline physical function status and covariates using linear regression models.

Results: In covariate-adjusted models without accounting for baseline physical function, every 1-unit (Nm/kg) increase in knee extensor strength was associated with physical function improvement of 17 WOMAC units (95% confidence interval (CI) −29 to −5). When accounting for baseline severity of physical function, every 1-unit increase in knee extensor strength was associated with physical function improvement of 24 WOMAC units (95% CI −42 to −7) in participants with severe physical dysfunction. There were no associations between change in strength and change in physical function in participants with mild or moderate physical dysfunction at baseline. The association between change in knee flexor strength and change in physical function was not significant, irrespective of baseline function status.

Conclusions: In patients with severe physical dysfunction, an increase in knee extensor strength and improved physical function were associated.

Keywords: Exercise, Knee muscle, Physical function, Knee osteoarthritis

* Correspondence: k.bennell@unimelb.edu.au
[1]Centre for Health, Exercise and Sports Medicine, Department of Physiotherapy, School of Health Sciences, The University of Melbourne, Melbourne, VIC 3010, Australia
Full list of author information is available at the end of the article

Background

People with knee osteoarthritis (OA) often have difficulty performing activities of daily living and physical dysfunction is a key driver for total knee arthroplasty eligibility [1]. Knee muscle weakness is a typical feature of knee OA [2] and is associated with physical dysfunction in people with the disease [3]. Clinical guidelines recommend knee muscle strengthening exercises to improve physical function [4, 5]. However, the amount of knee muscle strength increase needed for clinically relevant improvements in physical function is unclear. Understanding how much increase in knee muscle strength is associated with improved physical function could assist clinicians in providing appropriate strength gain targets for their patients in order to optimise outcomes from exercise.

In people with knee OA, deficits in knee extensor and flexor strength, relative to body mass, range between 20 and 40% compared to individuals without knee OA [6–10]. Evidence from observational [11, 12] and pre–post exercise [13, 14] studies supports an association between change in knee muscle strength and change in self-reported physical function in people with [11–14] or at risk for [11] knee OA. Although these study designs preclude causal inferences, these studies provide some insight into the magnitude of increase in knee muscle strength potentially associated with physical function improvement. However, interpretation is limited by the assumption that the relationship between change in strength and function is consistent across all patients, irrespective of baseline dysfunction. Previous research has determined that the magnitude of the minimal clinically important improvement (MCII) in physical function in people with knee OA depends on baseline physical function status [15]. Specifically, patients with less difficulty with physical function require less improvement in physical function to have a clinical meaningful improvement compared to patients with more severe physical dysfunction [15]. Therefore, it is possible that relationships between changes in knee muscle strength and physical function may be influenced by baseline physical function status. However, this has not been evaluated to date.

In a randomised controlled trial (RCT), we compared outcomes at 12 weeks from two exercise programmes (weight-bearing neuromuscular exercise versus non-weight-bearing quadriceps strengthening) in people with medial tibiofemoral knee OA and varus alignment [16]. Comparable between-group improvements in self-reported physical function and knee muscle strength over the 12-week study period were found with both exercise programmes [16]. Using pooled data from this RCT, the purpose of this exploratory study was to evaluate the association between change in knee muscle strength and change in self-reported physical function in patients following 12 weeks of exercise and to evaluate magnitudes of association according to baseline severity in physical dysfunction.

Methods

Participants

Data from people who participated in a RCT were used [16]. Between July 2010 and July 2011, 100 people aged > 50 years with medial tibiofemoral compartment knee OA and varus malalignment were recruited from the community. Individuals were eligible if they had: radiographic medial tibiofemoral knee OA (defined as Kellgren and Lawrence grade 2 or greater [17]) with greater medial tibiofemoral joint space narrowing compared to lateral tibiofemoral joint narrowing [18], and medial compartment osteophyte severity greater than or equal to lateral compartment osteophyte severity [18]; static varus alignment on radiograph (defined as a mechanical axis angle of $< 181°$ for females and $< 183°$ for males) [19]; and average knee pain over the past week of ≥ 25 on a 100-mm visual analogue scale (VAS). Exclusion criteria included: knee surgery or an intraarticular corticosteroid injection within the last 6 months; oral corticosteroid use current or within the past 4 weeks; systemic arthritic conditions; prior joint replacement (hip or knee) or tibial osteotomy surgery; other non-pharmacologic treatment within the past 6 months; or body mass index > 36 kg/m^2. The most symptomatic knee was deemed the study knee in cases of bilaterally eligible cases. Ethical approval was obtained from the University of Melbourne Human Ethics Committee and all participants provided written informed consent.

Interventions

Participants were randomised to one of two 12-week home-based exercise programmes (either neuromuscular exercise or traditional quadriceps strengthening exercises) [16]. Participants were supervised by a physiotherapist for 14 sessions and were instructed to exercise a minimum of 4 days per week [16]. Further detail on the exercise programmes and the trial protocol has been published previously [20].

Dependent variable (outcome)

Self-reported physical function was assessed using the WOMAC physical function subscale with knee-related questions on a scale from 0 ('none') to 4 ('extreme'). The total score was normalised to a 0–100 score, where higher scores indicate extreme difficulty [21]. The WOMAC has been demonstrated previously as reliable, valid and responsive [21]. Improvements of 5.3, 11.8 and 20.4 points on the WOMAC physical function scale have been associated previously with a MCII in people with knee OA with mild, moderate and severe physical dysfunction respectively [15].

Independent variables

A KinCom 125-AP isokinetic dynamometer (Chattecx, Chattanooga, TN, USA) was used to assess maximal isometric knee extensor and knee flexor strength at 60° knee flexion. Following submaximal efforts, participants performed three maximal trials while receiving strong verbal encouragement to "push/pull as hard as you can" for the knee extensor and knee flexor muscles respectively. The distance from the ankle cuff to the rotation axis of the dynamometer was used as the lever arm length. The peak force (Newtons) from three maximal contractions (gravity compensated) was multiplied by the lever arm length (m) and divided by body mass (kg). Muscle strength was normalised to body mass (kg) as a large proportion of the items on the WOMAC physical function subscale involve weight-bearing activities [21].

Other measures

Average overall knee pain during the past week was assessed using a 100-mm VAS with endpoints of "no pain" and "worst pain possible" [22]. Disease severity was assessed using the Kellgren and Lawrence grading scale [17]. Participants were graded as either grade 2 (definitive osteophytes with possible narrowing of joint space), grade 3 (moderate multiple osteophytes, definite narrowing of joint space and some sclerosis and possible deformity of bone ends) or grade 4 (large osteophytes, marked narrowing of joint space, severe sclerosis and definite deformity of bone ends). Anatomic knee alignment was assessed from radiographs according to previously described methods [23].

Statistical analysis

Analyses were performed using Stata software, version 13.1 (Statacorp, College Station, TX, USA) and significance was set at $p < 0.05$. Data from both exercise groups were pooled because no significant interactions between exercise group (i.e. neuromuscular exercise and quadriceps strengthening groups) and strength were observed (Additional file 1: Table S1). One-way analyses of variance and Pearson chi-squared tests were used to compare baseline participant characteristics across the three levels of physical dysfunction severity for continuous and categorical data respectively. For descriptive purposes, paired t tests were used to determine change in knee muscle strength and symptoms for the cohort and each category of each physical dysfunction.

Missing follow-up data were imputed ($n = 8$ self-reported physical function; $n = 20$ knee muscle strength) using chained equations with predictive mean matching and a neighbourhood size of three. The multiple imputation model included change in knee extensor strength, change in knee flexor strength, change in VAS pain, change in WOMAC pain, change in WOMAC physical function, sex, age, BMI and the baseline score of each measures of knee strength (extensor and flexor) and symptoms (pain and function). Estimates from 20 imputed data sets were combined using Rubin's rules. Sensitivity analyses were performed using complete case analyses ($n = 80$) (Additional file 2: Table S2). Using previously described cut-off points in WOMAC physical function (0–100) [15], scores ≤ 35.5 were classified as mild physical dysfunction, scores ranging between 35.4 and 51.5 were classified as moderate physical dysfunction and scores > 51.5 were classified as severe physical dysfunction.

Separate linear regression models for knee extensor strength and knee flexor strength were used to estimate the association between change in strength (independent variable) and change in physical function (dependent variable), initially without considering baseline physical dysfunction. In models that considered changes in strength by baseline physical dysfunction severity, baseline physical dysfunction severity and an interaction term between the change in muscle strength and baseline physical function severity (e.g. 12-week change in knee extensor strength × baseline physical function severity) were also included. Regression models were unadjusted, as well as adjusted for age, sex, exercise group, baseline strength and change in pain (VAS). For each measure of strength, the interaction term (change in knee extensor strength × baseline physical dysfunction severity) was interrogated to yield a coefficient for each level of physical dysfunction. Residuals of each linear model were inspected using plots of for normality (normal quantile–quantile plots) and constant variance (scatter plots).

Results

Descriptive statistics for the cohort, and according to baseline physical dysfunction severity, are presented in Table 1. In general, the cohort was middle-aged and overweight, with both sexes represented equally. Further to this, participants were relatively comparable when categorised by severity of baseline physical function (Table 1) with few exceptions. Pain assessed using the VAS was significantly greater in participants with severe physical dysfunction compared to participants with mild and moderate dysfunction (Table 1). Knee extensor strength significantly increased for participants with mild, moderate and severe physical dysfunction at baseline (Table 2) by 5%, 8% and 13% respectively. Knee flexor strength did not increase significantly according to baseline physical dysfunction severity (Table 2). Symptoms significantly improved for participants with mild, moderate and severe physical dysfunction (Table 2).

Table 1 Baseline participant characteristics in the entire cohort and when categorised based on baseline physical dysfunction severity

	Total cohort ($n = 100$)	Baseline physical dysfunction severity		
		Mild ($n = 38$)	Moderate ($n = 43$)	Severe ($n = 19$)
Age (years)	62.4 ± 7.3	62.4 ± 6.8	62.2 ± 7.8	63.0 ± 7.6
Women, n (%)	52 (52%)	20 (53%)	22 (51%)	10 (53%)
Height (m)	1.67 ± 0.10	1.67 ± 0.10	1.68 ± 0.09	1.65 ± 0.11
Mass (kg)	82.7 ± 14.3	82.6 ± 15.2	84.0 ± 14.7	79.8 ± 11.5
Body mass index (kg/m^2)	29.64 ± 4.08	29.67 ± 4.29	29.69 ± 4.08	29.50 ± 3.85
Knee alignment[a] (degrees)	176.8 ± 3.5	176.6 ± 3.7	176.5 ± 3.4	177.9 ± 3.0
Neuromuscular exercise: quadriceps strengthening group	50:50	20:18	24:19	6:13
Bilateral osteoarthritis, yes:no	47:53	15:23	23:20	9:10
Radiographic disease severity[b]				
Grade 2	22 (22%)	7 (18%)	11 (26%)	4 (21%)
Grade 3	43 (43%)	16 (42%)	17 (40%)	10 (53%)
Grade 4	35 (35%)	15 (39%)	15 (35%)	5 (26%)
VAS average knee pain in the past week, 0–100 mm[c]	54.1 ± 15.0	52.8 ± 15.1	51.3 ± 12.5	62.8 ± 17.7[d,e]
WOMAC physical function, 0–100[c]	39.8 ± 14.1	26.2 ± 8.5	43.2 ± 4.5[d]	59.3 ± 8.2[d,e]
Knee extensor strength (Nm/kg)	1.45 ± 0.45	1.49 ± 0.48	1.50 ± 0.43	1.27 ± 0.39
Knee flexor strength (Nm/kg)	0.69 ± 0.22	0.69 ± 0.19	0.70 ± 0.24	0.64 ± 0.23

WOMAC Western Ontario and McMaster Universities Osteoarthritis Index, *VAS* visual analogue scale
[a]Anatomic alignment, where neutral alignment is 181° for females and 183° for males. Varus is < 181° for females and < 183 ° for males [19]
[b]Kellgren and Lawrence grade
[c]Higher scores indicates greater pain/dysfunction
[d]Significantly different to mild physical dysfunction ($p < 0.05$)
[e]Significantly different to moderate physical dysfunction ($p < 0.05$)

Knee extensor strength

Without accounting for baseline physical function status, change in knee extensor muscle strength along with all covariates considered in this study explained 10% of the variation in the change in physical function. A 1-unit increase (Nm/kg) in peak knee extensor strength was associated with a 17-unit improvement (95% CI −29 to −5) in WOMAC physical function. In another model, accounting for baseline physical function status and an interaction with change in knee extensor strength along with all covariates, 33% of the variation in the change in physical function was explained. In this model, a 1-unit increase (Nm/kg) in peak isometric knee extensor strength corresponded to a 24-unit improvement (95% CI −42 to −7) in WOMAC physical function score in participants with severe baseline dysfunction. Notably, the association between change in knee extensor strength and change in physical function was not significant for participants with mild and moderate baseline physical dysfunction (Table 3). Sensitivity analyses using only complete cases ($n = 80$) demonstrated similar results for change in knee extensor strength as the independent variable (Additional file 2: Table S2).

Table 2 Change (follow-up minus baseline) in knee muscle strength

	Baseline physical dysfunction severity			
	Total group	Mild	Moderate	Severe
Knee extensor strength (Nm/kg)	0.12 (0.07 to 0.17)*	0.08 (0.02 to 0.15)*	0.12 (0.06 to 0.19)*	0.17 (0.00 to 0.33)*
Knee flexor strength (Nm/kg)	0.05 (0.02 to 0.07)*	0.03 (−0.02 to 0.07)	0.05 (0.01 to 0.09)	0.08 (0.01 to 0.15)
WOMAC physical function	−11.07 (−13.59 to −8.54)*	−3.92 (−7.26 to −0.57)*	−14.69 (−18.23 to −11.14)*	−17.18 (−23.04 to −11.32)*
WOMAC pain	−10.40 (−13.10 to − 7.70)*	−6.73 (−11.41 to −2.05)*	−10.91 (−14.83 to −6.98)*	−16.59 (−21.76 to −11.44)*
VAS pain	−20.80 (−25.33 to −16.27)*	−22.81 (−30.23 to −15.39)*	−18.68 (−25.16 to −12.21)*	−21.58 (−33.74 to −9.42)*

Data presented as mean (95% confidence interval)
WOMAC Western Ontario and McMaster Universities Osteoarthritis Index, *VAS* visual analogue scale
*$p < 0.05$

Table 3 Linear relationships between 12-week change in strength-related measures (independent variable) and 12-week change in WOMAC function (dependent variable) for the entire cohort and according to physical dysfunction severity at baseline using imputed data

	Univariable analysis			Multivariable analysis[a]			Multivariable analysis[b]			Multivariable analysis[c]		
	Regression coefficient (95% CI)	p value	Adj. R^2	Regression coefficient (95% CI)	p value	Adj. R^2	Regression coefficient (95% CI)	p value	Adj. R^2	Regression coefficient (95% CI)	p value	Adj. R^2
Entire cohort												
Δ Knee extensor strength (Nm/kg)	−17.3 (−29.5 to −5.2)	0.01	0.09	−17.7 (−30.0 to −5.3)	0.01	0.08	−17.9 (−30.5 to −5.3)	0.01	0.06	−17.2 (−29.4 to −4.9)	0.01	0.10
Δ Knee flexor strength (Nm/kg)	−19.6 (−44.4 to 5.3)	0.12	0.03	−19.0 (−44.0 to 6.0)	0.13	0.05	−19.3 (−44.6 to 6.0)	0.13	0.00	−22.0 (−46.4 to 2.5)	0.08	0.06
According to baseline physical dysfunction												
Δ Knee extensor strength (Nm/kg)			0.27^d			0.27^d			0.26^d			0.33^d
Mild	−2.7 (−26.1 to 20.8)	0.82		−1.7 (−25.9 to 22.5)	0.89		−2.2 (−26.7 to 22.2)	0.86		4.8 (−20.2 to 29.8)	0.70	
Moderate	−13.4 (−32.6 to 5.9)	0.17		−13.8 (−32.7 to 5.2)	0.15		−13.4 (−33.3 to 6.4)	0.18		−16.9 (−35.7 to 1.9)	0.08	
Severe	−24.0 (−42.2 to −5.7)	0.01		−24.8 (−43.1 to −6.4)	0.01		−24.9 (−43.1 to −6.5)	0.01		−24.2 (−41.7 to −6.7)	0.01	
Δ Knee flexor strength (Nm/kg)			0.22^d			0.21^d			0.20^d			0.27^d
Mild	0.01 (−34.8 to 35.0)	0.99		−2.8 (−33.2 to 38.8)	0.88		2.20 (−34.4 to 38.8)	0.90		−7.3 (−44.3 to 29.7)	0.69	
Moderate	−13.9 (−45.0 to 17.2)	0.38		−13.8 (−44.5 to 16.8)	0.37		−14.21 (−45.2 to 16.8)	0.36		−10.2 (−39.8 to 19.3)	0.49	
Severe	−42.0 (−99.6 to 15.6)	0.15		−42.7 (−101.3 to 16.0)	0.15		−42.00 (−100.8 to 16.8)	0.16		−47.6 (−100.7 to 5.6)	0.08	

Adj. adjusted, *CI* confidence interval, *WOMAC* Western Ontario and McMaster Universities Osteoarthritis Index

[a]Adjusted for sex, age

[b]Adjusted for sex, age, exercise group, baseline strength

[c]Adjusted for sex, age, exercise group, baseline strength, change in pain (visual analogue scale)

[d]Adjusted R^2 value for the entire model including all terms

Knee flexor strength

Without accounting for baseline physical function status, increased knee flexor muscle strength along with all covariates considered in this study explained 6% of the variation in the change in physical function. However, the association between change in knee flexor strength and change in physical function was not statistically significant in the model unadjusted for covariates or in the models adjusted for any or all covariates (Table 3). When accounting for baseline physical function status and an interaction with change in knee flexor strength along with all covariates, 27% of the variation in the change in physical function was explained. In this model, the association between change in knee flexor strength and change in physical function was not significant, irrespective of baseline physical function status. Sensitivity analyses using only complete cases ($n = 80$) demonstrated a statistically significant association between increased knee flexor strength and improvement in physical function without accounting for baseline physical function status. In the sensitivity analyses accounting for baseline physical function status and an interaction with change in knee flexor strength, there was a significant association between increased knee flexor strength and improved physical function in those with severe physical dysfunction only (Additional file 2: Table S2).

Discussion

We observed a statistically significant association between increased knee extensor strength and improved self-reported physical function in people with knee OA who underwent exercise therapy. However, when investigating the cohort according to baseline severity of physical dysfunction, there was limited evidence of associations between change in knee muscle strength and change in physical function for participants with mild and moderate physical dysfunction at baseline. Conversely, for participants with severe physical dysfunction at baseline, there was a significant association between increased knee extensor strength and improved self-reported physical function. Taken together, the findings of this study provide preliminary evidence to suggest that the relationship between increased knee extensor strength and self-reported physical function improvement may depend on baseline levels of physical dysfunction.

Understanding the association between change in muscle strength and improved physical function following exercise is important. Exercise is a cornerstone treatment for knee OA [4, 5] and self-reported physical function using the WOMAC is recommended as an end-point in OA clinical trials [22]. Similar to previous research [13, 14, 24] we observed a statistically significant association between increased knee extensor strength and improvement in physical function without accounting for physical dysfunction severity at baseline. Based on the regression equation,

the 0.12 Nm/kg (8%) average increase in knee extensor strength was associated with a 2.05-unit improvement (95% CI −3.5 to −0.6) in WOMAC physical function. In the context of strength gains in people with knee OA, the strength gains in the current study are lower than mean increases of 17% (range 10.5% decrease to 49.5% increase) in response to resistance training in people with knee OA reported in a systematic review [25]. Notably, the relationship between self-reported physical function and variables of knee muscle strength, age, sex, exercise group, baseline strength and change in pain (VAS) explained 6–10% of the variation in self-reported physical function. In contrast to a 38-week longitudinal study where participants performed exercise [14], we did not observe an association between increases in knee flexor strength and improved self-reported function on the WOMAC despite the significant improvement in knee flexor strength we reported previously [16]. Several between-study differences such as strength measurement protocols, study duration and participant characteristics may account for the inconsistent findings. Further to this, the exercise interventions used in the current study did not specifically target knee flexor strength. Thus, changes in knee flexor strength were relatively small (Table 2), which may have contributed to a lack of statistical power to detect a statically significant association. Nonetheless, we observed potential evidence to support an association between change in knee flexor strength and improvement in physical function (48.6-unit improvement (95% CI −100.7 to 5.6) in WOMAC physical function), and hence we are hesitant to disregard the potential for a relationship. There was a statistically significant association between increased knee flexor strength and physical function improvement when analysing complete cases (Additional file 2: Table S2).

Our study extends existing knowledge by describing the association between knee muscle strength and self-reported function according to three baseline categories of physical dysfunction. Interestingly, the amount of variation explained by the relationship between physical function and knee extensor strength, age, sex, exercise group, baseline strength and change in pain (VAS) increased from 10 to 33% for the regression models when the baseline level of physical dysfunction was considered. In participants with severe physical dysfunction at baseline, increased knee extensor strength significantly contributed to improved physical function. Specifically, for participants with severe physical dysfunction at baseline, the 0.17 Nm/kg (13%) average increase in knee extensor strength was associated with a 4.1-unit improvement (CI 95% −7.1 to −1.1) in WOMAC physical function. The MCII for WOMAC physical function in knee OA patients with severe physical dysfunction has been estimated to be 20.4 units [15]. Therefore, based on the regression equation, a much larger gain in knee extensor strength of 0.85 Nm/kg (67%) is associated with a MCII in physical function for patients with severe physical dysfunction at baseline. Interestingly, only one of the 19 participants with severe physical dysfunction at baseline increased knee extensor strength ≥ 0.85 Nm/kg over the 12 weeks. Overall, it appears that an increase in knee extensor strength associated with a clinically relevant improvement in physical function is potentially achievable for few patients. Our findings suggest that resistance programmes should aim for greater increases in knee extensor strength, as this may yield greater self-reported physical function improvement for people with severe physical dysfunction at baseline. It is important to acknowledge that a large proportion of the variation in physical function remains unexplained (67%) by a linear relationship between physical function and knee muscle strength together with covariates. Future research is required to validate whether these estimates of knee extensor strength increases yield a MCII in physical function for knee OA patients with severe physical dysfunction in response to exercise.

In contrast to participants with severe physical dysfunction, changes in knee muscle strength were not associated with changes in physical function for participants with mild or moderate physical dysfunction at baseline. Reasons for differences in the associations depending on severity of baseline physical dysfunction are unclear. Increases in knee muscle strength were not statistically different across the levels of physical dysfunction, when accounting for baseline level of knee muscle strength (data not shown). Thus, factors other than increased maximal isometric knee extension/flexion strength appear to contribute to a clinically relevant improvement in physical function [15] following exercise for many participants. Various clinical and psychological factors predict deterioration in self-reported physical function [26] in people with knee OA. However, little is known regarding the association of these factors to improved physical function following exercise. In people with OA, treatment expectation has been shown to moderate the effectiveness of cognitive behavioural therapy [27] and there is some evidence to suggest that treatment expectations are related to clinical outcomes from exercise and acupuncture [28]. A recent study suggests that knee OA patients with higher treatment expectancy for exercise have greater self-efficacy and fewer depressive symptoms compared to patients with lower treatment expectancy [29]. The unexplained variation in self-reported physical function change observed in the current study may in part be accounted for by treatment expectation, self-efficacy and depressive symptoms. Future research should consider whether improvement in these factors, among others [30], differs according to physical dysfunction.

From a clinical perspective, our data suggest that either exercise programme used in this study is beneficial to improve physical function, irrespective of baseline physical function. Post-hoc analyses confirmed that improvement in physical function was no different between exercise groups according to the baseline level of physical dysfunction (interaction $p = 0.39$). Hence, this study does not question the efficacy of knee strengthening interventions to improve physical function. Instead, this study generates the hypotheses that physical function improvement is associated with factors other than increased knee extensor strength for patients with mild or moderate physical dysfunction at baseline, and that gains in knee extensor strength only partially account for improved physical function in patients with severe physical dysfunction.

Evidently, a greater understanding of how physical function improves in patients with knee OA following strengthening exercise is needed so that exercise prescription can be improved to optimise treatments.

Strengths of our study include a relatively large cohort with excellent adherence to the exercise interventions (median percentage of home exercises completed was 82% by the neuromuscular exercise group and 91% by the quadriceps strengthening exercise group) [16]. Limitations of our study also warrant consideration. First, as exploratory analyses, our findings are preliminary and require validation with larger samples. Our small sample size limits the accuracy of estimates as reflected by the wide confidence intervals. Second, although our data suggest that increased maximal isometric knee extensor strength is a potential mechanism underpinning improvement in physical function due to exercise for those with severe physical dysfunction at baseline, effects of exercise can only be determined by analysing effect modification by group (exercise versus no exercise). Third, the cut-off points used to categorise the severity of physical dysfunction were based on knee OA literature demonstrating that a MCII in physical function in response to non-steroidal anti-inflammatory drugs was dependent on the severity of physical dysfunction at baseline [15]. Thus, the cut-off points used to categorise physical function severity may not necessarily apply to exercise treatments. However, findings from regression analyses remained unchanged when using baseline physical function cut-off points based on tertiles (Additional file 3: Table S3). Fourth, our results can only be generalised to the two 12-week exercise programmes evaluated in the original trial. Similarly, due to the patient selection criteria of the original clinical trial, our findings are only generalisable to patients with medial knee OA and varus malalignment who report moderate levels of knee pain. Hence our findings may not be applicable to all patients with knee OA. Also, participants in the current study volunteered to be in an exercise trial, and thus may be more motivated to exercise than the average patient with knee OA. Lastly, our results cannot be generalised to self-reported measures of physical function beyond the WOMAC or to objective measures of physical function.

Conclusions

Overall, we found preliminary evidence to suggest that the association between change in knee muscle strength and improvement in self-reported physical function following 12 weeks of exercise therapy differs according to baseline difficulty with physical function. This may facilitate future research to optimise treatment effects of exercise. Further research is required to investigate factors that associate with improvement in physical function for knee OA patients, particularly those with mild to moderate physical dysfunction.

Additional files

Additional file 1: Table S1. Linear relationships between measure of peak isokinetic knee muscle strength (independent variable) and WOMAC physical function 100 scale (dependent variable), including interaction between 'exercise program' and 'measure of strength'. (DOCX 20 kb)

Additional file 2: Table S2. Linear relationships between change in strength-related measures (independent variable) and change on WOMAC function (dependent variable) according to physical dysfunction severity at baseline (complete cases n =80). (DOCX 21 kb)

Additional file 3: Table S3. Linear relationships between 12-week change in strength-related measures (independent variable) and 12-week change on WOMAC physical function (dependent variable) according to tertiles of physical dysfunction severity at baseline. (DOCX 26 kb)

Abbreviations

MCII: Minimal clinical important improvement; OA: Osteoarthritis; RCT: Randomised controlled trial; VAS: Visual analogue scale; WOMAC: Western Ontario and McMaster Universities Osteoarthritis Index

Acknowledgements
Not applicable.

Funding
The study was funded by the Australian National Health and Medical Research Council (Project # 628644). MH is supported by a Sir Randal Heymanson Research Fellowship from The University of Melbourne. RSH is supported by a Future Fellowship from the Australian Research Council (FT130100175). KLB is supported by a NHMRC Principal Research Fellowship (APP1058440).

Authors' contributions
MH, RSH, MvdE, MvdL, TVW, JK, FD and KLB conceived the design of this study. BRM and MH acquired the data. MH and JK performed statistical analyses. MH, RSH, MvdE, MvdL, JK, TVW, FD and KLB interpreted the data. MH drafted the manuscript. All authors revised the manuscript for intellectual content and approved the final version.

Consent for publication
The authors obtained consent from each participant.

Competing interests
The authors declare that they have no competing interests.

Author details
[1]Centre for Health, Exercise and Sports Medicine, Department of Physiotherapy, School of Health Sciences, The University of Melbourne, Melbourne, VIC 3010, Australia. [2]Amsterdam Rehabilitation Research Center Reade, Amsterdam, The Netherlands. [3]Department of Epidemiology and Preventive Medicine, Monash University, Melbourne, VIC, Australia. [4]Department of Physiotherapy, School of Health Sciences, The University of Melbourne, Melbourne, VIC, Australia.

References

1. Skou ST, Roos EM, Laursen MB, et al. Criteria used when deciding on eligibility for total knee arthroplasty—between thinking and doing. Knee. 2016;23:300–5.
2. Roos EM, Herzog W, Block JA, et al. Muscle weakness, afferent sensory dysfunction and exercise in knee osteoarthritis. Nat Rev Rheumatol. 2011;7:57–63.
3. Berger MJ, Kean CO, Goela A, et al. Disease severity and knee extensor force in knee osteoarthritis: data from the Osteoarthritis Initiative. Arthritis Care Res. 2012;64:729–34.
4. Fernandes L, Hagen KB, Bijlsma JW, et al. EULAR recommendations for the non-pharmacological core management of hip and knee osteoarthritis. Ann Rheum Dis. 2013;72:1125–35.
5. McAlindon TE, Bannuru RR, Sullivan MC, et al. OARSI guidelines for the non-surgical management of knee osteoarthritis. Osteoarthritis Cartilage. 2014;22:363–88.
6. Cheing GL, Hui-Chan CW. The motor dysfunction of patients with knee osteoarthritis in a Chinese population. Arthritis Rheum. 2001;45:62–8.
7. Jan MH, Lai JS, Tsauo JY, et al. Isokinetic study of muscle strength in osteoarthritic knees of females. J Formos Med Assoc. 1990;89:873–9.
8. Liikavainio T, Lyytinen T, Tyrvainen E, et al. Physical function and properties of quadriceps femoris muscle in men with knee osteoarthritis. Arch Phys Med Rehabil. 2008;89:2185–94.
9. Messier SP, Loeser RF, Hoover JL, et al. Osteoarthritis of the knee: effects on gait, strength, and flexibility. Arch Phys Med Rehabil. 1992;73:29–36.
10. Palmieri-Smith RM, Thomas AC, Karvonen-Gutierrez C, et al. Isometric quadriceps strength in women with mild, moderate, and severe knee osteoarthritis. Am J Phys Med Rehabil. 2010;89:541–8.
11. Ruhdorfer A, Wirth W, Eckstein F. Longitudinal change in thigh muscle strength prior to and concurrent with minimum clinically important worsening or improvement in knee function: data from the Osteoarthritis Initiative. Arthritis Rheumatol. 2016;68:826–36.
12. Sanchez-Ramirez DC, van der Leeden M, van der Esch M, et al. Increased knee muscle strength is associated with decreased activity limitations in established knee osteoarthritis: two-year follow-up study in the Amsterdam osteoarthritis cohort. J Rehabil Med. 2015;47:647–54.
13. Baker KR, Nelson ME, Felson DT, et al. The efficacy of home based progressive strength training in older adults with knee osteoarthritis: a randomized controlled trial. J Rheumatol. 2001;28:1655–65.
14. Knoop J, Steultjens MP, Roorda LD, et al. Improvement in upper leg muscle strength underlies beneficial effects of exercise therapy in knee osteoarthritis: secondary analysis from a randomised controlled trial. Physiotherapy. 2015;101:171–7.
15. Tubach F, Ravaud P, Baron G, et al. Evaluation of clinically relevant changes in patient reported outcomes in knee and hip osteoarthritis: the minimal clinically important improvement. Ann Rheum Dis. 2005;64:29–33.
16. Bennell KL, Kyriakides M, Metcalf B, et al. Neuromuscular versus quadriceps strengthening exercise in patients with medial knee osteoarthritis and varus malalignment: a randomized controlled trial. Arithis Rhematol. 2014;66:950–9.
17. Kellgren JH, Lawrence JS. Radiological assessment of osteo-arthrosis. Ann Rheum Dis. 1957;16:494–502.
18. Altman RD, Gold GE. Atlas of individual radiographic features in osteoarthritis, revised. Osteoarthritis Cartilage. 2007;15(Suppl A):1–56.
19. Kraus VB, Vail TP, Worrell T, et al. A comparative assessment of alignment angle of the knee by radiographic and physical examination methods. Arthritis Rheum. 2005;52:1730–5.
20. Bennell KL, Egerton T, Wrigley TV, et al. Comparison of neuromuscular and quadriceps strengthening exercise in the treatment of varus malaligned knees with medial knee osteoarthritis: a randomised controlled trial protocol. BMC Musculoskelet Disord. 2011;12:276.

21. Bellamy N, Buchanan WW, Goldsmith CH, et al. Validation study of WOMAC: a health status instrument for measuring clinically important patient relevant outcomes to antirheumatic drug therapy in patients with osteoarthritis of the hip or knee. J Rheumatol. 1988;15:1833–40.

22. Bellamy N. Osteoarthritis clinical trials: candidate variables and clinimetric properties. J Rheumatol. 1997;24:768–78.

23. Moreland JR, Bassett LW, Hanker GJ. Radiographic analysis of the axial alignment of the lower extremity. J Bone Joint Surg Am. 1987;69:745–9.

24. Maurer BT, Stern AG, Kinossian B, et al. Osteoarthritis of the knee: isokinetic quadriceps exercise versus an educational intervention. Arch Phys Med Rehabil. 1999;80:1293–9.

25. Lange AK, Vanwanseele B, Fiatarone Singh MA. Strength training for treatment of osteoarthritis of the knee: a systematic review. Arthritis Rheum. 2008;59:1488–94.

26. de Rooij M, van der Leeden M, Heymans MW, et al. Prognosis of pain and physical functioning in patients with knee osteoarthritis: a systematic review and meta-analysis. Arthritis Care Res. 2016;68:481–92.

27. Broderick JE, Keefe FJ, Schneider S, et al. Cognitive behaviroal therapy for chronic pain is effective, but for whom? Pain. 2016;157:2115–23.

28. Foster NE, Thomas E, Hill JC, Hay EM. The relationship between patients and practitioner expectations and preferences and clinical outcomes in a trial of exercise and acupuncture for knee osteoarthritis. Eur J Pain. 2010;14:402–9.

29. Marszalet J, Price LL, Harvey WF, Driban JB, Wang C. Outcome expectations and osteoarthritis: association of percieved benefits of exercise with self-efficacy and depression. Arthritis Care Res. 2017;69:491–8.

30. Runhaar J, Luijsterburg P, Dekker J, Bierma-Zeinstra SM. Identifying potential working mechanisms behind the positive effects of exercise therapy on pain and function in osteoarthritis; a systematic review. Osteoarthritis Cartilage. 2015;23:1071–82.

Glucocorticoid-induced leucine zipper (GILZ) is involved in glucocorticoid-induced and mineralocorticoid-induced leptin production by osteoarthritis synovial fibroblasts

Olivier Malaise[1*†], Biserka Relic[1†], Edith Charlier[1], Mustapha Zeddou[1], Sophie Neuville[1], Céline Deroyer[1], Philippe Gillet[2], Edouard Louis[3], Michel G. Malaise[1†] and Dominique de Seny[1†]

Abstract

Background: Glucocorticoid-induced leucine zipper (GILZ) is a mediator of the anti-inflammatory activities of glucocorticoids. However, GILZ deletion does not impair the anti-inflammatory activities of exogenous glucocorticoids in mice arthritis models and GILZ could also mediate some glucocorticoid-related adverse events. Osteoarthritis (OA) is a metabolic disorder that is partly attributed to adipokines such as leptin, and we previously observed that glucocorticoids induced leptin secretion in OA synovial fibroblasts. The purpose of this study was to position GILZ in OA through its involvement in the anti-inflammatory activities of glucocorticoids and/or in the metabolic pathway of leptin induction. The influences of mineralocorticoids on GILZ and leptin expression were also investigated.

Methods: Human synovial fibroblasts were isolated from OA patients during knee replacement surgery. Then, the cells were treated with a glucocorticoid (prednisolone), a mineralocorticoid (aldosterone), a glucocorticoid receptor (GR) antagonist (mifepristone), a selective glucocorticoid receptor agonist (Compound A), mineralocorticoid receptor (MR) antagonists (eplerenone and spironolactone), TNF-α or transforming growth factor (TGF)-β. Cells were transfected with shRNA lentiviruses for the silencing of GILZ and GR. The leptin, IL-6, IL-8 and matrix metalloproteinase (MMP)-1 levels were measured by ELISA. Leptin, the leptin receptor (Ob-R), GR and GILZ expression levels were analyzed by western blotting and/or RT-qPCR.

Results: (1) The glucocorticoid prednisolone and the mineralocorticoid aldosterone induced GILZ expression dose-dependently in OA synovial fibroblasts, through GR but not MR. Similar effects on leptin and Ob-R were observed: leptin secretion and Ob-R expression were also induced by prednisolone and aldosterone through GR; (2) GILZ silencing experiments demonstrated that GILZ was involved in the glucocorticoid-induced and mineralocorticoid-induced leptin secretion and Ob-R expression in OA synovial fibroblasts; and (3) GILZ inhibition did not alter the production of pro-inflammatory cytokines by OA synovial fibroblast or the anti-inflammatory properties of glucocorticoids.

(Continued on next page)

---

* Correspondence: olivier.malaise@chu.ulg.ac.be
†Equal contributors
[1]Laboratory of Rheumatology, Arthropôle, GIGA Research, University and CHU of Liège, Liège, Belgium
Full list of author information is available at the end of the article

(Continued from previous page)

Conclusions: The absence of GILZ prevents corticoid-induced leptin and Ob-R expression without affecting the anti-inflammatory properties of glucocorticoids in OA synovial fibroblasts. Mineralocorticoids also induce leptin and Ob-R expression through GILZ.

Keywords: Leptin, GILZ, Osteoarthritis, Glucocorticoids, Mineralocorticoids, Synovial fibroblasts

Background

The glucocorticoid-induced leucine zipper (GILZ) protein is an intracellular protein that is induced by glucocorticoids. Recent studies have highlighted a major role of GILZ in the anti-inflammatory activities of glucocorticoids. GILZ inhibits the nuclear factor (NF)-kB pathway in human macrophage cells, epithelial respiratory cells and T lymphocytes [1–4]. GILZ also promotes T helper (Th)17 cell polarization toward a regulatory mesenchymal stem cell phenotype in arthritis [5], and it even displays additional functions in depression [6] and spermatogenesis [7]. Further, GILZ is expressed by synovial fibroblasts and is an endogenous anti-inflammatory mediator in rheumatoid arthritis [8]. Ngo et al. have reported the anti-inflammatory activity of exogenous GILZ in the treatment of collagen-induced arthritis [9]. However, GILZ depletion does not always impair the anti-inflammatory activities of exogenous glucocorticoids [9, 10]. Thus, evidence of a central role of GILZ as an anti-inflammatory agent is lacking and controversial, and requires further exploration, specifically with respect to osteoarthritis (OA), for which intra-articular glucocorticoid injections are used as a symptomatic treatment.

OA is characterized by cartilage breakdown, subchondral bone thickening, osteophyte formation and synovial inflammation. It was first considered to be a degenerative disease caused by aging and mechanical stress. However, obesity has also been identified as a risk factor for digital OA [11] (involving non-weight-bearing joints), suggesting a metabolic influence on OA pathogenesis [12]. The metabolic origin of OA can be partly attributed to the presence of adipokines, such as leptin [13–15], which has a well-established link with OA. For example, the synovial and serum leptin levels have both been correlated with the radiologic score for OA severity [14]; the leptin concentration in synovial fluid has been correlated with body mass index (BMI) [16]; higher leptin expression has been detected in vitro in OA cartilage tissues compared with healthy control tissues [13]; and obesity due to impaired leptin signaling in mice does not lead to OA, in contrast to what is observed in obesity due to overfeeding [15].

In vitro, leptin has pro-inflammatory properties; e.g., it induces interleukin-6 (IL-6) expression in synovial fibroblasts [17] and matrix metalloproteinase (MMP) production in human osteoarthritic cartilage [18]. We have previously demonstrated that OA synovial fibroblasts spontaneously produce leptin in vitro [19], suggesting their contribution to the intra-articular leptin level. Expression of leptin and its receptor (Ob-R) are strongly enhanced by glucocorticoids in OA synovial fibroblasts. Furthermore, we have previously demonstrated the involvement of transforming growth factor-β (TGF-β) signaling; prednisolone induces leptin secretion through the ALK1-Smad1/5 pathway, while TGF-β1 suppresses prednisolone-induced leptin secretion through ALK5-Smad2/3 [20].

Glucocorticoids bind to their native receptor, glucocorticoid receptor (GR), and mediate their effects through two different pathways: the "trans-repression" and the "trans-activation" [21]. Although this duality is more complex and although these two pathways are less separate than initially described, trans-repression is usually associated with anti-inflammatory effects, and trans-activation is typically correlated with adverse metabolic events. Selective glucocorticoid receptor agonists (SEGRAs) are GR agonists that are known to have a better benefit-risk ratio than glucocorticoids and do not induce adverse metabolic events. They only activate the trans-repression pathway without modulating trans-activation [21]. We previously observed that SEGRA compound A (CpdA), which is known to have a better benefit-risk ratio than glucocorticoids [22], does not induce leptin secretion or Ob-R expression [23]. Therefore, regarding the detrimental role of leptin in OA, we hypothesized that leptin and Ob-R induction could result from glucocorticoid-associated adverse events. However, the underlying mechanisms remain to be elucidated, and the link between GILZ and leptin is unknown.

GR is the native receptor of glucocorticoids. However, glucocorticoids can also act through mineralocorticoid receptor (MR) [24]. Conversely, mineralocorticoids act through GR [25] in addition to their native receptor, MR. Recent studies have suggested that components of metabolic syndrome are associated with abnormal aldosterone physiology [26]. Furthermore, leptin secretion is increased after aldosterone exposure in brown adipose tissue [27]. Of interest, GILZ expression is also induced by mineralocorticoids, e.g., its involvement in epithelial channel induction in the kidneys occurs through MR [28].

Therefore, in the present study, we investigated the following issues: (1) whether GILZ expression is also induced by mineralocorticoids in human OA synovial fibroblasts and whether this effect is dependent on either GR or MR; (2) whether GILZ and leptin expression are closely correlated; and (3) whether GILZ plays a central role as an anti-inflammatory agent in this type of cell.

Methods

Human synovial fibroblasts and cell culturing

Synovial tissue was obtained from patients with OA during knee replacement surgery. All patients (n = 16) presented with symptomatic knee OA without inflammatory disease or cancer. None of the patients had received oral or intra-articular glucocorticoids for at least one year. The mean patient age was 71 (58–82) years, and the mean BMI was 26.3 (22.2–32.7) kg/m^2. Seven patients were female (44 %).

Synovial fibroblasts were isolated as previously described [19]. Cells were cultured in DMEM (Cambrex Bio Science, USA) with 10 % FBS (Lonza, Switzerland), L-glutamine (2 mM), streptomycin (100 mg/mL) and penicillin (100 U/mL) (BioWhittaker, USA). A total of 5×10^5 synovial fibroblasts/well were plated in 24-well plates (BD Biosciences, USA). Cells were used at passages 3–7 and were stimulated with the glucocorticoid prednisolone (1 μM, unless stated otherwise), the mineralocorticoid aldosterone (1 and 10 μM, unless stated otherwise), the GR antagonist mifepristone (5 μM), the MR antagonist eplerenone (5 μM), the MR antagonist spironolactone (5 μM) (Sigma-Aldrich, USA), the SEGRA CpdA (1 and 10 μM) (Santa Cruz Biotechnology, USA), TGF-β1 (10 ng/mL) (Gibco-BRL, USA), tumor necrosis factor-α (TNF-α) (10 ng/mL) (Biosource, USA), and MG132 (10 μM) (Alexis Corporation, Switzerland). The proteasome inhibitor MG132 was added to the medium in the last 12 h to enhance GILZ visualization when GILZ was analyzed with western blot.

Transfection with lentiviruses expressing GILZ and GR small hairpin RNA (shRNA)

Lentiviral vectors were generated by co-transfecting Lenti-X 293 T cells (Clonetech, Belgium) with a pSPAX2 plasmid (Addgene, Plasmid #12260), a VSV-G-encoding vector, a GILZ (TSC22D3) shRNA plasmid (#TRCN0000013793 (GILZ shRNA1), #TRCN0000364625 (GILZ shRNA2) or #TRCN0000369187 (GILZ shRNA3), Sigma-Aldrich, USA), a GR (NR3C1) shRNA plasmid (#TRCN0000245007 (GR shRNA1), #TRCN0000245003 (GR shRNA2) or #TRCN0000245004 (GR shRNA3), Sigma-Aldrich, USA), or a non-target sequence-encoding plasmid (Sigma, Belgium, SHC002). At 72 h posttransfection, viral supernatants were collected, filtered, and concentrated 100 × by ultracentrifugation. Lentiviral vectors were then titrated using a quantitative polymerase chain reaction (PCR) Lentivirus Titration (Titer) Kit

(ABM, USA, LV900). A total of 5×10^5 synovial fibroblasts/well were plated in 24-well plates (BD Biosciences, USA) and infected with lentiviruses at a multiplicity of infection (MOI) of 30, unless otherwise indicated. After 72 h of incubation, the medium was removed, and the cells were stimulated.

Enzyme-linked immunosorbent assay (ELISA)

A commercially available sandwich ELISA kit (R&D Systems, USA) was used to quantify leptin, IL-6, IL-8 and MMP-1 expression in the culture supernatants. All experiments were performed in triplicate.

Western blotting

Total protein extracts were prepared as described previously [19]. Ob-R (B-3) (sc-8391), GR (41) (sc-136209), GILZ (sc-33780) (Santa Cruz Biotechnology, USA), and glyceraldehyde 3-phosphate dehydrogenase (GAPDH) (Sigma-Aldrich, USA) primary antibodies were used. Western blots were visualized with an anti-mouse or anti-rabbit secondary antibody (Cell Signaling, USA) diluted 1/1000 and enhanced chemiluminescence reagents (GE Healthcare, UK). Western blot band quantification was performed with Image Studio Lite software (USA), and protein expression levels were normalized to the GAPDH level.

Quantitative reverse transcription PCR (RT-qPCR)

Total RNA was isolated from synovial fibroblasts (either untreated or treated with the indicated concentration of prednisolone or aldosterone for 5 days) and purified using a Nucleospin RNA Kit, with rDNAse included (#740955,). Next, complementary DNA (Cdna) was synthesized by the reverse transcription of 1 μg RNA (in each reaction) with a RevertAid H Minus First Strand cDNA Synthesis Kit (#K1632, Thermo Scientific, Belgium) according to the manufacturer's instructions. The resulting cDNA was subsequently PCR amplified with a KAPA SYBR FAST detection system (#KK4611, Belgium). Real-time PCR was performed using a Light-Cycler 480 instrument (Roche, Belgium), and data were analyzed with LC480 software, release 1.5.0 SP4. cDNA dilution curves were generated for each gene and were used to calculate individual real-time PCR efficiencies ($E = 10^{[-1/\text{slope}]}$). The $2^{-\Delta\Delta CT}$ method was then used to calculate the relative gene expression levels between the untreated (calibrator sample) and treated synovial fibroblasts. Input amounts were normalized to the *β2-microglobulin* endogenous control gene. All primers were purchased from Eurogentec (Belgium). The following primer sequences were used: *leptin*, 5'-AACCCTGTGCGGATTCTTGT-3' (forward) and 5'-TCTTGGACTTTTTGGATGGGC-3' (reverse); *GILZ*, 5'-GCACAATTTCTCCATCTCCTTCTT-3' (forward)

Glucocorticoid-induced leucine zipper (GILZ) is involved in glucocorticoid-induced...

125

and 5'- TCAGATGATTCTTCACCAGATCCA-3' (reverse); β2-microglobulin, 5'-TTTCATCCATCCGACATTGA-3' (forward) and 5'-CCAGTCCTTGCTGAAAGACA-3' (reverse).

Statistical analysis

Log transformation was applied to all variables to normalize their distribution. Statistical analysis was performed using GraphPad Prism software (version 6) by one-way analysis of variance (ANOVA) for multiple comparisons, followed by Tukey's post hoc test. The results were considered significant at a p value <0.05. Graphs were constructed using the mean ± standard deviation (SD) calculated from three or more independent experimental replicates for the ELISA, RT-qPCR and western blot experiments. Independent experiments were performed using synovial fibroblasts from different patients (n = 3 or more).

Results

Prednisolone and aldosterone induced GILZ protein expression through GR in human OA synovial fibroblasts

Human OA synovial fibroblasts were stimulated for 5 days with prednisolone (1 μM) (a glucocorticoid) or aldosterone (1 or 10 μM) (a mineralocorticoid). Western blotting (Fig. 1a) revealed that prednisolone and aldosterone induced GILZ expression in these cells.

Glucocorticoids and mineralocorticoids have affinity for both GR and MR. Therefore, both receptors were investigated to determine which one is involved in GILZ expression. Cells were pre-incubated with a GR inhibitor (5 μM mifepristone) or MR inhibitor (5 μM eplerenone or 5 μM spironolactone) and were then stimulated for 5 days with prednisolone (1 μM) or aldosterone (1 or 10 μM). The GR inhibitor mifepristone strongly reduced both prednisolone- and aldosterone-induced GILZ protein expression (Fig. 1a). In contrast, the MR inhibitors eplerenone and spironolactone did not significantly modulate prednisolone-induced or aldosterone-induced GILZ expression in any experiments (Fig. 1a). These results suggest that mineralocorticoids and glucocorticoids induce GILZ expression through GR but not MR in OA synovial fibroblasts.

To further confirm the involvement of GR in prednisolone-induced and/or aldosterone-induced GILZ expression, we performed shRNA experiments to silence GR. Cells were infected with three different lentiviruses expressing GR shRNA or with a non-target control lentivirus. GR shRNA1, 2 and 3, but not the control shRNA, reduced endogenous GR expression (Fig. 1b). Two bands were observed: the antibody was raised against amino acids 176-289 of GR of human origin. It can therefore recognize both isoforms and probably other GRα transcript splice variants, which could explain the presence of

two large bands. Prednisolone-induced and aldosterone-induced GILZ expression was reduced when GR was silenced (Fig. 1c). The GR antagonist mifepristone was used as a positive control to demonstrate GR inactivation. Thus, we confirmed that glucocorticoid-induced and mineralocorticoid-induced GILZ expression was GR-dependent by the silencing of GR.

Leptin and GILZ were similarly modulated; leptin secretion and Ob-R expression were induced by prednisolone and aldosterone through GR

We have previously shown that glucocorticoids enhance leptin secretion and Ob-R expression in synovial fibroblasts ([19] and Fig. 2a: b* vs. a). Similar to prednisolone (Fig. 2a), the mineralocorticoid aldosterone also induced leptin secretion and Ob-R protein expression at 1 μM (Fig. 2b: b* vs. a) and 10 μM (Fig. 2c: b* vs. a). Moreover, using specific inhibitors (a GR inhibitor (mifepristone) and MR inhibitors (eplerenone and spironolactone)), we observed that the prednisolone-induced (Fig. 2a: c* vs. b*) and aldosterone-induced (Fig. 2b and c: c* vs. b*) leptin secretion and Ob-R expression were GR-dependent but not MR-dependent in all experiments, as observed with GILZ. These results suggest that aldosterone induces leptin secretion and Ob-R expression in OA synovial fibroblasts through GR but not MR, similar to glucocorticoids. The use of GR and MR antagonists did not modulate the endogenous level of leptin secretion or Ob-R expression. Human OA synovial fibroblasts were then infected with three different lentiviruses expressing GR shRNA or with a non-target control lentivirus. Prednisolone-induced and aldosterone-induced leptin secretion and Ob-R expression were abolished when GR was silenced (Fig. 3), confirming the involvement of GR signaling in the induction of these processes.

The induction of leptin by prednisolone and aldosterone was dose-dependent (Fig. 4a and b). A dose response was observed not only for leptin secretion in the cell culture supernatant (as measured by ELISA) (Fig. 4a) but also for leptin messenger RNA (mRNA) expression (as measured by RT-qPCR) (Fig. 4b). The induction of leptin by prednisolone was significant at concentrations of equal to or greater than 10 nM or 1000 nM for ELISA or RT-qPCR, respectively. However, it was not significant at 100 nM or 10 nM for RT-qPCR; although the mean value was higher than that for the control, the variance was high. Leptin induction by aldosterone was significant at concentrations of 100 nM and 1000 nM for ELISA and RT-qPCR, respectively. The induction of Ob-R (Fig. 4c) and GILZ (Fig. 4c for western blot and Fig. 5 for qRT-PCR) by prednisolone and aldosterone was also dose-dependent, with significant induction at a concentration equal to or greater than 100 nM.

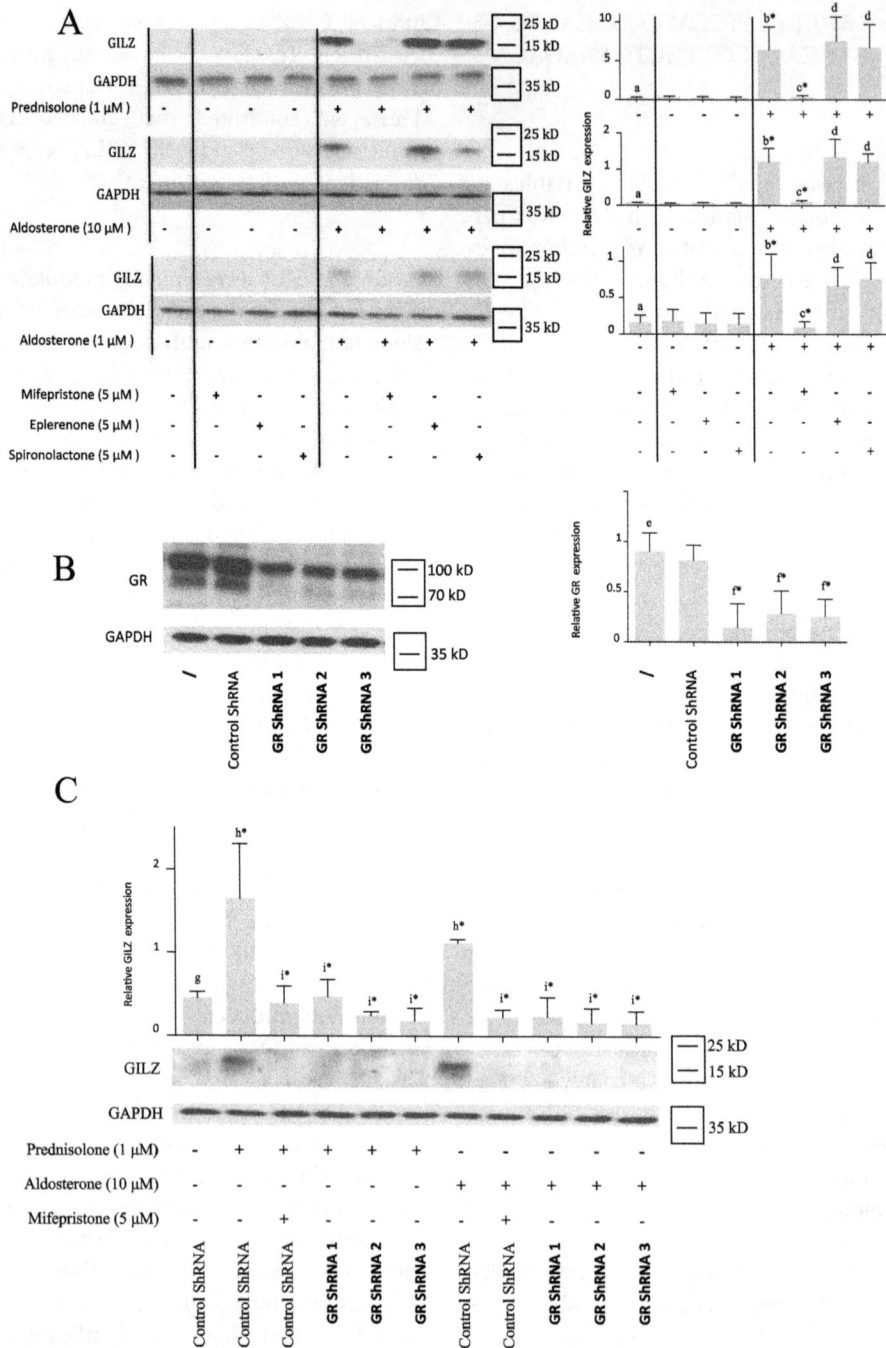

Fig. 1 Glucocorticoid-induced leucine zipper (*GILZ*) expression is induced by prednisolone and aldosterone through glucocorticoid receptor (*GR*). **a** Human osteoarthritis (OA) synovial fibroblasts were pre-incubated or not for 1 h with a GR inhibitor (mifepristone) or mineralocorticoid receptor (*MR*) inhibitors (eplerenone and spironolactone) and were then stimulated for 5 days with a glucocorticoid (prednisolone) or a mineralocorticoid (aldosterone). GILZ and glyceraldehyde 3-phosphate dehydrogenase (*GAPDH*) expression in whole-cell extracts were analyzed by western blotting. *Right panels*, quantification results of western blots shown in *left panels*. Protein levels were normalized to GAPDH. Graphs represent mean +/- SD (n = 4 patients). Significance was set at $p < 0.05$. *b**Significantly different from *a*; *c**significantly different from *b*; *d* not significantly different from *b*. **b, c** Synovial fibroblasts were infected with three different lentiviruses expressing GR shRNA or with a non-target control lentivirus and were stimulated or not for 5 days with prednisolone or aldosterone. A GR inhibitor (mifepristone) was used as a positive control for GR inactivation. GILZ, GR, and GAPDH expression in whole-cell extracts were analyzed by western blotting. *Right* (**b**) and *upper* (**c**) *panels*, quantification results of western blots shown in *left panels* and *lower panels*. Protein levels were normalized to GAPDH. Graphs represent mean +/- SD (n = 3 patients). Significance was set at $p < 0.05$. *f**Significantly different from *e*; *h**significantly different from *g*; *i**significantly different from *h*. *kD* kiloDalton, *shRNA* short hairpin RNA

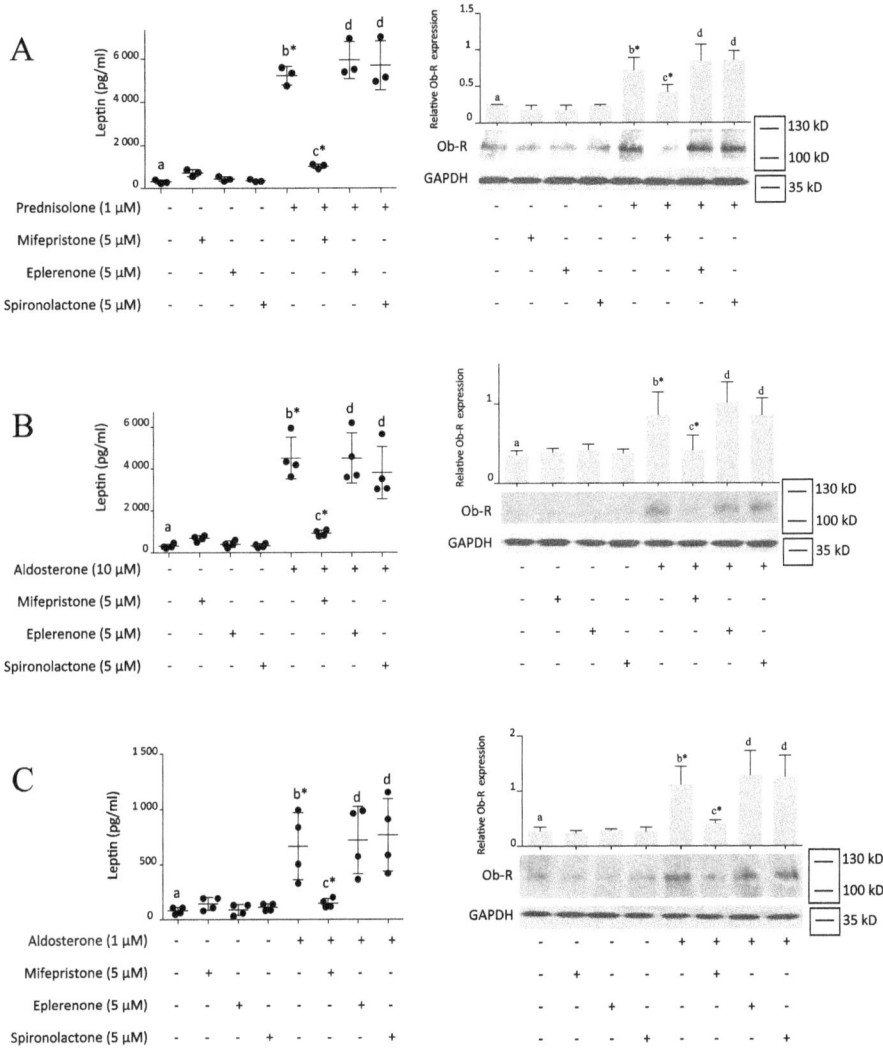

Fig. 2 Leptin secretion and leptin receptor (*Ob-R*) expression were induced by prednisolone and aldosterone through glucocorticoid receptor (GR) signaling. Human osteoarthritis (OA) synovial fibroblasts were pre-incubated or not for 1 h with a GR inhibitor (mifepristone) or mineralocorticoid receptor (MR) inhibitors (eplerenone and spironolactone) and were then stimulated for 5 days with a glucocorticoid (prednisolone) (**A**) or mineralocorticoid (aldosterone) (**B, C**). Leptin expression was measured in cell culture supernatants by ELISA. Ob-R and glyceraldehyde 3-phosphate dehydrogenase (*GAPDH*) expression in whole-cell extracts were analyzed by western blotting. *Upper panels* (*right*), quantification results of western blots shown in *bottom panels*. Proteins levels were normalized to GAPDH. Graphs represent mean +/- SD (n = 3 or 4 patients). Significance set at $p < 0.05$. b*Significantly different from *a*; c*significantly different from *b*; *d* not significantly different from *b*. *kD* kiloDalton

TGF-β did not induce GILZ expression, and it decreased prednisolone-induced GILZ expression (Fig. 6a), which is in accordance with our previous results demonstrating that TGF-β does not induce leptin secretion and that it decreases glucocorticoid-induced leptin secretion [20]. Moreover, the selective GR agonist CpdA, which does not induce leptin expression [23], also does not induce GILZ expression (Fig. 6b). Taken together, these results indicate that leptin and GILZ have similar expression profiles, suggesting correlation between their expression.

GILZ was involved in prednisolone-induced and aldosterone-induced leptin and Ob-R expression

ShRNA experiments for the silencing of GILZ expression were performed to determine whether GILZ is involved in prednisolone- and/or aldosterone-induced leptin secretion. Human OA synovial fibroblasts were infected with three different lentiviruses expressing GILZ shRNA or with a non-target control lentivirus. After 72 h of incubation, the medium was removed, and the cells were stimulated with prednisolone (1 μM) or aldosterone (1 or 10 μM). GILZ shRNA reduced GILZ

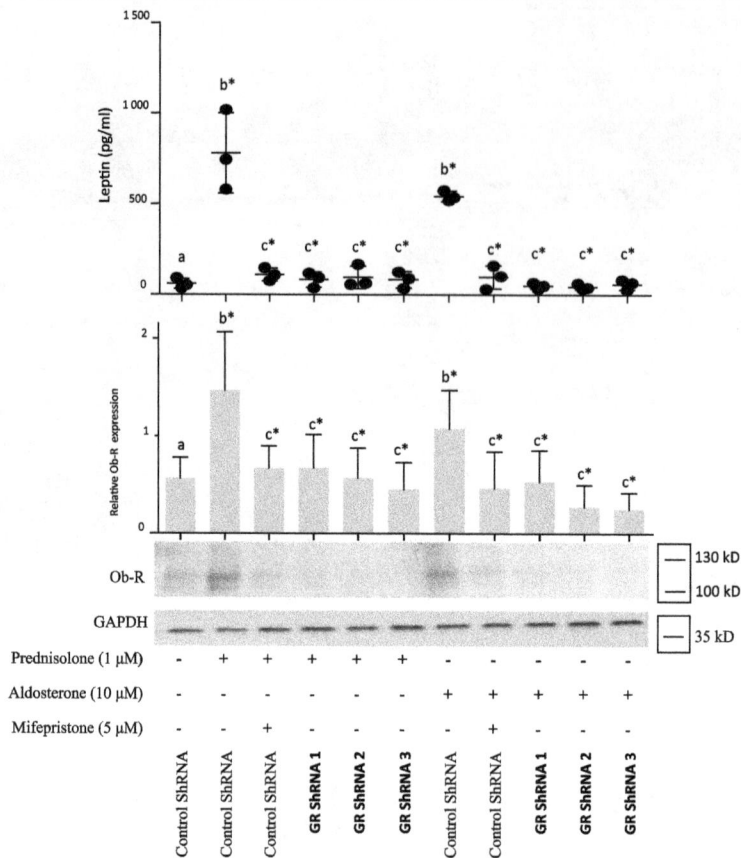

Fig. 3 Leptin secretion and leptin receptor (*Ob-R*) expression were induced by prednisolone and aldosterone through glucocorticoid receptor (GR) signaling. Synovial fibroblasts were infected with three different lentiviruses expressing GR short hairpin RNA (*shRNA*) or with a non-target control lentivirus and were stimulated for 5 days with prednisolone or aldosterone. The GR inhibitor mifepristone was used as a positive control for GR inhibition. Leptin expression was measured in the cell culture supernatants by ELISA. Ob-R and glyceraldehyde 3-phosphate dehydrogenase (*GAPDH*) expression were analyzed in whole-cell extracts by western blotting. *Middle panel*, quantification results of western blots shown in the *lower panel*. Protein levels were normalized to GAPDH. Graphs represent mean +/- SD (n = 3 patients). Significance was set at $p < 0.05$. *b**Significantly different from *a*; *c**significantly different from *b**. *kD* kiloDalton

expression following prednisolone (Fig. 7a) or aldosterone (Fig. 7b) stimulation. Downregulation of GILZ expression resulted in significant decreases in prednisolone-induced (Fig. 7a) and aldosterone-induced (Fig. 7b) leptin and Ob-R expression compared with the controls. These decreases were correlated with the shRNA MOI and with the degree of GILZ silencing (Fig. 7c). GILZ silencing did not alter GR expression or prednisolone-induced GR degradation (Fig. 8).

GILZ inhibition did not alter the anti-inflammatory properties of prednisolone

Synovial fibroblasts spontaneously produced the pro-inflammatory cytokines IL-6, IL-8 and MMP-1, and cell stimulation by TNF-α enhanced the secretion of these cytokines (Fig. 9a-c). Human OA synovial fibroblasts were infected with three different lentiviruses expressing GILZ shRNA or with a non-target control lentivirus. Cells were pre-incubated (Fig. 9d-f) or not (Fig. 9a-c) for

1 h with prednisolone (1 µM) and were then stimulated or not with TNF-α (10 ng/mL) for 12 h. GILZ-shRNA did not significantly alter TNF-α-induced IL-6, IL-8 and MMP-1 production (Fig. 9a-c). Moreover, GILZ inhibition did not alter the capacity for prednisolone to reduce the TNF-α-induced production of these cytokines (Fig. 9d-f). These results suggest that GILZ is not an essential mediator of the anti-inflammatory activities of glucocorticoids in OA synovial fibroblasts.

Discussion

Glucocorticoids are widely used by rheumatologists, either to treat a flare in inflammatory rheumatic diseases or to reduce pain and swelling through intra-articular injection into joints in OA [29]. Unfortunately, they also contribute to adverse events, such as diabetes mellitus and osteoporosis. Moreover, glucocorticoids enhance a catabolic reaction leading to the degradation of cartilage

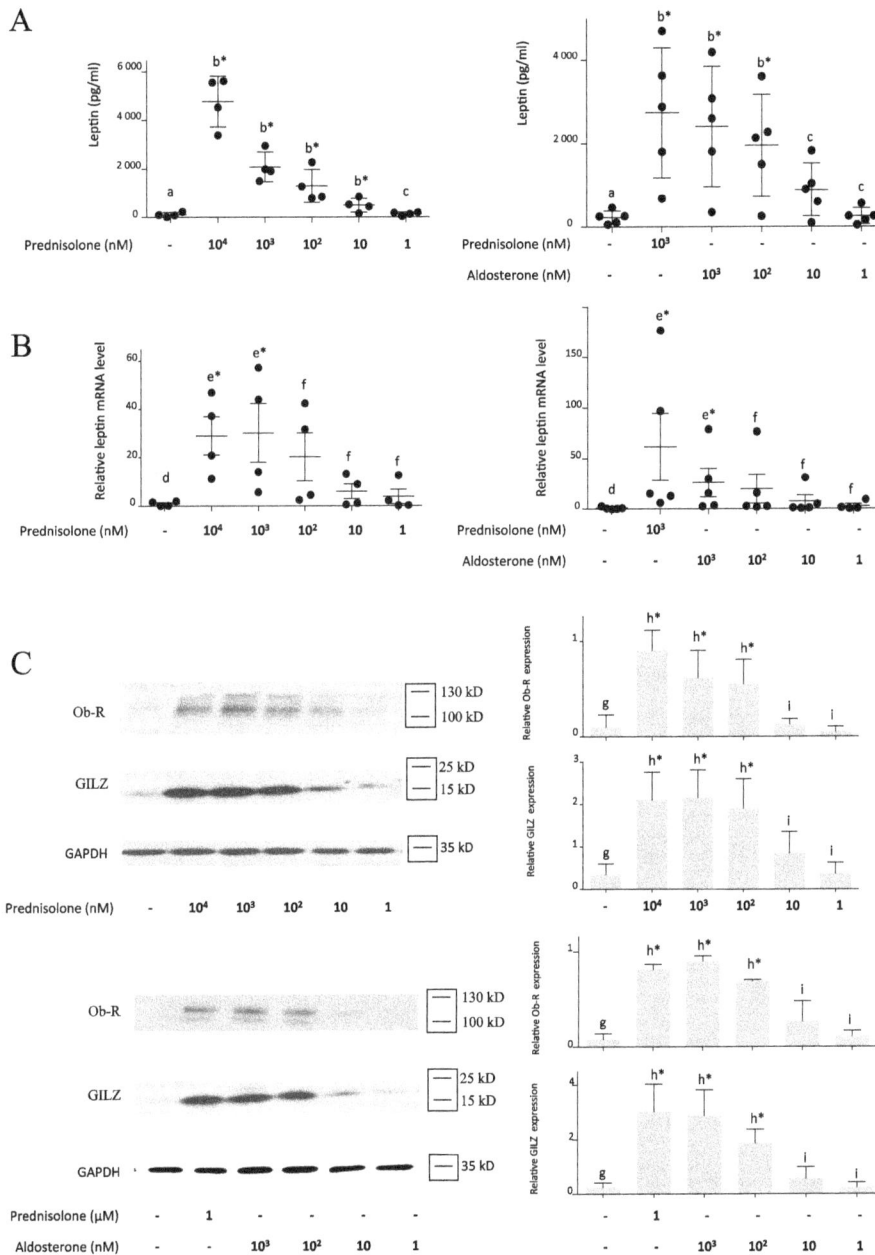

Fig. 4 Leptin secretion and leptin receptor (*Ob-R*) and glucocorticoid-induced leucine zipper (*GILZ*) expression were dose-dependent. **a**, **b** Human osteoarthritis (OA) synovial fibroblasts were stimulated for 5 days with increasing concentrations of a glucocorticoid (prednisolone) or mineralocorticoid (aldosterone). Leptin secretion was measured in the cell culture supernatants by ELISA, and leptin messenger RNA (mRNA) expression was measured by RT-qPCR. Graphs represent mean +/- SD (n = 4 or 5 patients). Significance was set at $p < 0.05$. *b**Significantly different from *a*; *c* not significantly different from *a*; *e**significantly different from *d*; *f* not significantly different from *d*. **c** Human OA synovial fibroblasts were stimulated for 5 days with increasing concentrations of a glucocorticoid (prednisolone) or mineralocorticoid (aldosterone). Ob-R, GILZ and glyceraldehyde 3-phosphate dehydrogenase (*GAPDH*) expression in whole-cell extracts were analyzed by western blotting. *Right panels*, quantification results of western blots shown in the *left panels*. Protein levels were normalized to GAPDH. Graphs represent mean +/- SD (n = 3 patients). Significance was set at $p < 0.05$. *h**Significantly different from *g*; *i* not significantly different from *g*

[30], and they suppress matrix protein markers of chondrogenic differentiation [31].

GILZ is an intracellular protein induced by glucocorticoids and is mainly present in immune cells [32–34]. It can also be induced by mineralocorticoids, as observed in kidney cells [28]. Beaulieu et al. have observed GILZ expression in the synovium of patients with rheumatoid arthritis and in cultured rheumatoid arthritis synovial fibroblasts and have found that its expression is enhanced by dexamethasone and significantly reduced

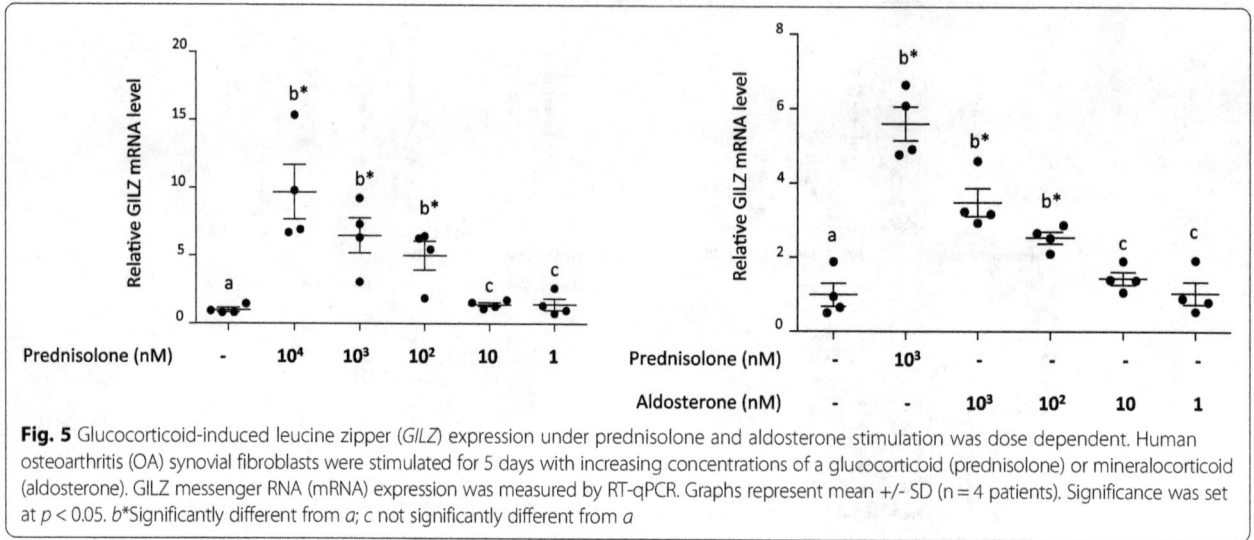

Fig. 5 Glucocorticoid-induced leucine zipper (*GILZ*) expression under prednisolone and aldosterone stimulation was dose dependent. Human osteoarthritis (OA) synovial fibroblasts were stimulated for 5 days with increasing concentrations of a glucocorticoid (prednisolone) or mineralocorticoid (aldosterone). GILZ messenger RNA (mRNA) expression was measured by RT-qPCR. Graphs represent mean +/- SD (n = 4 patients). Significance was set at $p < 0.05$. *b**Significantly different from *a*; *c* not significantly different from *a*

by mifepristone, suggestive of GR involvement [8]. Our work extends the presence of GILZ to human OA synovial fibroblasts and demonstrates for the first time that both the glucocorticoid prednisolone and the mineralocorticoid aldosterone induce GILZ expression in these cells in a dose-dependent and GR-dependent process, at the protein and the mRNA level.

We propose a novel role of GILZ in contributing to corticoid-induced leptin and Ob-R expression in OA synovial fibroblasts. Indeed, we have previously reported that human OA synovial fibroblasts produce leptin (a pro-inflammatory adipokine involved in OA pathogenesis) and its receptor, Ob-R, both spontaneously and after stimulation with glucocorticoids [19]. We have also

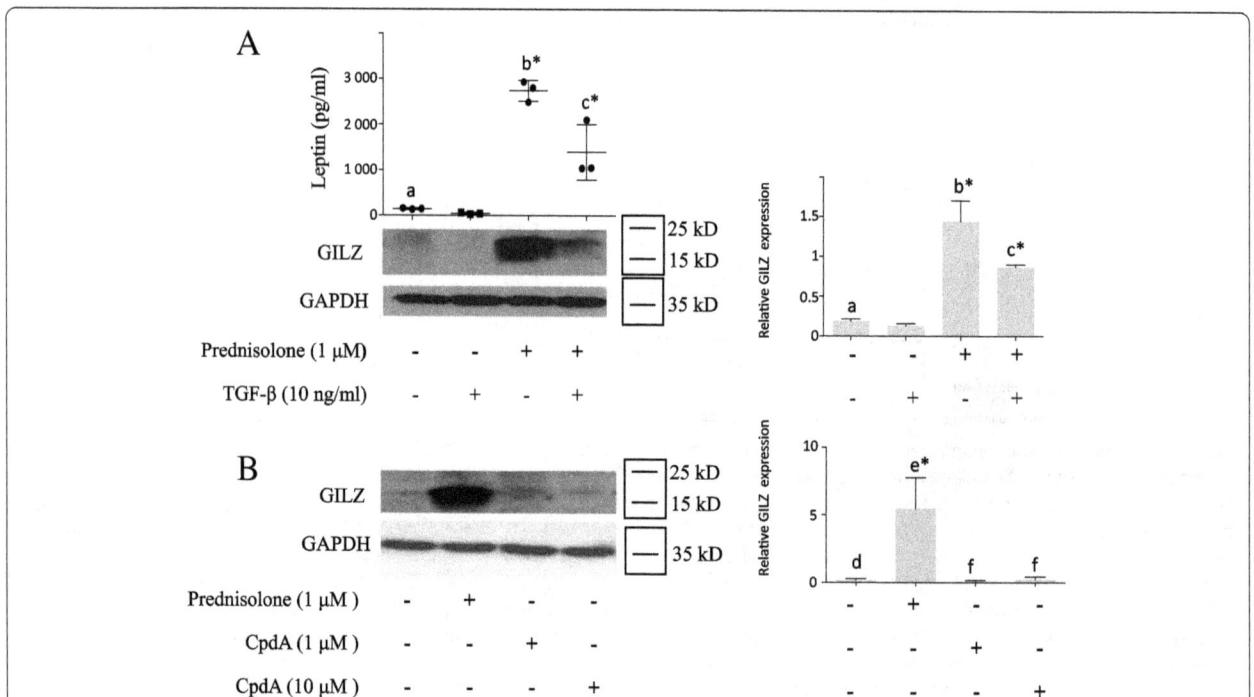

Fig. 6 Transforming growth factor-β (*TGF-β*) decreased both prednisolone-induced leptin secretion and glucocorticoid-induced leucine zipper (*GILZ*) expression; Compound A (*CpdA*) did not induce GILZ expression. Human osteoarthritis (OA) synovial fibroblasts were stimulated for 5 days with prednisolone, TGF-β (**A**), or CpdA (**B**). Leptin expression was measured in the cell culture supernatants by ELISA. GILZ and glyceraldehyde 3-phosphate dehydrogenase (*GAPDH*) expression in whole-cell extracts was analyzed by western blotting. *Right panels*, quantification results of western blots shown in the *left panels*. Protein levels were normalized to GAPDH. Graphs represent mean +/- SD (n = 3 patients). *b**Significantly different from *a*; *c**significantly different from *b*; *e**significantly different from *d*; *f* not significantly different from *d*

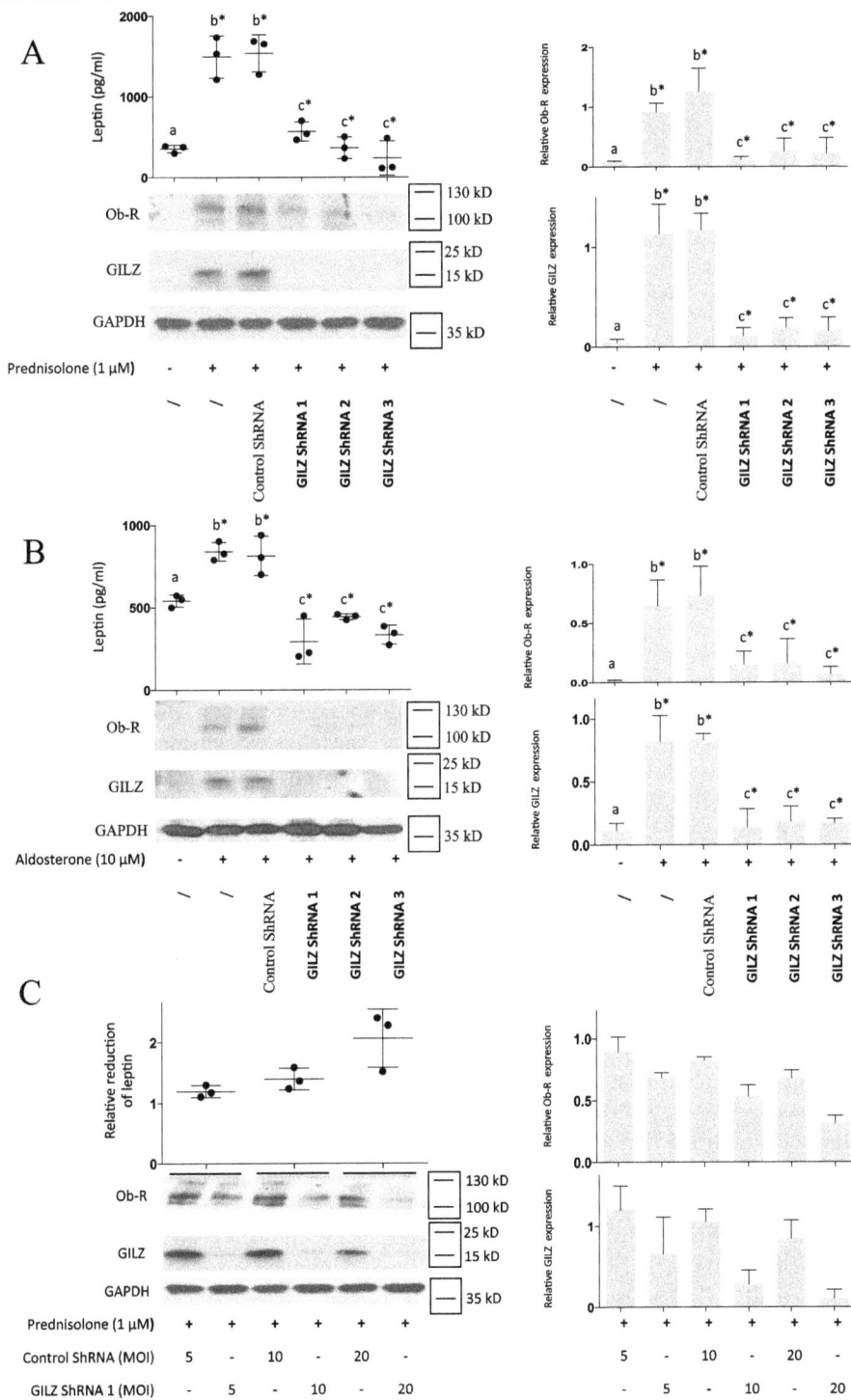

Fig. 7 Glucocorticoid-induced leucine zipper (*GILZ*) silencing inhibited glucocorticoid-induced and mineralocorticoid-induced leptin and leptin receptor (*Ob-R*) expression. Human osteoarthritis (OA) synovial fibroblasts were infected with three different lentiviruses expressing GILZ short hairpin RNA (*shRNA*) or with a control lentivirus (multiplicity of infection (MOI) 30 for **a** and **b**; MOI 5, 10 and 20 for **c**). After 72 h, the cells were stimulated for 5 days with a glucocorticoid (1 μM prednisolone) or mineralocorticoid (10 μM aldosterone). Leptin expression was measured in the cell culture supernatants by ELISA. Ob-R, GILZ and glyceraldehyde 3-phosphate dehydrogenase (*GAPDH*) expression in whole-cell extracts was analyzed by western blotting. *Right panels*, quantification results of western blots shown in the *left panels*. Protein levels were normalized to GAPDH. Graphs represent mean +/- SD (n = 5 patients). *b**Significantly different from *a*; *c**significantly different from *b*. *kD* kiloDalton

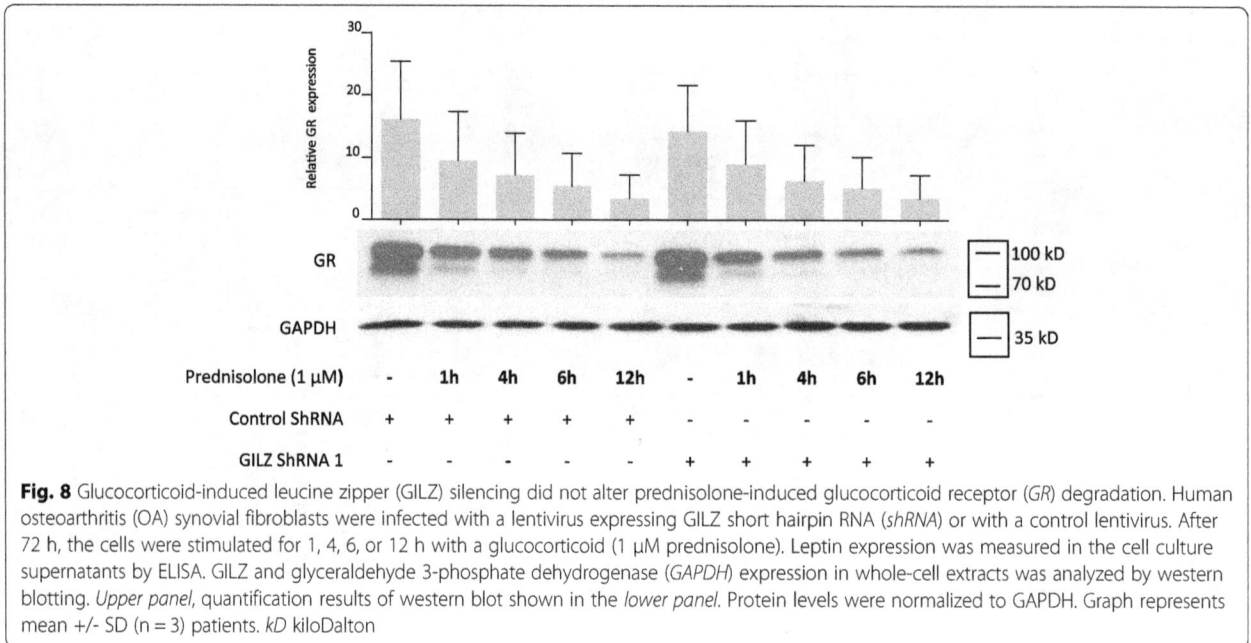

Fig. 8 Glucocorticoid-induced leucine zipper (GILZ) silencing did not alter prednisolone-induced glucocorticoid receptor (GR) degradation. Human osteoarthritis (OA) synovial fibroblasts were infected with a lentivirus expressing GILZ short hairpin RNA (shRNA) or with a control lentivirus. After 72 h, the cells were stimulated for 1, 4, 6, or 12 h with a glucocorticoid (1 μM prednisolone). Leptin expression was measured in the cell culture supernatants by ELISA. GILZ and glyceraldehyde 3-phosphate dehydrogenase (GAPDH) expression in whole-cell extracts was analyzed by western blotting. Upper panel, quantification results of western blot shown in the lower panel. Protein levels were normalized to GAPDH. Graph represents mean +/- SD (n = 3) patients. kD kiloDalton

previously demonstrated that leptin induction occurs independently of any adipogenesis-related processes by performing oil red staining and that it occurs in the absence of adipogenic mediators [19]. Among adipokines, leptin is of particular interest in metabolic OA, as we did not detect any endogenous or glucocorticoid-induced secretion of resistin or adiponectin in OA synovial fibroblasts [23]. The deleterious contribution of leptin to the pathogenesis of metabolic OA [15] indicates that leptin and Ob-R expression in synovial fibroblasts contribute to the adverse metabolic events caused by glucocorticoids. GILZ, leptin and Ob-R protein expression are closely correlated, as demonstrated by the significant reductions in leptin and Ob-R expression following GILZ silencing.

Moreover, we previously reported that TGF-β reduced the prednisolone-induced leptin secretion through ALK5-Smad2/3 [20]. In this work, we observed that TGF-β did not induce GILZ and reduced the prednisolone-induced GILZ expression, which is coherent with our previous results. This is also coherent with previous works in human bronchial epithelial cells, where TGF-β1 impaired the glucocorticoid trans-activation, did not induce GILZ mRNA and even reduced dexamethasone-induced GILZ expression also through ALK5-Smad2/3 [35].

GILZ is primarily described as a mediator of the anti-inflammatory activities of glucocorticoids in immune-related cells [32–34]. GILZ overexpression has significant anti-inflammatory effects in the treatment of collagen-induced arthritis [9, 10]. However, in the current study, GILZ depletion in OA synovial fibroblasts

did not alter either the TNF-α-induced pro-inflammatory protein levels (IL-6, IL-8, and MMP-1) or the capacity for glucocorticoids to downregulate the TNF-α-induced production of IL-6, IL-8, and MMP-1, supporting the notion that GILZ is not significantly involved in the anti-inflammatory regulation of glucocorticoids in OA. GILZ downregulation did not modulate GR expression or GR downregulation. A lack of inflammatory modulation in synovial cells following GILZ down-regulation has also been reported in mouse models of collagen-induced arthritis [9] and in human umbilical venous endothelial cells [10]. Last, although Beaulieu et al. [8] have previously shown that GILZ overexpression significantly inhibits the production of key pro-inflammatory cytokines, such as IL-6 and IL-8, in rheumatoid arthritis synovial fibroblasts, it has no effect on a panel of additional pro-inflammatory cytokines, such as IL-1β, TNF-α, and IL-12p70, which are produced by the same cells. Thus, involvement of GILZ in the inflammatory process appears to be cell-dependent.

In this study, we showed that the SEGRA CpdA (which activates only the trans-repression pathway and has a better benefit-risk ratio than glucocorticoids [22]) did not induce GILZ expression. This finding is consistent with our previous study showing that CpdA does not induce leptin secretion or Ob-R expression and that it exhibits similar anti-inflammatory effects to classical glucocorticoids [23], positioning the leptin secretion in the trans-activation pathway. While GILZ is not necessary for the glucocorticoid anti-inflammatory effect and is involved in leptin secretion, absence of GILZ induction by CpdA seems coherent. This result is also in

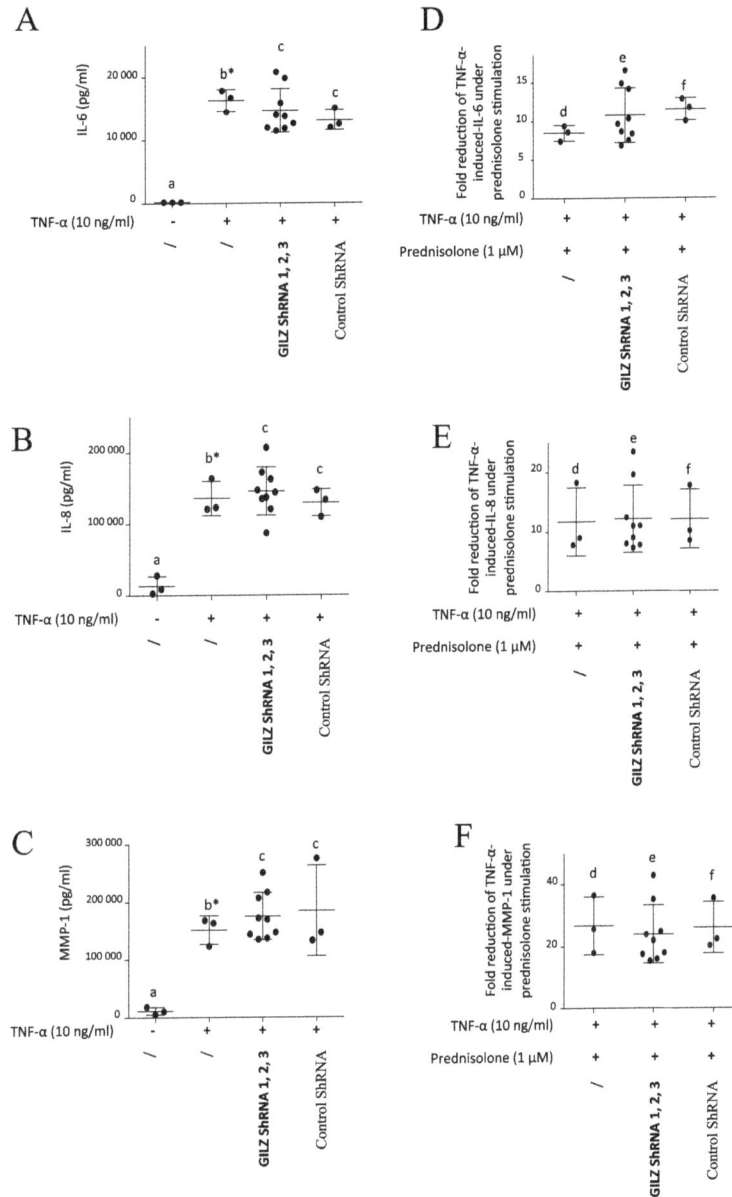

Fig. 9 Glucocorticoid-induced leucine zipper (*GILZ*) inhibition did not alter the capacity for prednisolone to reduce IL-6, IL-8 and matrix metalloproteinase-1 (*MMP-1*) production. Human osteoarthritis (OA) synovial fibroblasts were infected with three different lentiviruses expressing GILZ short hairpin RNA (*shRNA*) or with a control lentivirus (one sample was infected with one shRNA and the three results were pooled). Cells were pre-incubated (**D**, **E**, **F**) or not (**A**, **B**, **C**) for 1 h with prednisolone (1 μM) and were then stimulated or not with TNF-α (10 ng/mL) for 12 h. The IL-6, IL-8 and MMP-1 levels in the cell culture supernatants were measured by ELISA. Graphs represent mean +/- SD (n = 3 patients). Fold reductions in IL-6, IL-8, and MMP-1 induced by TNF-α were measured by comparing the levels in the presence or not of prednisolone (1 μM). *b**Significantly different from *a*; *c* not significantly different from *b*; *e f* not significantly different from *d*

agreement with Drebert et al., who have demonstrated a lack of GILZ induction under CpdA treatment in colon-cancer-derived myofibroblasts [36] and with Gavrila et al. using airway smooth muscle cells [37]. Moreover, other authors have demonstrated that CpdA does not in-duced DUSP1, which is another actor in the glucocortic-oid trans-activation [38].

From a metabolic point of view, it can be hypothesized that GILZ induction is deleterious in OA because it in-duces the adipokine leptin. Additional examples of the involvement of GILZ in glucocorticoid-associated ad-verse events have been reported. Dexamethasone and GILZ have been shown to inhibit the repair of respira-tory epithelial cells [39]. In addition, the long-term use

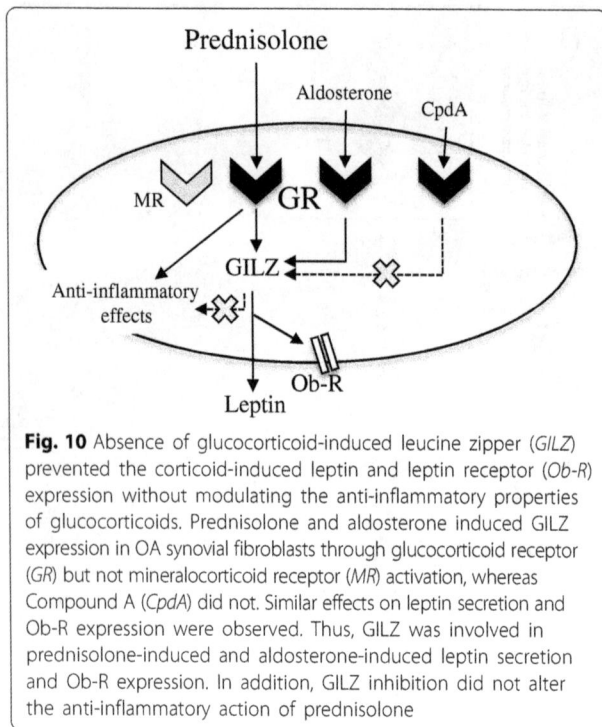

Fig. 10 Absence of glucocorticoid-induced leucine zipper (*GILZ*) prevented the corticoid-induced leptin and leptin receptor (*Ob-R*) expression without modulating the anti-inflammatory properties of glucocorticoids. Prednisolone and aldosterone induced GILZ expression in OA synovial fibroblasts through glucocorticoid receptor (*GR*) but not mineralocorticoid receptor (*MR*) activation, whereas Compound A (*CpdA*) did not. Similar effects on leptin secretion and Ob-R expression were observed. Thus, GILZ was involved in prednisolone-induced and aldosterone-induced leptin secretion and Ob-R expression. In addition, GILZ inhibition did not alter the anti-inflammatory action of prednisolone

of glucocorticoids has been demonstrated to have anti-myogenic effects due to the presence of GILZ as an effector [40].

In the present study, aldosterone, a mineralocorticoid, was also found to be a significant stimulator of GILZ, leptin, and Ob-R expressions. These results are in accordance with those of previous studies showing an in vitro increase in the leptin mRNA level in brown adipose tissue after aldosterone exposure [27] and higher circulating leptin levels in patients with primary hyperaldosteronism [41]. Aldosterone is known for its association with a bad metabolic profile (i.e., its association with the development of metabolic syndrome in humans) [42, 43] and for its aggravation of glucose intolerance by high fructose in rats [44]. It is also present in the synovial fluid of patients with OA [45]. Therefore, targeting the aldosterone pathway could be promising for the treatment of OA.

Corticoid concentrations in synovial fluid have not been well-described. With regard to glucocorticoids, human OA synovial fluid has been reported to contain 125 nM cortisol [45]. Significant induction of leptin, Ob-R, and GILZ expression has been observed at this concentration by prednisolone (a synthetic cortisol compound). Accordingly, the significant effect of glucocorticoids on leptin production in the joints in OA may be clinically relevant, even in the absence of exogenous glucocorticoid administration. However, the mineralocorticoid levels are 1000-fold decreased in biologic fluids compared to the glucocorticoid levels. Although 1 μM

aldosterone has been used in studies with mechanistic models [25], the physiological concentration is approximately 100 pM in OA synovial fluid [45], which was not sufficient to induce leptin or Ob-R expression in our model. Therefore, we cannot affirm that leptin and GILZ induction by aldosterone is clinically relevant. However, the use of 1 μM and 10 μM aldosterone in the current study confirmed the focus of our mechanistic model on the role of GILZ in leptin expression.

The influence of aldosterone on GILZ, leptin and Ob-R expressions is also GR-dependent; indeed, their induction remains unchanged in the presence of specific MR inhibitors, whereas it is abolished in the presence of specific GR inhibitors or after GR silencing. Lee et al. have observed that GR silencing blocks leptin induction by cortisol in human adipocytes, in contrast with MR silencing [46]. Leminen et al. have demonstrated in vivo downregulation of the expression of circulating leptin in humans with the GR inhibitor mifepristone [47]. However, the regulation of leptin by aldosterone appears to be tissue-dependent, and it requires further clarification. In mice with impaired leptin receptor signaling, MR blockade by eplerenone administration in vivo has been shown to reduce leptin mRNA expression in retroperitoneal adipose tissue [48].

Conclusion

In conclusion, we describe a new role for GILZ in the corticoid-induced leptin and Ob-R expression in OA synovial fibroblasts. Absence of GILZ prevents corticoid-induced leptin secretion and Ob-R expression without modulating the anti-inflammatory properties of glucocorticoids in OA synovial fibroblasts (Fig. 10). Regarding the deleterious involvement of leptin in OA pathogenesis, the use of GR agonists that do not activate GILZ pathways when using glucocorticoids should be evaluated.

Abbreviations
BMI: body mass index; CpdA: compound A; DMEM: Dulbecco's modified Eagle's medium; ELISA: enzyme-linked immunosorbent assay; FBS: fetal bovine serum; GAPDH: glyceraldehyde 3-phosphate dehydrogenase; GILZ: glucocorticoid-induced leucine zipper; GR: glucocorticoid receptor; IL: interleukin; MMP: matrix metalloproteinase; MOI: multiplicity of infection; MR: mineralocorticoid receptor; mRNA: messenger RNA; OA: osteoarthritis; Ob-R: leptin receptor; RT-qPCR: quantitative reverse transcription PCR; SD: standard deviation; SEGRA: selective glucocorticoid receptor agonist; shRNA: small hairpin RNA; TGF-β: transforming growth factor-β; TNF-α: tumor necrosis factor-α

Acknowledgements
The authors thank the associates at GIGA Viral Vectors for their expert technical assistance. We also thank the editing service "American Journal Experts" for the professional editing of this manuscript.

Funding
This study was supported by "Fonds Léon-Frédéricq", University of Liège, Belgium, and by "Fonds National pour la Recherche Scientifique" (FNRS), Belgium.

Authors' contributions

OM and BR designed the experiments and the manuscript, performed the *in vitro* experiments, and wrote the manuscript. EC, MZ, CD, and EL wrote the manuscript and made critical revision of the manuscript. SN performed the *in vitro* experiments. PG provided the synovial samples and performed critical revision of the manuscript. MGM and DdS designed the experiments and wrote the manuscript. All authors read and approved the final manuscript.

Authors' information

Not applicable.

Competing interests

All authors of this manuscript have disclosed any financial and personal relationships with other people or organizations that could have potentially and inappropriately influenced their work and conclusions with regard to the present study.

Consent for publication

Not applicable.

Author details

[1]Laboratory of Rheumatology, Arthropôle, GIGA Research, University and CHU of Liège, Liège, Belgium. [2]Department of Orthopedic Surgery, CHU of Liège, Liège, Belgium. [3]Laboratory of Gastroenterology, GIGA Research, University and CHU of Liège, Liège, Belgium.

References

1. Yang N, Zhang W, Shi XM. Glucocorticoid-induced leucine zipper (GILZ) mediates glucocorticoid action and inhibits inflammatory cytokine-induced COX-2 expression. J Cell Biochem. 2008;103(6):1760–71.
2. Yang YH, Aeberli D, Dacumos A, Xue JR, Morand EF. Annexin-1 regulates macrophage IL-6 and TNF via glucocorticoid-induced leucine zipper. J Immunol. 2009;183(2):1435–45.
3. Eddleston J, Herschbach J, Wagelie-Steffen AL, Christiansen SC, Zuraw BL. The anti-inflammatory effect of glucocorticoids is mediated by glucocorticoid-induced leucine zipper in epithelial cells. J Allergy Clin Immunol. 2007;119(1):115–22.
4. Esposito E, Bruscoli S, Mazzon E, et al. Glucocorticoid-induced leucine zipper (GILZ) over-expression in T lymphocytes inhibits inflammation and tissue damage in spinal cord injury. Neurotherapeutics. 2012;9(1):210–25.
5. Luz-Crawford P, Tejedor G, Mausset-Bonnefont AL, et al. Gilz governs the therapeutic potential of mesenchymal stem cells by inducing a switch from pathogenic to regulatory Th17 cells. Arthritis Rheum. 2015;67:1514–24.
6. Frodl T, Carballedo A, Frey EM, et al. Expression of glucocorticoid inducible genes is associated with reductions in cornu ammonis and dentate gyrus volumes in patients with major depressive disorder. Dev Psychopathol. 2014;26(4 Pt 2):1209–17.
7. Bruscoli S, Velardi E, Di Sante M, et al. Long glucocorticoid-induced leucine zipper (L-GILZ) protein interacts with ras protein pathway and contributes to spermatogenesis control. J Biol Chem. 2012;287(2):1242–51.
8. Beaulieu E, Ngo D, Santos L, et al. Glucocorticoid-induced leucine zipper is an endogenous antiinflammatory mediator in arthritis. Arthritis Rheum. 2010;62(9):2651–61.
9. Ngo D, Beaulieu E, Gu R, et al. Divergent effects of endogenous and exogenous glucocorticoid-induced leucine zipper in animal models of inflammation and arthritis. Arthritis Rheum. 2013;65(5):1203–12.
10. Cheng Q, Fan H, Ngo D, et al. GILZ overexpression inhibits endothelial cell adhesive function through regulation of NF-kappaB and MAPK activity. J Immunol. 2013;191(1):424–33.
11. Oliveria SA, Felson DT, Cirillo PA, Reed JI, Walker AM. Body weight, body mass index, and incident symptomatic osteoarthritis of the hand, hip, and knee. Epidemiology. 1999;10(2):161–6.
12. Yoshimura N, Muraki S, Oka H, et al. Accumulation of metabolic risk factors such as overweight, hypertension, dyslipidaemia, and impaired glucose tolerance raises the risk of occurrence and progression of knee osteoarthritis: a 3-year follow-up of the ROAD study. Osteoarthritis and cartilage/OARS, Osteoarthritis Research Society. 2012;20(11):1217–26.
13. Dumond H, Presle N, Terlain B, et al. Evidence for a key role of leptin in osteoarthritis. Arthritis Rheum. 2003;48(11):3118–29.
14. Stannus OP, Cao Y, Antony B, et al. Cross-sectional and longitudinal associations between circulating leptin and knee cartilage thickness in older adults. Ann Rheum Dis. 2015;74(1):82–8.
15. Griffin TM, Huebner JL, Kraus VB, Guilak F. Extreme obesity due to impaired leptin signaling in mice does not cause knee osteoarthritis. Arthritis Rheum. 2009;60(10):2935–44.
16. Vuolteenaho K, Koskinen A, Moilanen T, Moilanen E. Leptin levels are increased and its negative regulators, SOCS-3 and sOb-R are decreased in obese patients with osteoarthritis: a link between obesity and osteoarthritis. Ann Rheum Dis. 2012;71(11):1912–3.
17. Yang WH, Liu SC, Tsai CH, et al. Leptin induces IL-6 expression through OBRl receptor signaling pathway in human synovial fibroblasts. PLoS One. 2013;8(9), e75551.
18. Koskinen A, Vuolteenaho K, Nieminen R, Moilanen T, Moilanen E. Leptin enhances MMP-1, MMP-3 and MMP-13 production in human osteoarthritic cartilage and correlates with MMP-1 and MMP-3 in synovial fluid from OA patients. Clin Exp Rheumatol. 2011;29(1):57–64.
19. Relic B, Zeddou M, Desoroux A, Beguin Y, de Seny D, Malaise MG. Genistein induces adipogenesis but inhibits leptin induction in human synovial fibroblasts. Laboratory investigation; a journal of technical methods and pathology. 2009;89(7):811–22.
20. Zeddou M, Relic B, Malaise O, et al. Differential signalling through ALK-1 and ALK-5 regulates leptin expression in mesenchymal stem cells. Stem Cells Dev. 2012;21(11):1948–55.
21. Sundahl N, Bridelance J, Libert C, De Bosscher K, Beck IM. Selective glucocorticoid receptor modulation: new directions with non-steroidal scaffolds. Pharmacol Ther. 2015;152:28–41.
22. Schacke H, Berger M, Rehwinkel H, Asadullah K. Selective glucocorticoid receptor agonists (SEGRAs): novel ligands with an improved therapeutic index. Mol Cell Endocrinol. 2007;275(1-2):109–17.
23. Malaise O, Relic B, Quesada-Calvo F, et al. Selective glucocorticoid receptor modulator compound A, in contrast to prednisolone, does not induce leptin or the leptin receptor in human osteoarthritis synovial fibroblasts. Rheumatology. 2014;54:1087–92.
24. Sun B, Chamarthi B, Williams JS, et al. Different polymorphisms of the mineralocorticoid receptor gene are associated with either glucocorticoid or mineralocorticoid levels in hypertension. J Clin Endocrinol Metab. 2012;97(9):E1825–9.
25. Ren R, Oakley RH, Cruz-Topete D, Cidlowski JA. Dual role for glucocorticoids in cardiomyocyte hypertrophy and apoptosis. Endocrinology. 2012;153(11):5346–60.
26. Takahashi K, Murase T, Takatsu M, et al. Roles of oxidative stress and the mineralocorticoid receptor in cardiac pathology in a rat model of metabolic syndrome. Nagoya J Med Sci. 2015;77(1-2):275–89.
27. Kraus D, Jager J, Meier B, Fasshauer M, Klein J. Aldosterone inhibits uncoupling protein-1, induces insulin resistance, and stimulates proinflammatory adipokines in adipocytes. Horm Metab Res. 2005;37(7):455–9.
28. Ueda K, Fujiki K, Shirahige K, et al. Genome-wide analysis of murine renal distal convoluted tubular cells for the target genes of mineralocorticoid receptor. Biochem Biophys Res Commun. 2014;445(1):132–7.
29. Bellamy N, Campbell J, Robinson V, Gee T, Bourne R, Wells G. Intraarticular corticosteroid for treatment of osteoarthritis of the knee. Cochrane Database Syst Rev. 2006;(2):CD005328.
30. Celeste C, Ionescu M, Robin Poole A, Laverty S. Repeated intraarticular injections of triamcinolone acetonide alter cartilage matrix metabolism measured by biomarkers in synovial fluid. J Orthop Res. 2005;23(3):602–10.
31. Fubini SL, Todhunter RJ, Burton-Wurster N, Vernier-Singer M, MacLeod JN. Corticosteroids alter the differentiated phenotype of articular chondrocytes. J Orthop Res. 2001;19(4):688–95.
32. Riccardi C, Bruscoli S, Ayroldi E, Agostini M, Migliorati G. GILZ, a glucocorticoid hormone induced gene, modulates T lymphocytes activation and death through interaction with NF-kB. Adv Exp Med Biol. 2001;495:31–9.
33. Ayroldi E, Migliorati G, Bruscoli S, et al. Modulation of T-cell activation by the glucocorticoid-induced leucine zipper factor via inhibition of nuclear factor kappaB. Blood. 2001;98(3):743–53.
34. Berrebi D, Bruscoli S, Cohen N, et al. Synthesis of glucocorticoid-induced leucine zipper (GILZ) by macrophages: an anti-inflammatory and immunosuppressive mechanism shared by glucocorticoids and IL-10. Blood. 2003;101(2):729–38.

35. Keenan CR, Mok JS, Harris T, Xia Y, Salem S, Stewart AG. Bronchial epithelial cells are rendered insensitive to glucocorticoid transactivation by transforming growth factor-beta1. Respir Res. 2014;15:55.

36. Drebert Z, Bracke M, Beck IM. Glucocorticoids and the non-steroidal selective glucocorticoid receptor modulator, compound A, differentially affect colon cancer-derived myofibroblasts. J Steroid Biochem Mol Biol. 2015;149:92–105.

37. Gavrila A, Chachi L, Tliba O, Brightling C, Amrani Y. Effect of the plant derivative Compound A on the production of corticosteroid-resistant chemokines in airway smooth muscle cells. Am J Respir Cell Mol Biol. 2015; 53(5):728–37.

38. Reber LL, Daubeuf F, Plantinga M, et al. A dissociated glucocorticoid receptor modulator reduces airway hyperresponsiveness and inflammation in a mouse model of asthma. J Immunol. 2012;188(7):3478–87.

39. Liu J, Zhang M, Niu C, et al. Dexamethasone inhibits repair of human airway epithelial cells mediated by glucocorticoid-induced leucine zipper (GILZ). PLoS One. 2013;8(4), e60705.

40. Bruscoli S, Donato V, Velardi E, et al. Glucocorticoid-induced leucine zipper (GILZ) and long GILZ inhibit myogenic differentiation and mediate anti-myogenic effects of glucocorticoids. J Biol Chem. 2010;285(14):10385–96.

41. Iacobellis G, Petramala L, Cotesta D, et al. Adipokines and cardiometabolic profile in primary hyperaldosteronism. J Clin Endocrinol Metab. 2010;95(5): 2391–8.

42. Musani SK, Vasan RS, Bidulescu A, et al. Aldosterone, C-reactive protein, and plasma B-type natriuretic peptide are associated with the development of metabolic syndrome and longitudinal changes in metabolic syndrome components: findings from the Jackson Heart Study. Diabetes Care. 2013; 36(10):3084–92.

43. Cooper JN, Fried L, Tepper P, et al. Changes in serum aldosterone are associated with changes in obesity-related factors in normotensive overweight and obese young adults. Hypertens Res. 2013;36(10):895–901.

44. Sherajee SJ, Rafiq K, Nakano D, et al. Aldosterone aggravates glucose intolerance induced by high fructose. Eur J Pharmacol. 2013;720(1-3):63–8.

45. Rovensky J, Kvetnansky R, Radikova Z, et al. Hormone concentrations in synovial fluid of patients with rheumatoid arthritis. Clin Exp Rheumatol. 2005;23(3):292–6.

46. Lee MJ, Fried SK. The glucocorticoid receptor, not the mineralocorticoid receptor, plays the dominant role in adipogenesis and adipokine production in human adipocytes. Int J Obes (Lond). 2014;38(9):1228–33.

47. Leminen R, Raivio T, Ranta S, et al. Late follicular phase administration of mifepristone suppresses circulating leptin and FSH - mechanism(s) of action in emergency contraception? Eur J Endocrinol. 2005;152(3):411–8.

48. Guo C, Ricchiuti V, Lian BQ, et al. Mineralocorticoid receptor blockade reverses obesity-related changes in expression of adiponectin, peroxisome proliferator-activated receptor-gamma, and proinflammatory adipokines. Circulation. 2008;117(17):2253–61.

CCL17 blockade as a therapy for osteoarthritis pain and disease

Ming-Chin Lee[1], Reem Saleh[1], Adrian Achuthan[1], Andrew J. Fleetwood[1], Irmgard Förster[2], John A. Hamilton[1] and Andrew D. Cook[1*]

Abstract

Background: Granulocyte macrophage-colony stimulating factor (GM-CSF) has been implicated in the pathogenesis of a number of inflammatory diseases and in osteoarthritis (OA). We identified previously a new GM-CSF→Jmjd3→interferon regulatory factor 4 (IRF4)→chemokine (c-c motif) ligand 17 (CCL17) pathway, which is important for the development of inflammatory arthritis pain and disease. Tumour necrosis factor (TNF) can also be linked with this pathway. Here we investigated the involvement of the pathway in OA pain and disease development using the GM-CSF-dependent collagenase-induced OA (CiOA) model.

Methods: CiOA was induced in C57BL/6 wild-type (WT), $Irf4^{-/-}$, $Ccl17^{E/E}$, $Ccr4^{-/-}$, $Tnf^{-/-}$ and $GM\text{-}CSF^{-/-}$ mice. Additionally, therapeutic targeting of CCL17, Jmjd3 and cyclooxygenase 2 (COX-2) was evaluated. Development of pain (assessment of weight distribution) and OA disease (histologic scoring of synovitis, cartilage destruction and osteophyte size) were assessed. Synovial joint cells, including neutrophils, macrophages, fibroblasts and endothelial cells, were isolated (cell sorting) and gene expression analyzed (quantitative PCR).

Results: Studies in the gene-deficient mice indicated that IRF4, CCL17 and the CCL17 receptor, CCR4, but not TNF, were required for CiOA pain and optimal cartilage destruction and osteophyte size. Therapeutic neutralization of CCL17 and Jmjd3 ameliorated both pain and disease, whereas the COX-2 inhibitor only ameliorated pain. In the synovium $Ccl17$ mRNA was expressed only in the macrophages in a GM-CSF-dependent and IRF4-dependent manner.

Conclusions: The GM-CSF→Jmjd3→IRF4→CCL17 pathway is important for the development of CiOA, with CCL17 thus being a potential therapeutic target for the treatment of both OA pain and disease.

Keywords: Osteoarthritis, CCL17, Inflammation, Targeting, Animal models

Background

Osteoarthritis (OA) is the most common musculoskeletal disorder, characterized by chronic joint pain and substantial functional impairment [1]. Although OA has historically not been considered an inflammatory condition, a growing body of evidence supports the involvement of synovial inflammation in the observed cartilage degradation and bone erosion [2–6]. Proinflammatory cytokines are likely to be critical in driving such inflammation.

The collagenase-induced OA (CiOA) model involves the induction of joint instability by intra-articular injection of collagenase [7, 8] leading to joint damage, including cartilage matrix breakdown [9, 10], macrophage-mediated osteophyte formation [11, 12], as well as pain [8, 13], thereby mimicking features of the human disease [14]. We have previously demonstrated that granulocyte macrophage-colony stimulating factor (GM-CSF) is a key mediator in the CiOA model [8]. Both prophylactic, and notably therapeutic, blockade of GM-CSF using a neutralizing monoclonal antibody (mAb) have been shown to be effective at ameliorating CiOA-induced pain and disease [8]. As a result there is a current phase II trial in hand OA using this approach [15].

In addition to OA, GM-CSF has been implicated in the development of inflammatory pain and arthritic pain and disease [16–19], and blockade of GM-CSF and its receptor are currently showing promise in rheumatoid arthritis (RA) trials [15]. Regarding the mode of action

* Correspondence: adcook@unimelb.edu.au
[1]The University of Medicine, Department of Medicine, Royal Melbourne Hospital, Parkville, VIC 3050, Australia
Full list of author information is available at the end of the article

of GM-CSF, we have recently reported that GM-CSF induces the chemokine, chemokine (c-c motif) ligand 17 (CCL17), via Jmjd3-regulated interferon regulatory factor 4 (IRF4), to mediate inflammation, and that blockade of CCL17 can ameliorate GM-CSF-dependent inflammatory pain and arthritic pain and disease [18]. Furthermore, models in which tumour necrosis factor (TNF) is necessary can utilize this pathway [20].

In the current study we provide evidence that the GM-CSF→Jmjd3→IRF4→CCL17 pathway, originally identified in human and murine monocytes/macrophages [18], is required for CiOA pain and optimal arthritis development; however TNF is not involved.

Methods

Mice

The following were used: $Tnf^{-/-}$ [21], $Ccr4^{-/-}$ [22], GM-$CSF^{-/-}$ (from Ludwig Institute for Cancer Research) [23], $Irf4^{-/-}$ (from TW Mak) [24] and $Ccl17$ gene-deficient ($Ccl17^{E/E}$) mice (in which both copies of $Ccl17$ have been replaced by enhanced green fluorescent protein (EGFP)) [25], all backcrossed onto the C57BL/6 background (from the Walter and Eliza Hall Institute). Mice were fed standard rodent chow and water ad libitum. Mice of both sexes (8–12 weeks) were used; experiments were approved by The University of Melbourne Animal Ethics Committee.

CiOA

CiOA was induced as published [8, 26]. Briefly, mice received an intra-articular injection of one unit of collagenase type VII (Sigma-Aldrich) on days 0 and 2 to induce joint instability. At various time points, knee joints were collected for histology or cell isolation.

Pain reading

As a validated indicator of arthritic knee pain, the differential distribution of weight between the inflamed limb relative to the non-inflamed limb was measured using an incapacitance meter (IITC Life Science Inc, USA) [8, 17, 18, 27, 28]. Three measurements were taken for each time point and averaged.

Therapeutic treatment

Mice with CiOA were treated therapeutically, beginning once pain was evident (days 20–23), with (i) anti-mouse CCL17 mAb (150 μg intraperitoneal (i.p.), clone 110,904, R&D Systems) or isotype control mAb (GL117.41, Schering BioPharma) given twice weekly, (ii) the Jmjd3 inhibitor, GSK-J4 (0.5 mg/kg i.p., Santa Cruz Biotechnology), or vehicle (dimethyl sulfoxide (DMSO)) given daily for 5 days followed by twice weekly or (iii) the cyclooxygenase 2 (COX-2) inhibitor, SC58125 (1 mg/kg i.p., Tocris), or vehicle (DMSO) given weekly.

Histologic assessment

At termination, the knee joints were removed, fixed, decalcified and paraffin embedded as described previously [8, 18, 28]. Week-2 frontal sections (7 μm) were cut at various depths, stained with H&E and scored for synovitis from 0 (normal) to 3 (severe), as described before [8]. As previously published [8, 26, 29], week-6 sections were cut at various depths, stained with safranin O and fast green and scored for cartilage damage in terms of the OA depth into cartilage (grade) from 0 (normal) to 6 (bone loss, remodelling, deformation), and amount of cartilage affected (stage), from 0 (< 10% involvement) to 5 (> 75% involvement), in the lateral tibia (LT), lateral femur (LF), medial tibia (MT) and medial femur (MF) — the grade and stage values were multiplied to give an OA score. Three sections per knee joint at different depths were scored and the average OA score per joint region was calculated. This scoring is a more detailed version of the Osteoarthritis Research Society International (OARSI) scoring system for the mouse [30]. Finally, for each mouse, the OA scores from the LT, LF, MT and MF were also averaged to give a mean histologic score. Osteophyte size was assessed using ImageJ software (National Institutes of Health, Bethesda, MD, USA) [8].

Cell sorting

Joint tissues were harvested from CiOA mice and digested with 1 mg/kg collagenase IV (Worthington, USA), 0.5 mg/kg dispase (Worthington) and 1 μg/ml DNase (Sigma-Aldrich) in serum-free medium for 1 h at 37 °C. Fc receptors on isolated cells were blocked with normal mouse serum (1/4 dilution) and cells were stained with fluorochrome-conjugated mAbs specific for mouse CD45-PerCP-Cy5.5 (clone OX-1) and CD11b-APC-Cy7 (clone M1/70) (BD Biosciences), Ly6G-PE-Cy7 (clone 1A8), CD64-PE (clone X54-5/7.1), F4/80-BV421 (clone BM8) and CD31-BV605™ (clone 390) (Biolegend), MEFSK-4-APC (clone mEF-SK4) (Miltenyi Biotec) and the corresponding isotype controls. Cells were sorted on a fluorescence-activated cell sorting (FACS) Aria II (BD Biosciences) directly into RLY lysis buffer (Bioline) for mRNA expression analysis.

Quantitative PCR

Quantitative PCR was performed as previously described [18, 28]. Briefly, total RNA was extracted from sorted joint cells using Isolate II RNA Mini Kit (Bioline) and reverse transcribed using Tetro Reverse Transcriptase (Bioline). Quantitative PCR (qPCR) was performed using the ABI Prism 7900HT sequence detection system (Applied Biosystems) and pre-developed TaqMan probe/primer combinations for murine $Col1a1$, $Ccl17$, $Ccr4$, $Mmp3$, $Mmp13$ and Ubc (Life Technologies). Threshold cycle numbers were transformed to difference in cycle threshold

(ΔCt) values, and the results expressed relative to the reference gene, *Ubc*.

Statistics

Pain readings were analyzed using two-way analysis of variance (ANOVA). Histologic scores and osteophyte size were analyzed using one-way ANOVA or the Mann-Whitney two-sample rank test. Gene expression was analyzed using one-way ANOVA. Data are expressed as mean $\pm$ SEM; $p \leq 0.05$ was considered statistically significant.

Results

Both IRF4 and CCL17 are required for CiOA pain and optimal disease development

We have shown that CiOA pain and disease development are GM-CSF dependent [8]. We have also reported that both GM-CSF-driven inflammatory pain and arthritis models (using exogenous GM-CSF) [17, 18], and GM-CSF-dependent inflammatory pain and arthritis models

(e.g. zymosan-induced arthritis (ZIA)) are dependent on IRF4 and CCL17 [18], and on TNF [20]. Given these prior observations, we first determined whether arthritic pain and disease in the CiOA model are also dependent on TNF, IRF4 and/or CCL17.

CiOA was induced in *Tnf*$^{-/-}$, *Irf4*$^{-/-}$ and *Ccl17* gene-deficient (*Ccl17*$^{E/E}$) mice and pain monitored over a 6-week period as previously described [8, 17, 18], by a change in weight distribution (using an incapacitance meter). As before [8], C57BL/6 WT mice developed pain around 3 weeks post collagenase injection; *Tnf*$^{-/-}$ mice developed a similar degree of pain with similar kinetics, whereas neither *Irf4*$^{-/-}$ nor *Ccl17*$^{E/E}$ mice had any detectable pain (Fig. 1a). The collagenase-injected joints were evaluated histologically at 6 weeks (Fig. 1b) and disease was scored according to the published protocol [8]. While *Tnf*$^{-/-}$ and WT mice had comparable scores, both *Irf4*$^{-/-}$ and *Ccl17*$^{E/E}$ mice had less arthritis compared to WT mice, with the mean score significantly

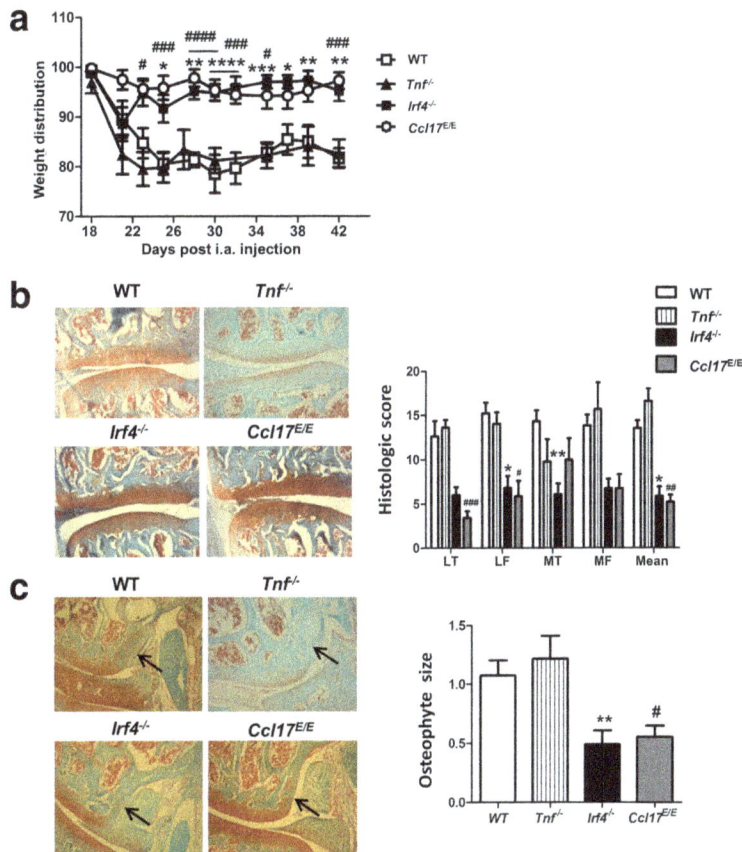

Fig. 1 Interferon regulatory factor 4 (IRF4) and chemokine (c-c motif) ligand 17 (CCL17), but not TNF, are required for collagenase-induced osteoarthritis (CiOA) pain and optimal disease development. CiOA was induced in wild-type (WT), *Tnf*$^{-/-}$, *Irf4*$^{-/-}$ and *Ccl17*$^{E/E}$ mice by intra-articular collagenase injection (see "Methods"). **a** Pain (change in weight distribution; see "Methods") was monitored over time. **b** Representative histologic pictures of knee joints (Safranin O/fast green stain, original magnification ×100) and quantification of arthritis at day 42. **c** Representative histologic pictures of osteophytes (indicated by arrow) (Safranin O/fast green stain; original magnification ×100) and quantification of osteophyte size. Results are expressed as the mean $\pm$ SEM; n = 5–10 mice per strain (from two independent experiments). i.a., intra-articular; LT, lateral tibia; LF, lateral femur; MT, medial tibia; MF, medial femur. *$p < 0.05$, **$p < 0.01$, ***$p < 0.001$, ****$p < 0.0001$, WT vs. *Irf4*$^{-/-}$ mice. #$p < 0.05$, ##$p < 0.01$, ###$p < 0.001$, WT vs. *Ccl17*$^{E/E}$ mice

lower for both strains compared to that observed in WT mice (Fig. 1b). Likewise, osteophyte size was similar in $Tnf^{-/-}$ and WT mice, and was reduced in both $Irf4^{-/-}$ and $Ccl17^{E/E}$ mice (Fig. 1c).

Since C-C motif chemokine receptor 4 (CCR4) is usually considered to be the receptor for CCL17 [31], we also examined whether $Ccr4^{-/-}$ mice are resistant to CiOA pain and disease development. $Ccr4^{-/-}$ mice did not develop CiOA-induced arthritic pain (Fig. 2a) and also had

significantly less overall disease and a reduction in osteophyte size (Fig. 2b and c, respectively) than WT mice.

The data above indicate that in addition to GM-CSF [8], both IRF4 and CCL17, the latter acting via CCR4, are required for CiOA pain and disease development and are consistent with our GM-CSF→IRF4→CCL17 pathway [18] being important in the CiOA model; however, TNF is not required.

Therapeutic neutralization of CCL17 ameliorates CiOA pain and disease development

We evaluated next whether targeting CCL17 therapeutically, and therefore of potential clinical relevance, would suppress CiOA-induced pain and disease as we found previously for GM-CSF [8]. Following CiOA induction, once pain was evident (day 20), WT mice were treated with either PBS, isotype mAb or anti-CCL17 mAb until week 6. PBS-treated or isotype-treated mice continued to exhibit pain whereas pain was rapidly reversed in mice receiving anti-CCL17 mAb (Fig. 3a). This abolition of pain was maintained until week 6 (Fig. 3a). By histologic assessment, at 6 weeks the anti-CCL17 mAb-treated mice also had significantly milder disease and a reduction in osteophyte size compared to isotype-treated mice (Fig. 3b and c, respectively).

Therapeutic inhibition of Jmjd3 ameliorates both CiOA pain and disease development

GM-CSF [8] and IRF4 (Fig. 1) are required for the development of CiOA arthritic pain and disease; also GM-CSF regulates IRF4 expression via Jmjd3 in human monocytes [18], $Irf4$ being a direct target of Jmjd3-mediated demethylation [18, 32]. We thus examined whether the Jmjd3 inhibitor, GSK-J4 [18], could also reverse CiOA pain and disease. Following CiOA induction, when pain was evident (day 20), mice were treated with either PBS, vehicle (DMSO) or GSK-J4 until week 6. Treatment with PBS or DMSO had no effect on CiOA-induced pain; however, GSK-J4 treatment reversed it (Fig. 4a). Likewise, on histologic assessment arthritis development was lower and osteophyte size reduced in the GSK-J4-treated mice compared to vehicle-treated mice (Fig. 4b and c, respectively).

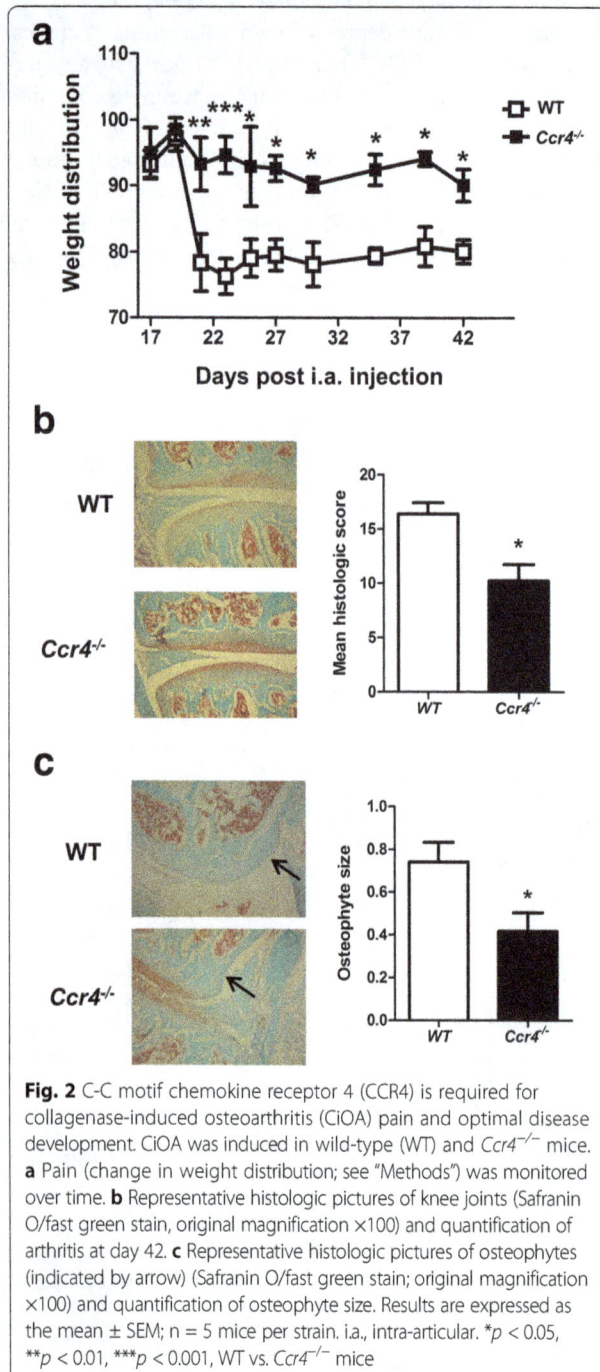

Fig. 2 C-C motif chemokine receptor 4 (CCR4) is required for collagenase-induced osteoarthritis (CiOA) pain and optimal disease development. CiOA was induced in wild-type (WT) and $Ccr4^{-/-}$ mice. **a** Pain (change in weight distribution; see "Methods") was monitored over time. **b** Representative histologic pictures of knee joints (Safranin O/fast green stain, original magnification ×100) and quantification of arthritis at day 42. **c** Representative histologic pictures of osteophytes (indicated by arrow) (Safranin O/fast green stain; original magnification ×100) and quantification of osteophyte size. Results are expressed as the mean ± SEM; n = 5 mice per strain. i.a., intra-articular. *$p < 0.05$, **$p < 0.01$, ***$p < 0.001$, WT vs. $Ccr4^{-/-}$ mice

Therapeutic inhibition of COX-2 ameliorates CiOA pain but not disease development

Given that inflammatory arthritis models requiring the GM-CSF→IRF4→CCL17 pathway were COX-dependent [18], we assessed whether CiOA was COX-2-dependent. When CiOA-induced pain was evident (day 23), mice were treated with the COX-2 inhibitor, SC58128, or vehicle (DMSO). SC58128 rapidly reversed the pain (Fig. 5a); however, by histology it had no effect on arthritis development or osteophyte size at 6 weeks (Fig. 5b and c, respectively).

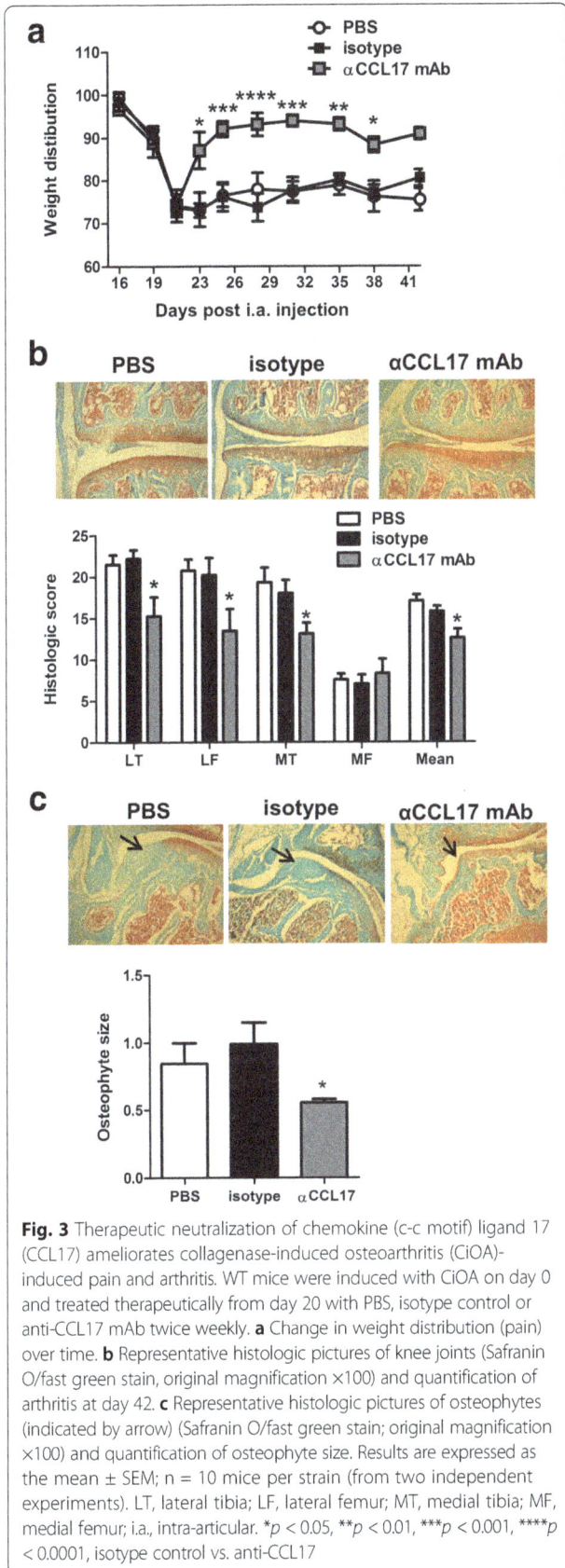

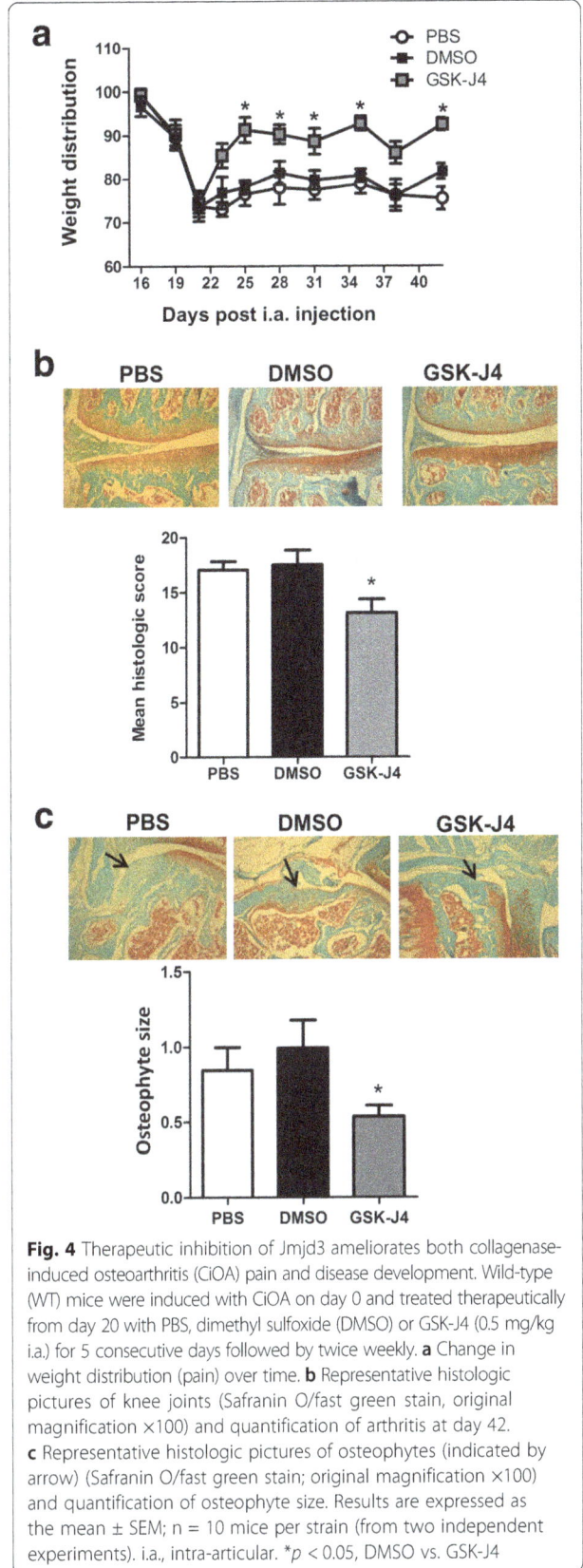

Fig. 3 Therapeutic neutralization of chemokine (c-c motif) ligand 17 (CCL17) ameliorates collagenase-induced osteoarthritis (CiOA)-induced pain and arthritis. WT mice were induced with CiOA on day 0 and treated therapeutically from day 20 with PBS, isotype control or anti-CCL17 mAb twice weekly. **a** Change in weight distribution (pain) over time. **b** Representative histologic pictures of knee joints (Safranin O/fast green stain, original magnification ×100) and quantification of arthritis at day 42. **c** Representative histologic pictures of osteophytes (indicated by arrow) (Safranin O/fast green stain; original magnification ×100) and quantification of osteophyte size. Results are expressed as the mean ± SEM; n = 10 mice per strain (from two independent experiments). LT, lateral tibia; LF, lateral femur; MT, medial tibia; MF, medial femur; i.a., intra-articular. *$p < 0.05$, **$p < 0.01$, ***$p < 0.001$, ****$p < 0.0001$, isotype control vs. anti-CCL17

Fig. 4 Therapeutic inhibition of Jmjd3 ameliorates both collagenase-induced osteoarthritis (CiOA) pain and disease development. Wild-type (WT) mice were induced with CiOA on day 0 and treated therapeutically from day 20 with PBS, dimethyl sulfoxide (DMSO) or GSK-J4 (0.5 mg/kg i.a.) for 5 consecutive days followed by twice weekly. **a** Change in weight distribution (pain) over time. **b** Representative histologic pictures of knee joints (Safranin O/fast green stain, original magnification ×100) and quantification of arthritis at day 42. **c** Representative histologic pictures of osteophytes (indicated by arrow) (Safranin O/fast green stain; original magnification ×100) and quantification of osteophyte size. Results are expressed as the mean ± SEM; n = 10 mice per strain (from two independent experiments). i.a., intra-articular. *$p < 0.05$, DMSO vs. GSK-J4

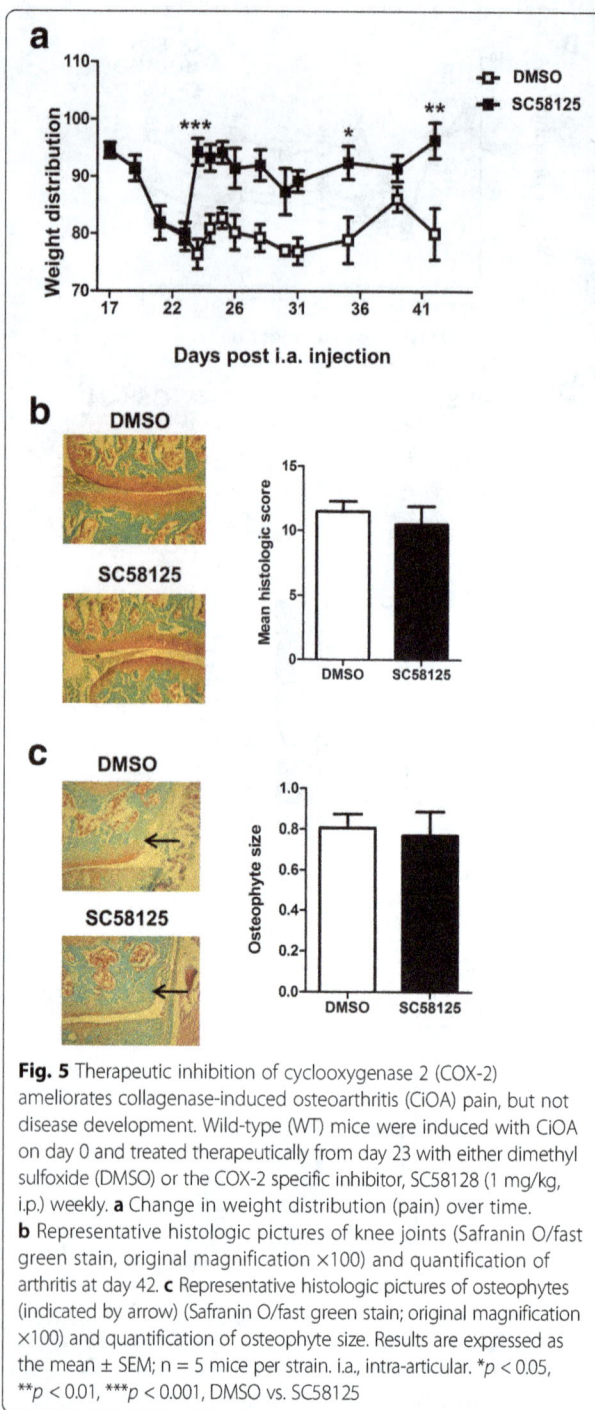

Fig. 5 Therapeutic inhibition of cyclooxygenase 2 (COX-2) ameliorates collagenase-induced osteoarthritis (CiOA) pain, but not disease development. Wild-type (WT) mice were induced with CiOA on day 0 and treated therapeutically from day 23 with either dimethyl sulfoxide (DMSO) or the COX-2 specific inhibitor, SC58128 (1 mg/kg, i.p.) weekly. **a** Change in weight distribution (pain) over time. **b** Representative histologic pictures of knee joints (Safranin O/fast green stain, original magnification ×100) and quantification of arthritis at day 42. **c** Representative histologic pictures of osteophytes (indicated by arrow) (Safranin O/fast green stain; original magnification ×100) and quantification of osteophyte size. Results are expressed as the mean ± SEM; n = 5 mice per strain. i.a., intra-articular. *$p < 0.05$, **$p < 0.01$, ***$p < 0.001$, DMSO vs. SC58125

CCL17 is expressed in CiOA synovial macrophages and regulated by IRF4 and GM-CSF

Since synovitis in OA is often associated with greater symptoms such as pain and joint dysfunction and may promote more rapid cartilage degeneration [33] we explored a role for IRF4 and CCL17 in early synovitis in CiOA. The transient synovitis in CiOA was previously found to be GM-CSF dependent, being virtually absent in $GM\text{-}CSF^{-/-}$ mice [8]. As expected, mild synovitis was

observed in WT mice at 1 (data not shown) and 2 (Fig. 6a) weeks post CiOA induction [8]; interestingly, $Irf4^{-/-}$ mice, but not $Ccl17^{E/E}$ mice, had a slight reduction in synovitis (Fig. 6a).

In order to examine whether there was a difference in cell populations present during synovitis in the absence of IRF4 or CCL17, the synovial cell populations present at day 7 post CiOA induction from WT, $Irf4^{-/-}$ and $Ccl17^{E/E}$ mice were analysed by flow cytometry; $GM\text{-}CSF^{-/-}$ mice were also included. Cells were identified as follows: CD45$^+$ cells - neutrophils (CD11b$^+$Ly6G$^+$) and macrophages (CD11b$^+$Ly6G$^-$F4/80$^+$CD64$^+$); CD45$^-$ cells - endothelial cells (CD31$^+$mEF-SK4$^-$), fibroblasts (CD31$^-$mEF-SK4$^+$) and other cells (CD31$^-$mEF-SK4$^-$) (Additional file 1 A) [34, 35]. The percentage of synovial neutrophils, but not of the other cell populations defined above, was reduced in the synovial cell populations from both $Irf4^{-/-}$ and $GM\text{-}CSF^{-/-}$ mice compared to WT mice, whereas no differences were seen in $Ccl17^{E/E}$ mice compared to WT mice (Additional file 2).

The synovial cells were sorted to determine which populations were producing CCL17 at the mRNA level. To confirm CD45$^-$CD31$^-$mEF-SK4$^+$ cells were fibroblasts, the fibroblast-associated $Col1a1$ gene was found only in this population (Additional file 1 B). Consistent with our prior in vitro and in vivo data [18]), $Ccl17$ mRNA was detected exclusively in macrophages from WT mice but was not present in the macrophages from $Irf4^{-/-}$ or $GM\text{-}CSF^{-/-}$ mice (Fig. 6b); $Ccr4$ mRNA expression was widely expressed but predominantly in fibroblasts and endothelial cells (data not shown).

To determine whether the synovial cells from the different gene-deficient mice also had reduced mRNA expression for other genes compared to the synovial cells from WT mice, we examined certain genes implicated in the breakdown of extracellular matrices [36]. $Mmp3$ (stromelysin-1) mRNA and $Mmp13$ (collagenase-3) mRNA (Additional file 1 C and D, respectively) were exclusively expressed in fibroblasts, with lower expression seen in fibroblasts from $Irf4^{-/-}$, $Ccl17^{E/E}$ and $GM\text{-}CSF^{-/-}$ mice compared to fibroblasts from WT mice.

These data indicate that while the degree of synovitis present early in CiOA in the absence of CCL17 is not affected, the gene expression of mediators potentially important for joint damage was. Furthermore CCL17 is produced by synovial macrophages in a GM-CSF-dependent and IRF4-dependent manner, consistent with our proposed pathway being active in these cells [18].

Discussion

We have previously reported the importance of GM-CSF in the progression of pain and disease in the CiOA model [8]. Here we demonstrate that IRF4, CCL17 and CCR4 are also required. Therapeutic inhibition of

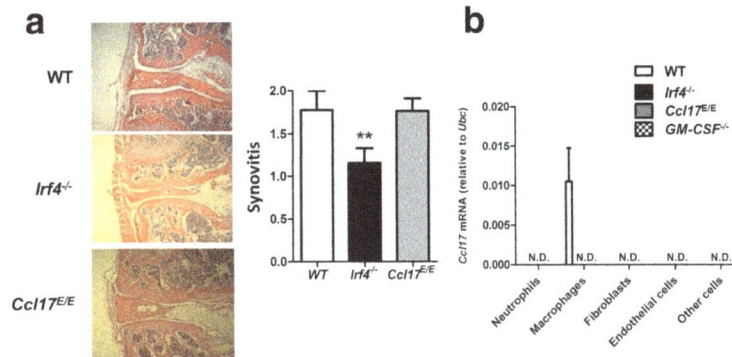

Fig. 6 Chemokine (c-c motif) ligand 17 (CCL17) is expressed in collagenase-induced osteoarthritis (CiOA) synovial macrophages and regulated by interferon regulatory factor 4 (IRF4) and granulocyte macrophage-colony stimulating factor (GM-CSF). **a** CiOA was induced in wild-type (WT), $Irf4^{-/-}$ and $Ccl17^{E/E}$ mice and the joints were histologically assessed at week 2. Representative histologic pictures of knee joints (H&E stain, original magnification ×100) and quantification of synovitis; n = 5–10 mice per strain. **b** Synovial cell populations were sorted from joints at week 1 from WT, $Irf4^{-/-}$, $Ccl17^{E/E}$ and GM-$CSF^{-/-}$ mice undergoing CiOA and $Ccl17$ mRNA expression was measured; n = 3–6 mice per strain; Results are expressed as the mean ± SEM. N.D., not detected. **p < 0.01, WT vs. $Irf4^{-/-}$ mice

CCL17 or Jmjd3 was successful in ameliorating the already established arthritic pain and disease. Thus our previously proposed GM-CSF→Jmjd3→IRF4→CCL17 pathway, first identified in human and murine monocytes/macrophages, appears to be important not only in the context of inflammatory arthritis and pain (e.g. ZIA) [18], but also in a model of OA, including in the development of the associated pain. However, TNF, which we have found before to be important for the initiation of ZIA pain and disease and mechanistically can use the same pathway leading to CCL17 formation via GM-CSF and JMJD3-regulated IRF4 formation [20], was not required for the development of CiOA pain or disease. CiOA pain, first detected at 3 weeks, was rapidly reversed by treatment with a specific COX-2 inhibitor but there was no effect on histologic scoring or osteophyte size.

CiOA shares some features with human OA, such as the development of synovitis, cartilage erosion and osteophytes [8, 11], which we have shown to be GM-CSF dependent [8]; there are a number of studies using this macrophage-dependent model in rodents (see, for example [8–13, 37, 38]). Interestingly, the proportion of synovial macrophages was not altered in the absence of GM-CSF, although there was a reduction in the proportion of neutrophils. A lack of IRF4 resulted in a slight reduction in early synovitis, with once again a reduction in the proportion of synovial neutrophils, while a lack of CCL17 had no effect; however, in the absence of either GM-CSF [8], IRF4 or CCL17 there was no pain development at week 3 and significantly reduced histologic scores and osteophyte size at week 6 (Fig. 1a-c). Thus, the degree of early synovitis observed upon deletion of IRF4 and CCL17, in contrast to that observed upon deletion of GM-CSF, does not correlate with the subsequent pain levels and histologic changes. In line with these observations, in OA the degrees of joint pain and structural change do not always overlap [5]. In the absence of IRF4 or CCL17, the activation states of the cells and the levels of associated inflammatory mediators present during synovitis may differ, which are likely important for the subsequent pathologic changes. In support of this mechanism, our gene expression analysis indicated that $Ccl17$ mRNA is expressed in the CiOA synovial macrophages from WT mice, but not in those from GM-$CSF^{-/-}$ and $IRF4^{-/-}$ mice, data consistent with the involvement of the GM-CSF→IRF4→CCL17 pathway in the CiOA synovial macrophages, a cell type considered to be important in OA pathogenesis [2–6, 33, 39].

Importantly, therapeutic blockade of CCL17 ameliorated both CiOA pain and disease. CCL17 was originally considered to be a M2 cytokine due to its preferential attraction of T_H2 lymphocytes [25, 40]. It can be produced by certain macrophage/dendritic cell populations [18, 23, 41, 42] and is elevated in many inflammatory conditions [18, 43–45] and in synovial fluid in OA [46]. CiOA synovitis in the absence of CCL17 suggests that CCL17 has other functions, apart from a chemotactic role [18]. In this connection, we have also observed in models of inflammatory arthritis, including lymphocyte-independent models, that a lack of CCL17 has more profound effects on cartilage damage and bone erosion than on cellular infiltration [18]. We have reported that systemic administration of CCL17 can drive arthritic pain in an inflamed joint in a COX-dependent manner [18]. Our data showing the therapeutic efficacy of a COX-2 inhibitor on CiOA pain (Fig. 5) is consistent with CCL17 being able to regulate joint eicosanoid levels in some manner. There are conflicting data as to whether the CCL17 receptor, CCR4, is expressed in neurons [47–50] as such expression would indicate the possibility of their direct activation by CCL17. Human microglial cells have been reported to express CCR4 [51], suggesting CCL17 could also act at this level in pain development. However, the blockade of CiOA pain by systemic anti-CCL17 mAb administration suggests a peripheral algesic action for CCL17, at least in this model.

The clinical syndrome of "OA" affects not only the composition, structure and function of articular cartilage but also the integrity of multiple joint tissues such as synovium, bone, etc., i.e. an appreciation has emerged that OA is a "whole joint" disease (see, for example, previous work [2–6, 33]). Also, as adult articular cartilage is avascular and aneural, pathogenic changes to non-cartilaginous joint tissues are of particular interest in understanding the source of pain generation in OA [33]. During OA progression, the synovial membrane is one source of proinflammatory and catabolic products, including matrix metalloproteinases (MMPs) and aggrecanases, which potentially contribute to articular matrix breakdown [33]. The synovial cell gene expression analysis described here indicated that $Ccr4$ mRNA was expressed in a number of cell types, including fibroblasts, in the CiOA model while only fibroblasts appeared to express MMP3 and MMP13 which have been shown to be important for macrophage-mediated cartilage breakdown in experimental OA, including in CiOA [8, 52–54]. We found that, compared to WT mice, synovial fibroblasts from $GM\text{-}CSF^{-/-}$, $Irf4^{-/-}$ and $Ccl17^{E/E}$ mice all had reduced mRNA expression of these MMPs and these gene-deficient mice also had reduced joint destruction and osteophyte size at 6 weeks post CiOA induction. As one possible mechanism, it could be that macrophage-derived CCL17 activates directly CCR4-expressing fibroblasts, which in turn augment MMP3 and MMP13 expression, leading to joint damage - both MMPs are expressed in synovial tissue from patients with early symptomatic OA [55]. Notably, CCL17-mediated CCR4 activation in other models is reported to up-regulate MMP13 [56, 57]. Importantly, cells in both cartilage and bone are also likely to express MMPs [58] and whether CCL17 acts directly on cartilage and bone requires further investigation, as does the relative contribution of the synovium, cartilage and bone to pain and joint destruction in this model.

Blockade of TNF has revolutionized RA treatment. We have recently shown that TNF can be linked to the GM-CSF→IRF4→CCL17 pathway, with the actions of TNF and GM-CSF being interdependent [20]. Interestingly, TNF is not required for CiOA pain and disease. It is not the only proinflammatory cytokine capable of associating with GM-CSF biology nor does GM-CSF-initiated inflammation necessarily involve TNF. For example, IL-1 can induce GM-CSF in a number of cell populations [59–61] and an IL-1-driven monoarticular arthritis model is GM-CSF dependent [62]. However, IL-1 is also not required for CiOA development [37]. How collagenase initiates the

GM-CSF-dependent pathway in the CiOA model is unknown, as is the relationship of the pathway to other mediators important in this model, for example, the alarmins, S100A8 and S100A9 [38]. Consistent with our findings, anti-TNF treatment in the destabilization of the medial meniscus model did not ameliorate late-stage OA pain [63]. Some studies have assessed the benefit of anti-TNF therapies in patients with hand or knee OA with variable results [4, 6, 64, 65]. Better patient stratification and large, randomized, placebo-controlled trials would appear to be needed [4].

Conclusions

From the findings described, we have evidence consistent with the GM-CSF→Jmjd3→IRF4→CCL17 pathway being important in CiOA, regulating both pain and disease. Whether the pathway is relevant to other experimental OA models is being explored. As for GM-CSF [8], therapeutic blockade of CCL17 was effective at ameliorating both pain and disease. As mentioned, low-grade inflammation is now being recognized as important in OA pathogenesis and progression [2–6, 33, 66] and pain has the highest impact on its burden [65]. Targeting GM-CSF or its receptor in RA is yielding promising results [15] and, as a result of prior findings in the CiOA model [8], a phase II trial in hand OA is currently underway [15]; however, given the possible adverse side effects associated with GM-CSF/GM-CSFR blockade, such as pulmonary alveolar proteinosis and infections [16, 67], targeting CCL17, which is elevated in the synovial fluid of patients with OA [46] and which we have found to be downstream of GM-CSF [18], may have some advantages for the treatment of not only inflammatory arthritis but also at least for some patients with OA.

Additional files

Additional file 1: Synovial cell populations from joints at week 1 from WT, $Irf4^{-/-}$, $Ccl17^{E/E}$ and $GM\text{-}CSF^{-/-}$ mice undergoing CiOA were sorted and gene expression measured. (A) Representative FACS plots showing synovial cell sorting strategy. CD45$^+$ cells (II) were sorted into neutrophils (CD11b$^+$Ly6G$^+$) (III) and macrophages (CD11b$^+$Ly6G$^-$F4/80$^+$CD64$^+$) (IV); CD45$^-$ cells (I) were sorted into endothelial cells (CD31$^+$mEF-SK4$^-$) (V), fibroblasts (CD31$^-$mEF-SK4$^+$) (VII) and other cells (CD31$^-$mEF-SK4$^-$) (VI). (B-D) mRNA expression in sorted synovial cell populations. (B) $Col1a1$, (C) $Mmp3$ and (D) $Mmp13$. Results are expressed as the mean ± SEM; n = 3–6 mice per strain. N.D. not detected. $^*p < 0.05$, $^{**}p < 0.01$, WT vs. $Irf4^{-/-}$, $Ccl17^{E/E}$ or $GM\text{-}CSF^{-/-}$ mice. (PDF 257 kb)

Additional file 2: Proportions of synovial cell populations in knee joints from CiOA mice at day 7. (PDF 85 kb)

Abbreviations

ANOVA: Analysis of variance; CCL17: Chemokine (c-c motif) ligand 17; CCR4: C-C motif chemokine receptor 4; CiOA: Collagenase-induced osteoarthritis; COX-2: Cyclooxygenase 2; DMSO: Dimethyl sulfoxide; Fc: Crystallisable fragment; GM-CSF: Granulocyte macrophage-colony stimulating factor; GM-CSFR: Granulocyte macrophage-colony stimulating factor receptor; IL: Interleukin; IRF4: Interferon regulatory factor 4; LF: Lateral femur; LT: Lateral tibia; mAb: Monoclonal antibody;

MF: Medial femur; MMP: Matrix metalloproteinase; mRNA: Messenger RNA; MT: Medial tibia; OA: Osteoarthritis; PBS: Phosphate-buffered saline; RA: Rheumatoid arthritis; TNF: Tumour necrosis factor; WT: Wild-type; ZIA: Zymosan-induced arthritis

Acknowledgements
We thank members of Melbourne Brain Centre Parkville Flow Cytometry Facility for flow cytometry assistance.

Funding
This work was supported by grants from Arthritis Australia (1757679) and the National Health and Medical Research Council (NHMRC) (1043147), and by a NMHRC Senior Principal Research Fellowship (JAH). IF was supported by the Deutsche Forschungsgemeinschaft IRTG 2168 (DFG).

Authors' contributions
JAH and ADC conceived, designed and coordinated the study. M-CL, RS, AA, AJF and ADC performed the experiments. IF provided materials. M-CL, JH and ADC analysed and interpreted the data. M-CL and ADC drafted the manuscript. AJF, IF and JAH provided critical revision of the manuscript. All authors read and approved the final manuscript.

Consent for publication
Not applicable.

Competing interests
The authors declare that they have no competing interests.

Author details
[1]The University of Medicine, Department of Medicine, Royal Melbourne Hospital, Parkville, VIC 3050, Australia. [2]Immunology and Environment, Life and Medical Sciences Institute, University of Bonn, 53115 Bonn, Germany.

References
1. Chen D, Shen J, Zhao W, Wang T, Han L, Hamilton JL, Im HJ. Osteoarthritis: toward a comprehensive understanding of pathological mechanism. Bone Res. 2017;5:16044.
2. Benito MJ, Veale DJ, FitzGerald O, van den Berg WB, Bresnihan B. Synovial tissue inflammation in early and late osteoarthritis. Ann Rheum Dis. 2005;64:1263–7.
3. Liu-Bryan R, Terkeltaub R. Emerging regulators of the inflammatory process in osteoarthritis. Nat Rev Rheumatol. 2015;11:35–44.
4. Wenham CY, McDermott M, Conaghan PG. Biological therapies in osteoarthritis. Curr Pharm Des. 2015;21:2206–15.
5. Mathiessen A, Conaghan PG. Synovitis in osteoarthritis: current understanding with therapeutic implications. Arthritis Res Ther. 2017;19:18.
6. Robinson WH, Lepus CM, Wang Q, Raghu H, Mao R, Lindstrom TM, Sokolove J. Low-grade inflammation as a key mediator of the pathogenesis of osteoarthritis. Nat Rev Rheumatol. 2016;12:580–92.
7. Kamekura S, Hoshi K, Shimoaka T, Chung U, Chikuda H, Yamada T, Uchida M, Ogata N, Seichi A, Nakamura K, Kawaguchi H. Osteoarthritis development in novel experimental mouse models induced by knee joint instability. Osteoarthr Cartil. 2005;13:632–41.
8. Cook AD, Pobjoy J, Steidl S, Durr M, Braine EL, Turner AL, Lacey DC, Hamilton JA. Granulocyte-macrophage colony-stimulating factor is a key mediator in experimental osteoarthritis pain and disease development. Arthritis Res Ther. 2012;14:R199.
9. Blom AB, van Lent PL, Libregts S, Holthuysen AE, van der Kraan PM, van Rooijen N, van den Berg WB. Crucial role of macrophages in matrix metalloproteinase-mediated cartilage destruction during experimental osteoarthritis: involvement of matrix metalloproteinase 3. Arthritis Rheum. 2007;56:147–57.
10. Botter SM, van Osch GJ, Waarsing JH, van der Linden JC, Verhaar JA, Pols HA, van Leeuwen JP, Weinans H. Cartilage damage pattern in relation to subchondral plate thickness in a collagenase-induced model of osteoarthritis. Osteoarthr Cartil. 2008;16:506–14.
11. Blom AB, van Lent PL, Holthuysen AE, van der Kraan PM, Roth J, van Rooijen N, van den Berg WB. Synovial lining macrophages mediate osteophyte formation during experimental osteoarthritis. Osteoarthr Cartil. 2004;12:627–35.
12. van Lent PL, Blom AB, van der Kraan P, Holthuysen AE, Vitters E, van Rooijen N, Smeets RL, Nabbe KC, van den Berg WB. Crucial role of synovial lining macrophages in the promotion of transforming growth factor beta-mediated osteophyte formation. Arthritis Rheum. 2004;50:103–11.
13. Adaes S, Mendonca M, Santos TN, Castro-Lopes JM, Ferreira-Gomes J, Neto FL. Intra-articular injection of collagenase in the knee of rats as an alternative model to study nociception associated with osteoarthritis. Arthritis Res Ther. 2014;16:R10.
14. McGonagle D, Hermann KG, Tan AL. Differentiation between osteoarthritis and psoriatic arthritis: implications for pathogenesis and treatment in the biologic therapy era. Rheumatology. 2015;54:29–38.
15. Hamilton JA, Cook AD, Tak PP. Anti-colony-stimulating factor therapies for inflammatory and autoimmune diseases. Nat Rev Drug Discov. 2017;16:53–70.
16. Hamilton JA. Colony-stimulating factors in inflammation and autoimmunity. Nat Rev Immunol. 2008;8:533–44.
17. Cook AD, Pobjoy J, Sarros S, Steidl S, Durr M, Lacey DC, Hamilton JA. Granulocyte-macrophage colony-stimulating factor is a key mediator in inflammatory and arthritic pain. Ann Rheum Dis. 2013;72:265–70.
18. Achuthan A, Cook AD, Lee MC, Saleh R, Khiew HW, Chang MW, Louis C, Fleetwood AJ, Lacey DC, Christensen AD, Frye AT, Lam PY, Kusano H, Nomura K, Steiner N, Forster I, Nutt SL, Olshansky M, Turner SJ, Hamilton JA. Granulocyte macrophage colony-stimulating factor induces CCL17 production via IRF4 to mediate inflammation. J Clin Invest. 2016;126:3453–66.
19. Cook AD, Braine EL, Campbell IK, Rich MJ, Hamilton JA. Blockade of collagen-induced arthritis post-onset by antibody to granulocyte-macrophage colony-stimulating factor (GM-CSF): requirement for GM-CSF in the effector phase of disease. Arthritis Res. 2001;3:293–8.
20. Cook AD, Lee MC, Saleh R, Khiew HW, Christensen AD, Achuthan A, Fleetwood AJ, Lacey DC, Smith JE, Förster I, Hamilton JA. TNF and granulocyte macrophage-colony stimulating factor interdependence mediates inflammation via CCL17. JCI Insight 2018;3:e99249.
21. Korner H, Cook M, Riminton DS, Lemckert FA, Hoek RM, Ledermann B, Kontgen F, Fazekas de St Groth B, Sedgwick JD. Distinct roles for lymphotoxin-alpha and tumor necrosis factor in organogenesis and spatial organization of lymphoid tissue. Eur J Immunol. 1997;27:2600–9.
22. Chvatchko Y, Hoogewerf AJ, Meyer A, Alouani S, Juillard P, Buser R, Conquet F, Proudfoot AE, Wells TN, Power CA. A key role for CC chemokine receptor 4 in lipopolysaccharide-induced endotoxic shock. J Exp Med. 2000;191:1755–64.
23. Stanley E, Lieschke GJ, Grail D, Metcalf D, Hodgson G, Gall JA, Maher DW, Cebon J, Sinickas V, Dunn AR. Granulocyte/macrophage colony-stimulating factor-deficient mice show no major perturbation of hematopoiesis but develop a characteristic pulmonary pathology. Proc Natl Acad Sci USA. 1994;91:5592–6.
24. Mittrucker HW, Matsuyama T, Grossman A, Kundig TM, Potter J, Shahinian A, Wakeham A, Patterson B, Ohashi PS, Mak TW. Requirement for the transcription factor LSIRF/IRF4 for mature B and T lymphocyte function. Science. 1997;275:540–3.
25. Alferink J, Lieberam I, Reindl W, Behrens A, Weiss S, Huser N, Gerauer K, Ross R, Reske-Kunz AB, Ahmad-Nejad P, Wagner H, Forster I. Compartmentalized production of CCL17 in vivo: strong inducibility in peripheral dendritic cells contrasts selective absence from the spleen. J Exp Med. 2003;197:585–99.
26. van den Bosch MH, Blom AB, Kram V, Maeda A, Sikka S, Gabet Y, Kilts TM, van den Berg WB, van Lent PL, van der Kraan PM, Young MF. WISP1/CCN4 aggravates cartilage degeneration in experimental osteoarthritis. Osteoarthr Cartil. 2017;25:1900–11.
27. Inglis JJ, McNamee KE, Chia SL, Essex D, Feldmann M, Williams RO, Hunt SP, Vincent T. Regulation of pain sensitivity in experimental osteoarthritis by the endogenous peripheral opioid system. Arthritis Rheum. 2008;58:3110–9.
28. Lee MC, McCubbin JA, Christensen AD, Poole DP, Rajasekhar P, Lieu T, Bunnett NW, Garcia-Caraballo S, Erickson A, Brierley SM, Saleh R, Achuthan

A, Fleetwood AJ, Anderson RL, Hamilton JA, Cook AD. G-CSF Receptor Blockade Ameliorates Arthritic Pain and Disease. The Journal of Immunology 2017;198(9):3565–575.

29. ter Huurne M, Schelbergen R, Blattes R, Blom A, de Munter W, Grevers LC, Jeanson J, Noel D, Casteilla L, Jorgensen C, van den Berg W, van Lent PL. Antiinflammatory and chondroprotective effects of intraarticular injection of adipose-derived stem cells in experimental osteoarthritis. Arthritis Rheum. 2012;64:3604–13.

30. Glasson SS, Chambers MG, Van Den Berg WB, Little CB. The OARSI histopathology initiative - recommendations for histological assessments of osteoarthritis in the mouse. Osteoarthr Cartil. 2010;18(Suppl 3):S17–23.

31. Santulli-Marotto S, Boakye K, Lacy E, Wu SJ, Luongo J, Kavalkovich K, Coelho A, Hogaboam CM, Ryan M. Engagement of two distinct binding domains on CCL17 is required for signaling through CCR4 and establishment of localized inflammatory conditions in the lung. PLoS One. 2013;8:e81465.

32. Satoh T, Takeuchi O, Vandenbon A, Yasuda K, Tanaka Y, Kumagai Y, Miyake T, Matsushita K, Okazaki T, Saitoh T, Honma K, Matsuyama T, Yui K, Tsujimura T, Standley DM, Nakanishi K, Nakai K, Akira S. The Jmjd3-Irf4 axis regulates M2 macrophage polarization and host responses against helminth infection. Nat Immunol. 2010;11:936–44.

33. Scanzello CR, Goldring SR. The role of synovitis in osteoarthritis pathogenesis. Bone. 2012;51:249–57.

34. Cook AD, Louis C, Robinson MJ, Saleh R, Sleeman MA, Hamilton JA. Granulocyte macrophage colony-stimulating factor receptor alpha expression and its targeting in antigen-induced arthritis and inflammation. Arthritis Res Ther. 2016;18:287.

35. Anzai A, Choi JL, He S, Fenn AM, Nairz M, Rattik S, McAlpine CS, Mindur JE, Chan CT, Iwamoto Y, Tricot B, Wojtkiewicz GR, Weissleder R, Libby P, Nahrendorf M, Stone JR, Becker B, Swirski FK. The infarcted myocardium solicits GM-CSF for the detrimental oversupply of inflammatory leukocytes. J Exp Med. 2017;214:3293–310.

36. Rose BJ, Kooyman DL. A Tale of Two Joints: The role of matrix metalloproteases in cartilage biology. Dis Markers. 2016;2016:4895050.

37. van Dalen SC, Blom AB, Sloetjes AW, Helsen MM, Roth J, Vogl T, van de Loo FA, Koenders MI, van der Kraan PM, van den Berg WB, van den Bosch MH, van Lent PL. Interleukin-1 is not involved in synovial inflammation and cartilage destruction in collagenase-induced osteoarthritis. Osteoarthr Cartil. 2017;25:385–96.

38. van Lent PL, Blom AB, Schelbergen RF, Sloetjes A, Lafeber FP, Lems WF, Cats H, Vogl T, Roth J, van den Berg WB. Active involvement of alarmins S100A8 and S100A9 in the regulation of synovial activation and joint destruction during mouse and human osteoarthritis. Arthritis Rheum. 2012;64:1466–76.

39. Scanzello CR, Plaas A, Crow MK. Innate immune system activation in osteoarthritis: is osteoarthritis a chronic wound? Curr Opin Rheumatol. 2008; 20:565–72.

40. Iellem A, Mariani M, Lang R, Recalde H, Panina-Bordignon P, Sinigaglia F, D'Ambrosio D. Unique chemotactic response profile and specific expression of chemokine receptors CCR4 and CCR8 by CD4(+)CD25(+) regulatory T cells. J Exp Med. 2001;194:847–53.

41. Katakura T, Miyazaki M, Kobayashi M, Herndon DN, Suzuki F. CCL17 and IL-10 as effectors that enable alternatively activated macrophages to inhibit the generation of classically activated macrophages. J Immunol. 2004;172:1407–13.

42. Stutte S, Quast T, Gerbitzki N, Savinko T, Novak N, Reifenberger J, Homey B, Kolanus W, Alenius H, Forster I. Requirement of CCL17 for CCR7- and CXCR4-dependent migration of cutaneous dendritic cells. Proc Natl Acad Sci USA. 2010;107:8736–41.

43. Heiseke AF, Faul AC, Lehr HA, Forster I, Schmid RM, Krug AB, Reindl W. CCL17 promotes intestinal inflammation in mice and counteracts regulatory T cell-mediated protection from colitis. Gastroenterology. 2012;142:335–45.

44. Weber C, Meiler S, Doring Y, Koch M, Drechsler M, Megens RT, Rowinska Z, Bidzhekov K, Fecher C, Ribechini E, van Zandvoort MA, Binder CJ, Jelinek I, Hristov M, Boon L, Jung S, Korn T, Lutz MB, Forster I, Zenke M, Hieronymus T, Junt T, Zernecke A. CCL17-expressing dendritic cells drive atherosclerosis by restraining regulatory T cell homeostasis in mice. J Clin Invest. 2011;121:2898–910.

45. Okamoto H, Koizumi K, Yamanaka H, Saito T, Kamatani N. A role for TARC/CCL17, a CC chemokine, in systemic lupus erythematosus. J Rheumatol. 2003;30:2369–73.

46. Hillen MR, Moret FM, van der Wurff-Jacobs K, Radstake T, Hack CE, Lafeber F, van Roon J. Targeting CD1c-expressing classical dendritic cells to prevent thymus and activation-regulated chemokine (TARC)-mediated T-cell chemotaxis in rheumatoid arthritis. Scand J Rheumatol. 2017;46:11–6.

47. Oh SB, Tran PB, Gillard SE, Hurley RW, Hammond DL, Miller RJ. Chemokines and glycoprotein120 produce pain hypersensitivity by directly exciting primary nociceptive neurons. J Neurosci. 2001;21:5027–35.

48. Thakur M, Crow M, Richards N, Davey GI, Levine E, Kelleher JH, Agley CC, Denk F, Harridge SD, McMahon SB. Defining the nociceptor transcriptome. Front Mol Neurosci. 2014;7:87.

49. Li CL, Li KC, Wu D, Chen Y, Luo H, Zhao JR, Wang SS, Sun MM, Lu YJ, Zhong YQ, Hu XY, Hou R, Zhou BB, Bao L, Xiao HS, Zhang X. Somatosensory neuron types identified by high-coverage single-cell RNA-sequencing and functional heterogeneity. Cell Res. 2016;26:83–102.

50. Cook AD, Christensen AD, Tewari D, SB MM, Hamilton JA. Immune Cytokines and Their Receptors in Inflammatory Pain. Trends Immunol. 2018;10:29-38.

51. Etemad S, Zamin RM, Ruitenberg MJ, Filgueira L. A novel in vitro human microglia model: characterization of human monocyte-derived microglia. J Neurosci Methods. 2012;209:79–89.

52. Neuhold LA, Killar L, Zhao W, Sung ML, Warner L, Kulik J, Turner J, Wu W, Billinghurst C, Meijers T, Poole AR, Babij P, DeGennaro LJ. Postnatal expression in hyaline cartilage of constitutively active human collagenase-3 (MMP-13) induces osteoarthritis in mice. J Clin Invest. 2001;107:35–44.

53. van den Berg WB. Osteoarthritis year 2010 in review: pathomechanisms. Osteoarthr Cartil. 2011;19:338–41.

54. Bondeson J, Blom AB, Wainwright S, Hughes C, Caterson B, van den Berg WB. The role of synovial macrophages and macrophage-produced mediators in driving inflammatory and destructive responses in osteoarthritis. Arthritis Rheum. 2010;62:647–57.

55. van den Bosch MH, Blom AB, van de Loo FA, Koenders MI, Lafeber FP, van den Berg WB, van der Kraan PM, van Lent PL. Brief report: induction of matrix metalloproteinase expression by synovial wnt signaling and association with disease progression in early symptomatic osteoarthritis. Arthritis Rheumatol. 2017;69:1978–83.

56. Ou B, Zhao J, Guan S, Feng H, Wangpu X, Zhu C, Zong Y, Ma J, Sun J, Shen X, Zheng M, Lu A. CCR4 promotes metastasis via ERK/NF-kappaB/MMP13 pathway and acts downstream of TNF-alpha in colorectal cancer. Oncotarget. 2016;7:47637–49.

57. Li CM, Hou L, Zhang H, Zhang WY. CCL17 Induces trophoblast migration and invasion by regulating matrix metalloproteinase and integrin expression in human first-trimester placenta. Reprod Sci. 2014; https://doi.org/10.1177/1933719113519170.

58. Lee AS, Ellman MB, Yan D, Kroin JS, Cole BJ, van Wijnen AJ, Im HJ. A current review of molecular mechanisms regarding osteoarthritis and pain. Gene. 2013;527:440–7.

59. Leizer T, Cebon J, Layton JE, Hamilton JA. Cytokine regulation of colony-stimulating factor production in cultured human synovial fibroblasts: I. Induction of GM-CSF and G-CSF production by interleukin-1 and tumor necrosis factor. Blood. 1990;76:1989–96.

60. Campbell IK, Novak U, Cebon J, Layton JE, Hamilton JA. Human articular cartilage and chondrocytes produce hemopoietic colony-stimulating factors in culture in response to IL-1. J Immunol. 1991;147:1238–46.

61. Lawlor KE, Wong PK, Campbell IK, van Rooijen N, Wicks IP. Acute CD4+ T lymphocyte-dependent interleukin-1-driven arthritis selectively requires interleukin-2 and interleukin-4, joint macrophages, granulocyte-macrophage colony-stimulating factor, interleukin-6, and leukemia inhibitory factor. Arthritis Rheum. 2005;52:3749–54.

62. Yang YH, Hamilton JA. Dependence of interleukin-1-induced arthritis on granulocyte-macrophage colony-stimulating factor. Arthritis Rheum. 2001; 44:111–9.

63. McNamee KE, Burleigh A, Gompels LL, Feldmann M, Allen SJ, Williams RO, Dawbarn D, Vincent TL, Inglis JJ. Treatment of murine osteoarthritis with TrkAd5 reveals a pivotal role for nerve growth factor in non-inflammatory joint pain. Pain. 2010;149:386–92.

64. Chevalier X, Eymard F, Richette P. Biologic agents in osteoarthritis: hopes and disappointments. Nat Rev Rheumatol. 2013;9:400–10.

65. Schaible HG. Mechanisms of chronic pain in osteoarthritis. Curr Rheumatol Rep. 2012;14:549–56.

66. Rahmati M, Mobasheri A, Mozafari M. Inflammatory mediators in osteoarthritis: a critical review of the state-of-the-art, current prospects, and future challenges. Bone. 2016;85:81–90.

67. Hamilton JA. GM-CSF as a target in inflammatory/autoimmune disease: current evidence and future therapeutic potential. Expert Rev Clin Immunol. 2015;11:457–65.

Accuracy of magnetic resonance imaging to detect cartilage loss in severe osteoarthritis of the first carpometacarpal joint: comparison with histological evaluation

Michael S. Saltzherr[1,2,3*], J. Henk Coert[4], Ruud W. Selles[2,5], Johan W. van Neck[2], Jean-Bart Jaquet[6], Gerjo J. V. M. van Osch[7], Edwin H. G. Oei[1], Jolanda J. Luime[3] and Galied S. R. Muradin[1]

Abstract

Background: Magnetic resonance imaging (MRI) is increasingly used for research in hand osteoarthritis, but imaging the thin cartilage layers in the hand joints remains challenging. We therefore assessed the accuracy of MRI in detecting cartilage loss in patients with symptomatic osteoarthritis of the first carpometacarpal (CMC1) joint.

Methods: Twelve patients scheduled for trapeziectomy to treat severe symptomatic osteoarthritis of the CMC1 joint underwent a preoperative high resolution 3D spoiled gradient (SPGR) MRI scan. Subsequently, the resected trapezium was evaluated histologically. The sections were scored for cartilage damage severity (Osteoarthritis Research Society International (OARSI) score), and extent of damage (percentage surface area). Each MRI scan was scored for the area of normal cartilage, partial cartilage loss and full cartilage loss. The percentages of the total surface area with any cartilage loss and full-thickness cartilage loss were calculated using MRI and histological evaluation.

Results: MRI and histological evaluation both identified large areas of overall cartilage loss. The median (IQR) surface area of any cartilage loss on MRI was 98% (82–100%), and on histological assessment 96% (87–98%). However, MRI underestimated the extent of full-thickness cartilage loss. The median (IQR) surface area of full-thickness cartilage loss on MRI was 43% (22–70%), and on histological evaluation 79% (67–85%). The difference was caused by a thin layer of high signal on the articulating surface, which was interpreted as damaged cartilage on MRI but which was not identified on histological evaluation.

Conclusions: Three-dimensional SPGR MRI of the CMC1 joint demonstrates overall cartilage damage, but underestimates full-thickness cartilage loss in patients with advanced osteoarthritis.

Keywords: Magnetic resonance imaging, First carpometacarpal joint, Cartilage, Histology, Osteoarthritis

Background

Osteoarthritis (OA) of the hand is the most prevalent disease of the hand joint, which can lead to pain and functional impairment. The disease is characterized by cartilage loss, subchondral bone changes and inflammation of the synovium. Despite the fact that changes in bone only are directly visible on conventional radiography (CR), and that joint damage on CR is only weakly associated with symptoms [1], it is the most widely used imaging method for assessing structural changes in hand OA in both clinical practice and clinical trials [2, 3].

Magnetic resonance imaging (MRI) is gaining popularity in studies of hand OA [4, 5] as it depicts bone, cartilage, and soft tissue changes, and images the complete joint in multiple planes. As a result, MRI has given us new insights into hand OA, such as the involvement of collateral ligaments [6, 7], the high prevalence of synovitis [8] and significant associations of joint pain with bone marrow lesions (BML) and synovitis [9, 10].

* Correspondence: m.saltzherr@erasmusmc.nl
[1]Department of Radiology, Erasmus MC, University Medical Center Rotterdam, Rotterdam, The Netherlands
[2]Department of Plastic, Reconstructive and Hand Surgery, Erasmus MC, University Medical Center Rotterdam, Rotterdam, The Netherlands
Full list of author information is available at the end of the article

MRI of cartilage in hand OA has been less well-explored, yet accurate cartilage assessment would be a valuable addition to other pathological change detected by MRI in the assessment and follow up monitoring of the whole joint in hand OA. In studies of knee OA, quantification of cartilage using MRI is often an outcome measure in clinical trials, but cartilage imaging in the small joints of the hand is more challenging, as smaller voxel sizes are needed to depict the thin cartilage layer. Previous studies have reported that reliable quantitative evaluation of the cartilage layer in the small joints of the hand can be performed using conventional MRI and small dedicated coils [11, 12].

While in-vivo cartilage quantification with MRI in knee OA correlates well with histological findings [13, 14], to our knowledge, there are no reports in the literature of a comparison between in-vivo MRI cartilage assessment of the hand joints and histological evaluation. As surgery in hand OA is only regularly performed for treatment of OA at the base of the thumb, comparison between MRI and histological evaluation is only feasible in patients with symptomatic thumb base OA.

The aim of this study was therefore to quantitatively compare MRI-detected cartilage loss in patients with OA in the first carpometacarpal (CMC1) joint with histological evaluation.

Methods
Patients
We recruited 20 symptomatic patients who had been scheduled for trapeziectomy or hemitrapeziectomy to treat OA in the CMC1 joint. From April 2010 until October 2011 consecutive eligible patients at a University hospital and two teaching hospitals in the Netherlands were invited to participate in the study. The indication for surgery was based on severe pain and/or loss of function. Prior to surgery, patients underwent MRI and functional assessment of the thumb. Patients with previous surgery to the base of the thumb, or patients with contra-indications to undergoing MRI were excluded.

Patients were operated on by the surgeon treating them for hand OA. Additionally two healthy controls were included for comparison of MRI images only. This study was approved by the local ethics committees of the participating hospitals. All patients provided written informed consent prior to the investigation.

MRI acquisition
MRI was performed using 3.0 T scanners (GE HD and GE Discovery MR750, GE healthcare, Milwaukee, Wisconsin). Patients were placed in the prone position with the arm extended above the head, the hand placed in the center of the magnet, and the thumb fully extended on a custom-made platform to stabilize and immobilize the hand. A custom-

made 4.0-mm loop coil was placed on the dorsal side of the CMC1 joint and taped to the hand. Sagittal 3D fast spoiled gradient (SPGR) sequences with fat saturation (FS) were obtained with a spatial resolution of 0.1 by 0.2 mm (echo time (TE) minimal; field of view (FOV) 3–4 cm; frequency 256–320; phase 128–224; slice thickness 0.7 mm; bandwidth 15.6 kHz; two signals acquired). Proton density (PD)-weighted, fast recovery fast spin echo (FRFSE) sequences were acquired in the coronal and sagittal plane (repetition time (TR) 2400; TE 30; echo train length (ETL) 6; FOV 3–4 cm; frequency 256–320; phase 128–160; slice thickness 1.0 mm; bandwidth 15.6 kHz; three signals acquired). T2-weighted FRFSE sequences with fat saturation were obtained in the coronal direction (TR 3000; TE 68; ETL 6; FOV 4 cm; frequency 192; phase 128; slice thickness 2.0 mm; bandwidth 15.6 kHz; four signals acquired). The scanning acquisition time was 25 minutes.

MRI evaluation
A series of evaluations were made of the MR images from patients in whom histological evaluation was not possible. In the first evaluation, we tested a scoring method for cartilage assessment similar to the MRI OA knee score (MOAKS) [15]. However, we decided not to use this scoring method as the cases tested all received the highest score possible, even though clear differences in cartilage damage were visible on the images. In the second evaluation we tested the currently used scoring method, which uses the same definitions as MOAKS for identification of partial-thickness cartilage loss and full-thickness cartilage loss, but the extent of the cartilage damage is not scored on an ordinal scale from 0–3, but on a ratio scale from 0–100%. After the second evaluation we decided to score a thin layer of one or two voxels of high signal intensity (comparable to cartilage) on the bony surface area as partial-thickness loss, not full-thickness loss.

All images were evaluated by two musculoskeletal radiologists and a hand surgeon (GM, EO and HC) together in consensus. The readers were blinded to patient data, clinical data, histological findings and other imaging results. The anonymized images were read using the open source software ClearCanvas Workstation (ClearCanvas Inc., Toronto, Canada). Using all available sequences, the articular surface of the trapezium was evaluated for grade of cartilage loss as normal cartilage thickness, partial-thickness loss of cartilage, or full-thickness loss of cartilage. On each 0.7-mm SPGR FS slice the readers indicated the surface corresponding to each grade.

Measurements from all slices per patient were summed to compute the total articular surface, total area of normal thickness, total area of partial-thickness loss, total area of full-thickness loss, and total area of any thickness loss (full and partial loss combined). Percentages of these were calculated for comparison with histological findings. The image quality of the SPGR images was scored as either low, sufficient for evaluation, or good. Low means that there is a reasonable chance that error was introduced because of the poor image quality.

The CMC1 joints were scored for presence or absence of osteophytes, erosions/cysts, and subluxation. Osteophytes were defined as abnormal bone formation in the peri-articular region on the SPGR and PD images. Erosions/cysts were considered as a single feature and were defined as sharply marginated bone lesions with increased signal intensity on SPGR images, and intermediate signal on PD images, which were visible in two planes. The joint was considered to be subluxated when 33% or more of the metacarpal surface area was not aligned with the trapezial surface area in the coronal or sagittal plane. Synovitis was not scored as we did not use a contrast agent.

Tissue preparation

During surgery the trapezium bone was extracted as a whole or in multiple parts. If the trapezium was not extracted in one piece, care was taken that the articular area of the trapezium facing the first metacarpal bone was kept intact by splitting the trapezium horizontally leaving at least 5 mm of the distal trapezium intact. The resected trapezium was fixed in neutral buffered 10% formalin in the operating room. Trapezium bones were decalcified in formic acid. Large decalcified specimens were cut in half and all samples were embedded in paraffin. Each millimeter, a 5-μm-thick section was cut in the sagittal direction of the bone, mounted and stained with thionin [16].

Histological evaluation

All histological sections were scored for cartilage damage by a trained researcher (MS). To determine the reproducibility of these scores, 10 patients were also scored by GvO, an experienced cartilage researcher. The scorers were blinded to the results of the MRI evaluation.

All available sections were scored for severity and extent of cartilage damage. Severity of cartilage damage was scored according to the semi-quantitative grading and staging system devised by the Osteoarthritis Research Society International (OARSI) Working Group [17]. Grade, defined by depth of cartilage damage, and stage defined by the extent of horizontal cartilage damage were assessed. The OARSI grading system consists of six grades that describe increasing depth of damage to the cartilage damage. Grades 1–4 are subsequently described as: grade 1, edema or cell changes with an intact surface; grade 2, small surface discontinuities; grade 3, vertical fissures; and grade 4, delamination of the superficial zone. For comparison with MRI we defined grades 1–4 together as "cartilage with (near) normal thickness". Grade 4.5 is described as mid-zone excavation, and was defined by us as "partial thickness loss of cartilage" for comparison with MRI. Grades 5 and 6 are described as: grade 5, complete erosion of hyaline cartilage to the level of mineralized bone; and grade 6, deformation and change in the contour of the articular surface. For comparison with MRI we defined grades 5 and 6 together as "full-thickness cartilage loss" (see Fig. 1 for examples).

Each histological section was scored for the amount of the articular surface that corresponded to each grade in

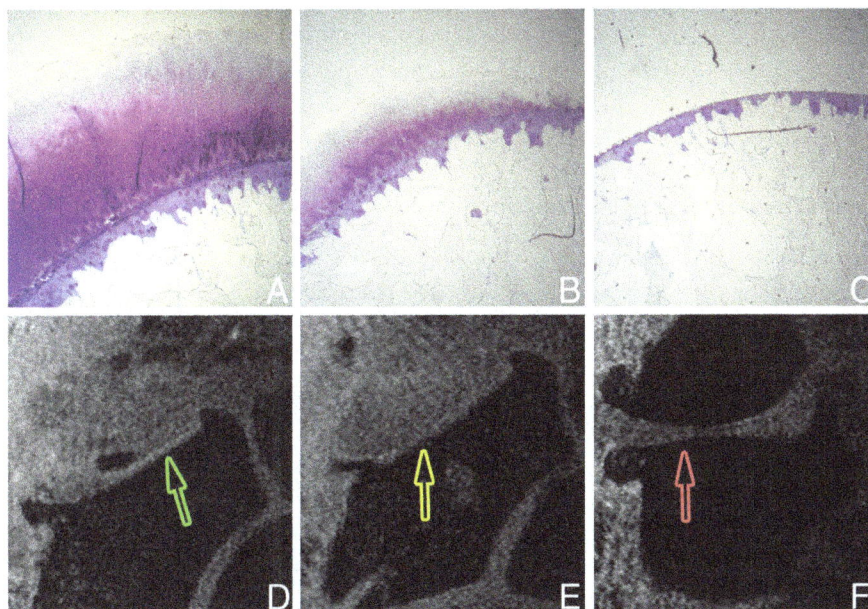

Fig. 1 Example images of histological grading (**a-c**) and magnetic resonance imaging scoring (**d-f**), all from one patient. *Arrows* (**d-f**) indicate locations shown in **a-c**. **a**, **d** Cartilage of (near) normal thickness. **b**, **e** Partial-thickness loss of cartilage. **c**, **f** Full-thickness loss of cartilage. Due to subluxation in the joint, the metacarpal base is not seen in **d** and **e**. The quality of the magnetic resonance images was rated as good

decimals of percentage (i.e., either 0%, 10%, 20%, etc). The sum of the scores for each section had to be 100%. If there was no identifiable articular surface in a section, then no score was assigned to that section. Finally, all section scores per patient were averaged to calculate the total percentage area of (near) normal cartilage thickness, partial loss of cartilage thickness, and full loss of cartilage thickness.

Statistical analysis

Descriptive statistics were used to describe the results of MRI and histological evaluation. Inter-reader reliability of the histology scores was calculated using the intra-class correlation coefficient (ICC). The ICC values were calculated as two-way random, single measures of absolute agreement [18].

Results

Patients

Twenty patients and two healthy controls were included in the study. In five patients, the trapezium was very deformed and could not be extracted without severely damaging the distal articular surface. We were therefore unable to obtain histological specimens from these patients. During histological analysis of the 15 specimens, we noticed that a considerable part of the articular surface was missing in the specimens of 3 patients. These patients were excluded from further analysis. The MRI scans of the excluded patients were used for training and calibration of the MRI score.

The final patient group consisted of 12 patients; two were male and 10 were female, with an average age of 60 (range 46–77) years. The median number of days between MRI and surgery was 8 (range 1–39). Mean grip strength (SD) was 23 (11) kg and mean pinch strength (SD) was 3.8 (0.9) kg. Self-reported pain assessed by visual analog score (possible range 0–100) varied widely between patients. The median (IQR) pain score at rest was 19 (5–31), and the median pain score during thumb movement was 57 (37–67).

MRI

The image quality in 8 out of our 12 patients was adequate or higher, but was low in the other 4 patients. All patients had one or more osteophytes at the trapezium. All but one patient had cysts and/or erosions on the trapezium, and 7 out of 12 CMC1 joints were malaligned or subluxated. Overall cartilage damage was severe (Table 1). All patients had at least one small area with full-thickness cartilage loss; 5 out of 12 patients did not have any remaining area of cartilage of normal thickness. The median (IQR) surface area of trapezial cartilage damage was 98% (82–100%). The percentage area with full-thickness loss of cartilage was 43% (22–70%). The image quality in both healthy controls was good, and they both had normal cartilage layers, without any damage.

Histological evaluation

The mean number of histological sections acquired from each trapezium containing articular surface was 10 (range 9–14). Ten patients were scored independently by both readers. For inter-reader reliability of the detection of any cartilage loss over all scored sections containing articular surface ($n = 100$) was ICC = 0.70 (95%CI = 0.53-0.81), and the inter-reader reliability over all sections for full cartilage loss, the ICC was 0.84 (95% CI 0.76–0.90). Overall cartilage quality was poor (Table 1). No patient had any normal healthy

Table 1 Histological and MRI scores for each individual patient

Patient	Histological evaluation			MRI			
	Normal	Partial-thickness loss	Full-thickness loss	Normal	Partial-thickness loss	Full-thickness loss	Image quality
1	0	0	100	28	45	27	Adequate
2	6	9	85	0	44	56	Low
3	0	25	75	0	77	23	Adequate
4	2	10	88	17	68	15	Adequate
5	22	30	48	37	54	9	Good
6	0	15	85	14	15	71	Adequate
7	4	17	79	2	31	68	Adequate
8	25	22	53	35	22	43	Good
9	10	31	59	19	61	20	Adequate
10	1	18	82	0	74	26	Low
11	3	11	86	0	26	74	Low
12	16	10	74	0	7	93	Low

For both histological evaluation and magnetic resonance imaging (MRI) the percentages of the articular surface that were normal, had partial-thickness loss of cartilage, or had full-thickness loss of cartilage, and MRI image quality are shown

cartilage remaining. The best cartilage observed had a histological grade of 3, with vertical fissures extending from the surface into the mid zone and depletion of matrix staining in the upper half of the cartilage. In 11 out of 12 patients there was complete erosion of the cartilage on more than half of the articulating surface. The median (IQR) surface area of trapezial cartilage damage was 96% (87–98%). The percentage area with full-thickness loss of cartilage was 79% (67–85%).

After analysis, the largest differences between histological scores were in areas near osteophytes, which were sometimes partly covered with cartilage (Fig. 2). For scoring purposes osteophytes were excluded from the articular surface, and the cartilage formed on top of osteophytes was ignored. The lack of a clear anatomical landmark between the articular surface and osteophytes was the main cause of variations in scoring, as the region where the articular surface stopped and the osteophyte began was inconsistently scored.

MRI vs histological evaluation

Both MRI and histological evaluation identified large areas of cartilage loss, with histological evaluation identifying slightly larger areas compared with MRI. The individual scores for each patient obtained by the two modalities are represented in Fig. 3. Histological evaluation identified substantially larger areas with full loss of cartilage than MRI (Fig. 4). Retrospective direct comparison of SPGR images and histological sections showed that the difference between MRI and histological evaluation in scoring any cartilage loss could in most cases be attributed to a thin layer of high signal intensity on the bony surface, which was scored as cartilage on MRI, but was not identified as cartilage on histological evaluation (Fig. 5).

Image quality for MRI was scored as low in 4 out of 12 patients due to motion artifacts and inability to place the surface coil in the optimal position because of disfigurement of the joint. However, we did not find a relationship between image quality and discrepancies between MRI and histological evaluation.

Discussion

Our study showed that the overall extent of cartilage loss in small joints of the hand could be detected with 3D SPGR MRI. However, MRI underestimated the area of full-thickness loss of cartilage.

Previous studies have shown that the SPGR sequence is an accurate sequence to image cartilage in the knee joint [19, 20]. While it has been shown that SPGR may overestimate cartilage damage in early OA due to magnetic field inhomogeneity artifacts, considerable underestimation of cartilage damage has not been reported.

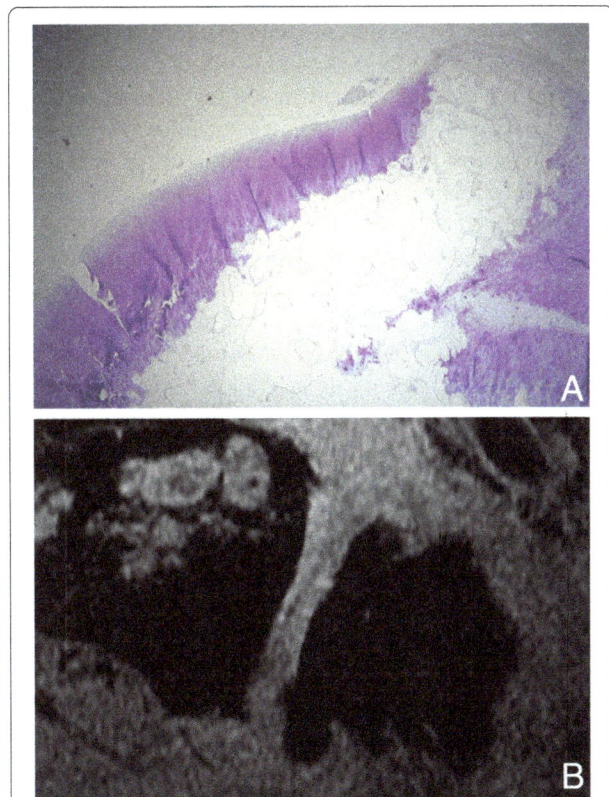

Fig. 2 a Part of a histological section obtained from one of the patients. An osteophyte is visible on the right side. The remaining cartilage partially continues to cover the articulating surfaces of the osteophyte. **b** Spoiled gradient magnetic resonance image of the same patient, where the same osteophyte is on the upper side of the trapezium. Cartilage is visible in the center of the articulating surface of the trapezium and partially continues to cover the osteophyte, comparable with the histological image

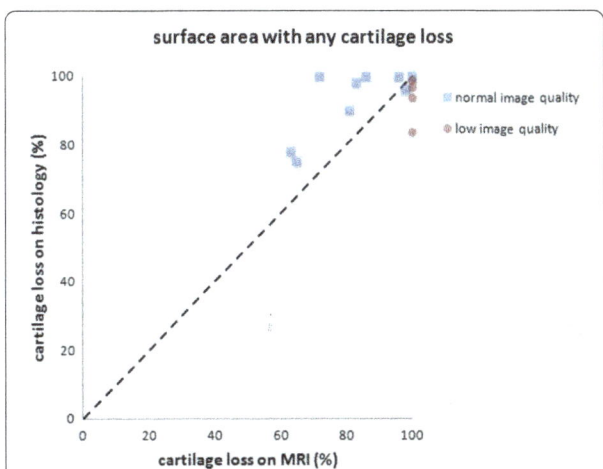

Fig. 3 Relative area of the trapezial articular surface with any loss of cartilage identified. Each *dot* represents one patient measured by magnetic resonance imaging (*MRI*) and histological evaluation. Perfect agreement would result in all dots being positioned on the *diagonal line*

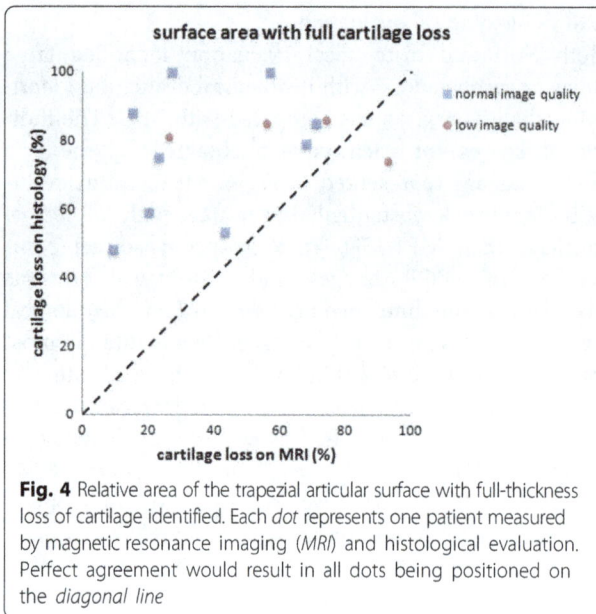

Fig. 4 Relative area of the trapezial articular surface with full-thickness loss of cartilage identified. Each *dot* represents one patient measured by magnetic resonance imaging (*MRI*) and histological evaluation. Perfect agreement would result in all dots being positioned on the *diagonal line*

In previous studies assessing the accuracy of detection of cartilage defects and/or cartilage volume in the knee using MRI, the patient group either consisted of patients with relatively little damage, [19, 21–23] or the areas with severe cartilage damage were not analyzed [14, 24]. In the studies of patients with knee OA and relatively little cartilage damage, SPGR MRI had high sensitivity and specificity for detecting cartilage lesions in comparison with arthroscopy [19, 23] and very good correlation with cartilage thickness in comparison with histological evaluation [22].

The underestimation of full cartilage loss with MRI was caused by the thin layers of high signal on the articular surface that were visible on SPGR MRI, which were interpreted as thin layers of damaged cartilage. On retrospective comparison of the acquired SPGR and PD images and histological evaluation, the thin layers of high signal intensity on SPGR images were not identifiable on the PD images, and histological examination identified bare bone at the corresponding locations. These thin lines of high signal intensity adjacent to subchondral bone have previously received little attention in knee OA, as the line is very thin compared to the thicker knee cartilage, and has been counted as full loss of cartilage thickness in MRI knee OA studies [25]. The same kind of thin lines were previously described by Yoshioka et al. [26] in healthy volunteers on the posterior region of the femoral condyle within normal cartilage. The origin of this line is unclear. In our study it may have been caused by an artifact, but we cannot exclude the possibility that it represents a real anatomical substrate, such as a loose-lying layer of thin soft tissue, which may be lost during histological preparation.

We recognize that our study has limitations. First, the study design required patients to be scheduled for trapeziectomy, limiting the spectrum of disease severity. However, this is the only feasible method for acquiring in vivo histological specimens of cartilage from the small joints of the hand. To maximize the variation in cartilage status between our subjects, we included all patients undergoing trapeziectomy for treatment of pain and functional impairment, irrelevant of the severity of OA as determined radiographically. While we expected to also include some patients with mild cartilage damage, all our patients had severe cartilage damage on histological evaluation. Patients with milder OA or pre-clinical OA will have less damaged cartilage, but as mild thinning of the cartilage was also detectable in the less damaged areas of

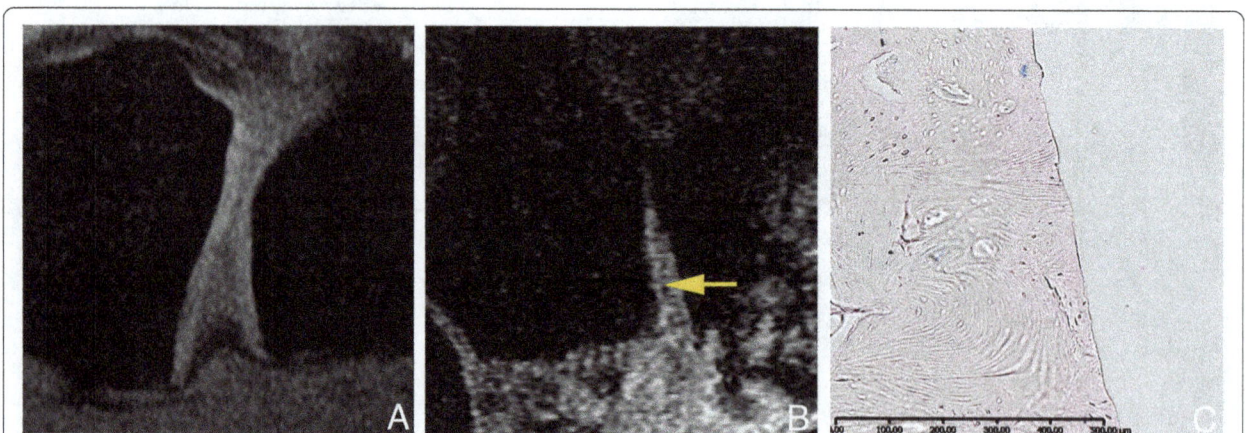

Fig. 5 a Zoomed spoiled gradient, magnetic resonance image with fat saturation, of the first carpometacarpal joint (CMC1) in a healthy volunteer, showing a thick cartilage layer with high signal intensity. **b** Image of the CMC1 joint in a patient. *Arrow* indicates a thin band of high signal intensity, which was scored as partial loss of cartilage thickness (there appears to be some cartilage remaining). The image quality was rated as adequate. **c** Magnification of a histological section from the same patient; each *tick* on the *scale bar* represents 50 μm. The whole articular surface area in this patient had the same appearance, with only bare bone apparent

the joints in our patients, we expect that the imaging method can be used in patients with less severe OA.

The second limitation concerns image quality. Four out of twelve of our MRI examinations were of poor image quality, which may have impacted the MRI results of these four patients. Our coil was a loop coil with a diameter of 40 mm, which was optimal for imaging the CMC1 joint in healthy volunteers. However, in our patients with CMC1 OA, the distance between the coil and the center of the joint was larger because of the presence of osteophytes and subluxation, and the inability of patients to hold the thumb in full extension for optimal coil placement, reducing signal-to-noise ratio. Motion artIfacts also had a big impact on image quality. Improvements in either patient/coil positioning or the coil itself should be able to increase overall image quality.

The third limitation concerns the chosen MRI pulse sequence. We chose to assess cartilage with a 3D SPGR fat-suppressed pulse sequence for its high in-plane resolution with thin 0.7-mm slices, to be able to detect small cartilage lesions. This pulse sequence has previously shown promising results in the small joints of the finger [11, 27]. In healthy volunteers this sequence clearly delineated high-signal cartilage layers. In our study population of patients with advanced osteoarthritis only and with histologically proven abnormal cartilage, the signal intensity of cartilage was lower than expected based on MRI in healthy volunteers. Our MRI readers, therefore, sometimes had trouble delineating the cartilage from the joint fluid, which is a known disadvantage of this pulse sequence [28, 29]. While this will have introduced some error in the results, this was often resolved after cross-checking with the PD and T2 FSE sequences to make the distinction between fluid and cartilage. In this study we did not detect any small focal areas of cartilage loss, raising the question whether such thin slices are required to evaluate cartilage damage in advanced OA. Other pulse sequences such as dual-echo steady state (DESS), SPGR with iterative decomposition of water and fat with echo asymmetry and least-squares estimation (IDEAL), and true fast imaging with steady state precession (TrueFISP) have been found to have better cartilage-to-fluid contrast in the knee joints in healthy volunteers [28, 29]. If these sequences can be adequately optimized for the small FOV and high resolution, they may improve accuracy for detecting cartilage damage in the small joints of the hand.

Our MRI scoring method worked in a small number of patients, but is too time-consuming for larger studies. We chose this method to be as accurate as possible, but would not advise it for use in larger studies; instead, either automated segmentation for detailed detection of cartilage damage or a semi-quantitative score would probably be better.

Conclusion

Three-dimensional SPGR MRI of the carpometacarpal joint of the thumb is able to detect the overall extent of cartilage damage. However, in severe cartilage damage, a layer of high signal intensity on the bone can be seen on 3D SPGR MRI, which does not always correspond to cartilage on histological evaluation, and could therefore lead to overestimation of the remaining cartilage.

Abbreviations

BML: Bone marrow lesions; CMC1: First carpometacarpal joint; CR: Conventional radiology; ETL: Echo train length; FOV: Field of view; FRFSE: Fast recovery fast spin echo; FS: Fat suppression; ICC: Intraclass correlation coefficient; MOAKS: Magnetic resonance imaging osteoarthritis knee score; MRI: Magnetic resonance imaging; OA: Osteoarthritis; OARSI: Osteoarthritis Research Society International; PD: Proton density; SPGR: Spoiled gradient; TE: Echo time; TR: Repetition time

Acknowledgements

We would like to thank participating hand surgeons Professor SER Hovius, Dr ET Walbeehm and Dr CA van Nieuwenhoven for their effort during surgery to keep the trapezium intact; Nicole Kops of the department of orthopedics for preparing the histological sections; Professor JMW Hazes, chair of the department of rheumatology, for her part in acquiring funding; and Professor GP Krestin, chair of the department of radiology, for use of the department's MRI facilities.

Funding

This study was funded by an internal Erasmus MC grant, aimed at promoting cooperation of multiple internal research departments. The funding source had no active role in the study.

Authors' contributions

MS contributed to the design, collected the MRI data, performed histological scoring, performed the analysis, and drafted the manuscript. HC contributed to the design, provided some of the patients, scored the MRI data, and revised the manuscript. RS, JvN, and JL obtained the funding, conceived the study, helped with design, and revised the manuscript. JJ provided most of the patients and revised the manuscript. GvO contributed to design, performed histological scoring, and critically revised the manuscript. EO scored the MRI data and critically revised the manuscript. GM contributed to design, scored the MRI data, helped with interpretation of data, and helped draft the manuscript. All authors read and approved the final manuscript.

Competing interests

The authors declare that they have no competing interests.

Consent for publication

Written consent was acquired from the patients for the use of their histological and magnetic resonance images in this paper.

Author details

[1]Department of Radiology, Erasmus MC, University Medical Center Rotterdam, Rotterdam, The Netherlands. [2]Department of Plastic, Reconstructive and Hand Surgery, Erasmus MC, University Medical Center Rotterdam, Rotterdam, The Netherlands. [3]Department of Rheumatology, Erasmus MC, University Medical Center Rotterdam, Rotterdam, The Netherlands. [4]Department of Plastic, Reconstructive and Hand Surgery, University Medical Center Utrecht, Utrecht, The Netherlands. [5]Department of Rehabilitation Medicine, Erasmus MC, University Medical Center Rotterdam,

Rotterdam, The Netherlands. [6]Department of Plastic, Reconstructive and Hand surgery, Maasstad Hospital, Rotterdam, The Netherlands. [7]Department of Orthopaedics and Department of Otorhinolaryngology, Erasmus MC, University Medical Center Rotterdam, Rotterdam, The Netherlands.

References

1. Dahaghin S, Bierma-Zeinstra SM, Ginai AZ, et al. Prevalence and pattern of radiographic hand osteoarthritis and association with pain and disability (the Rotterdam study). Ann Rheum Dis. 2005;64(5):682–7.

2. Maheu E, Altman RD, Bloch DA, et al. Design and conduct of clinical trials in patients with osteoarthritis of the hand: recommendations from a task force of the Osteoarthritis Research Society International. Osteoarthritis Cartilage. 2006;14(4):303–22.

3. Kloppenburg M, Bøyesen P, Smeets W, et al. Report from the OMERACT Hand Osteoarthritis Special Interest Group: advances and future research priorities. J Rheumatol. 2014;41(4):810–8.

4. Haugen IK, Lillegraven S, Slatkowsky-Christensen B, et al. Hand osteoarthritis and MRI: development and first validation step of the proposed Oslo hand osteoarthritis MRI score. Ann Rheum Dis. 2011;70(6):1033–8.

5. Haugen IK, Ostergaard M, Eshed I, et al. Iterative development and reliability of the OMERACT hand osteoarthritis MRI scoring system. J Rheumatol. 2014; 41(2):386–91.

6. Tan AL, Grainger AJ, Tanner SF, et al. High-resolution magnetic resonance imaging for the assessment of hand osteoarthritis. Arthritis Rheum. 2005; 52(8):2355–65.

7. Tan AL, Toumi H, Benjamin M, et al. Combined high-resolution magnetic resonance imaging and histological examination to explore the role of ligaments and tendons in the phenotypic expression of early hand osteoarthritis. Ann Rheum Dis. 2006;65(10):1267–72.

8. Wittoek R, Jans L, Lambrecht V, et al. Reliability and construct validity of ultrasonography of soft tissue and destructive changes in erosive osteoarthritis of the interphalangeal finger joints: a comparison with MRI. Ann Rheum Dis. 2011;70(2):278–83.

9. Haugen IK, Boyesen P, Slatkowsky-Christensen B, et al. Associations between MRI-defined synovitis, bone marrow lesions and structural features and measures of pain and physical function in hand osteoarthritis. Ann Rheum Dis. 2012;71(6):899–904.

10. Haugen IK, Slatkowsky Christensen B, Boyesen P, et al. Increasing synovitis and bone marrow lesions are associated with incident joint tenderness in hand osteoarthritis. Ann Rheum Dis. 2016;75(4):702–8. doi:10.1136/annrheumdis-2014-2068292015.

11. Peterfy CG, van Dijke CF, Lu Y, et al. Quantification of the volume of articular cartilage in the metacarpophalangeal joints of the hand: accuracy and precision of three-dimensional MR imaging. AJR Am J Roentgenol. 1995;165(2):371–5.

12. Lazovic-Stojkovic J, Mosher TJ, Smith HE, et al. Interphalangeal joint cartilage: high-spatial-resolution in vivo MR T2 mapping–a feasibility study. Radiology. 2004;233(1):292–6.

13. Dupuy DE, Spillane RM, Rosol MS, et al. Quantification of articular cartilage in the knee with three-dimensional MR imaging. Acad Radiol. 1996;3(11):919–24.

14. Saadat E, Jobke B, Chu B, et al. Diagnostic performance of in vivo 3-T MRI for articular cartilage abnormalities in human osteoarthritic knees using histology as standard of reference. Eur Radiol. 2008;18(10):2292–302.

15. Hunter DJ, Guermazi A, Lo GH, et al. Evolution of semi-quantitative whole joint assessment of knee OA: MOAKS (MRI osteoarthritis knee score). Osteoarthritis Cartilage. 2011;19(8):990–1002.

16. Bulstra SK, Drukker J, Kuijer R, et al. Thionin staining of paraffin and plastic embedded sections of cartilage. Biotech Histochem. 1993;68(1):20–8.

17. Pritzker KP, Gay S, Jimenez SA, et al. Osteoarthritis cartilage histopathology: grading and staging. Osteoarthritis Cartilage. 2006;14(1):13–29.

18. Shrout PE, Fleiss JL. Intraclass correlations: uses in assessing rater reliability. Psychol Bull. 1979;86(2):420–8.

19. Disler DG, McCauley TR, Kelman CG, et al. Fat-suppressed three-dimensional spoiled gradient-echo MR imaging of hyaline cartilage defects in the knee: comparison with standard MR imaging and arthroscopy. AJR Am J Roentgenol. 1996;167(1):127–32.

20. Recht MP, Piraino DW, Paletta GA, et al. Accuracy of fat-suppressed three-dimensional spoiled gradient-echo FLASH MR imaging in the detection of patellofemoral articular cartilage abnormalities. Radiology. 1996;198(1):209–12.

21. McGibbon CA, Trahan CA. Measurement accuracy of focal cartilage defects from MRI and correlation of MRI graded lesions with histology: a preliminary study. Osteoarthritis Cartilage. 2003;11(7):483–93.

22. Kladny B, Martus P, Schiwy-Bochat KH, et al. Measurement of cartilage thickness in the human knee-joint by magnetic resonance imaging using a three-dimensional gradient-echo sequence. Int Orthop. 1999;23(5):264–7.

23. Yoshioka H, Stevens K, Hargreaves BA, et al. Magnetic resonance imaging of articular cartilage of the knee: comparison between fat-suppressed three-dimensional SPGR imaging, fat-suppressed FSE imaging, and fat-suppressed three-dimensional DEFT imaging, and correlation with arthroscopy. J Magn Reson Imaging. 2004;20(5):857–64.

24. Burgkart R, Glaser C, Hyhlik-Durr A, et al. Magnetic resonance imaging-based assessment of cartilage loss in severe osteoarthritis: accuracy, precision, and diagnostic value. Arthritis Rheum. 2001;44(9):2072–7.

25. Frobell RB, Wirth W, Nevitt M, et al. Presence, location, type and size of denuded areas of subchondral bone in the knee as a function of radiographic stage of OA - data from the OA initiative. Osteoarthritis Cartilage. 2010;18(5):668–76.

26. Yoshioka H, Stevens K, Genovese M, et al. Articular cartilage of knee: normal patterns at MR imaging that mimic disease in healthy subjects and patients with osteoarthritis. Radiology. 2004;231(1):31–8.

27. Kwok WE, You Z, Monu J, et al. High-resolution uniform MR imaging of finger joints using a dedicated RF coil at 3 T. J Magn Reson Imaging. 2010;31(1):240–7.

28. Siepmann DB, McGovern J, Brittain JH, et al. High-resolution 3D cartilage imaging with IDEAL SPGR at 3 T. AJR Am J Roentgenol. 2007;189(6):1510–5.

29. Friedrich KM, Reiter G, Kaiser B, et al. High-resolution cartilage imaging of the knee at 3 T: Basic evaluation of modern isotropic 3D MR-sequences. Eur J Radiol. 2011;78(3):398–405.

Curcumin slows osteoarthritis progression and relieves osteoarthritis-associated pain symptoms in a post-traumatic osteoarthritis mouse model

Zhuo Zhang[1,2,3†], Daniel J. Leong[1,2†], Lin Xu[1,2], Zhiyong He[1,2], Angela Wang[1,2], Mahantesh Navati[4,5], Sun J. Kim[1], David M. Hirsh[1], John A. Hardin[1], Neil J. Cobelli[1], Joel M. Friedman[4,5] and Hui B. Sun[1,2*]

Abstract

Background: Curcumin has been shown to have chondroprotective potential in vitro. However, its effect on disease and symptom modification in osteoarthritis (OA) is largely unknown. This study aimed to determine whether curcumin could slow progression of OA and relieve OA-related pain in a mouse model of destabilization of the medial meniscus (DMM).

Methods: Expression of selected cartilage degradative-associated genes was evaluated in human primary chondrocytes treated with curcumin and curcumin nanoparticles and assayed by real-time PCR. The mice subjected to DMM surgery were orally administered curcumin or topically administered curcumin nanoparticles for 8 weeks. Cartilage integrity was evaluated by Safranin O staining and Osteoarthritis Research Society International (OARSI) score, and by immunohistochemical staining of cleaved aggrecan and type II collagen, and levels of matrix metalloproteinase (MMP)-13 and ADAMTS5. Synovitis and subchondral bone thickness were scored based on histologic images. OA-associated pain and symptoms were evaluated by von Frey assay, and locomotor behavior including distance traveled and rearing.

Results: Both curcumin and nanoparticles encapsulating curcumin suppressed mRNA expression of pro-inflammatory mediators IL-1β and TNF-α, MMPs 1, 3, and 13, and aggrecanase ADAMTS5, and upregulated the chondroprotective transcriptional regulator CITED2, in primary cultured chondrocytes in the absence or presence of IL-1β. Oral administration of curcumin significantly reduced OA disease progression, but showed no significant effect on OA pain relief. Curcumin was detected in the infrapatellar fat pad (IPFP) following topical administration of curcumin nanoparticles on the skin of the injured mouse knee. Compared to vehicle-treated controls, topical treatment led to: (1) reduced proteoglycan loss and cartilage erosion and lower OARSI scores, (2) reduced synovitis and subchondral plate thickness, (3) reduced immunochemical staining of type II collagen and aggrecan cleavage epitopes and numbers of chondrocytes positive for MMP-13 and ADAMTS5 in the articular cartilage, and (4) reduced expression of adipokines and pro-inflammatory mediators in the IPFP. In contrast to oral curcumin, topical application of curcumin nanoparticles relieved OA-related pain as indicated by reduced tactile hypersensitivity and improved locomotor behavior.

Conclusion: This study provides the first evidence that curcumin significantly slows OA disease progression and exerts a palliative effect in an OA mouse model.

Keywords: Post-traumatic osteoarthritis, Curcumin, Nutraceuticals, Chondroprotection, MMPs, ADAMTS5

* Correspondence: herb.sun@einstein.yu.edu
†Equal contributors
[1]Department of Orthopaedic Surgery, Albert Einstein College of Medicine, Bronx, NY, USA
[2]Department of Radiation Oncology, Albert Einstein College of Medicine, Bronx, NY, USA
Full list of author information is available at the end of the article

Background

Osteoarthritis (OA) is a progressive and degenerative disease of the articular joints involving the articular cartilage, synovium, and subchondral bone, and is a leading cause of pain and disability in the adult population [1]. Despite the high prevalence of OA, there is currently no cure or effective treatment that halts or reverses disease progression [2]. While current pharmacologic treatments such as analgesics and nonsteroidal anti-inflammatory drugs (NSAIDs) provide symptomatic relief, such as relieving pain, they do not exert a clear clinical effect on OA disease prevention or modification [3]. In most cases, long-term use of these treatments has been associated with substantial gastrointestinal, renal, and cardiovascular side effects [3]. There is a clear and urgent need for new therapeutic strategies that are effective and safe for OA treatment.

Curcumin, the principal curcuminoid and the most active component in turmeric, is a biologically active phytochemical [4, 5]. Evidence from several recent in vitro studies suggests that curcumin may exert a chondroprotective effect through actions such as anti-inflammatory, anti-oxidative stress, and anti-catabolic activity that are critical for mitigating OA disease pathogenesis and symptoms. For example, curcumin has been shown to mitigate the inflammatory process by decreasing synthesis of inflammatory mediators such as interleukin (IL)-1β, tumor necrosis factor (TNF)-α, IL-6, IL-8, prostaglandin E2 (PGE$_2$), and cyclooxygenase-2 (COX-2) [6–8], inhibit IL-1β-induced extracellular matrix degradation [9] and chondrocyte apoptosis [10, 11], and mitigate the overproduction of reactive oxygen and nitrogen species [12, 13]. Moreover, curcumin, by inhibiting the activator protein 1 (AP-1) pathway [14] and nuclear factor kappa B (NF-kB) activation [14–16], suppresses the gene expression of a number of matrix metalloproteinases (MMPs), which play critical roles in the breakdown of the cartilage extracellular matrix [7, 14–17].

Despite the recent progress, the effect of curcumin on OA disease progression and pain relief is largely unknown. Moon et al. showed that following intraperitoneal injection of curcumin every other day for 2 weeks, expression of TNF-α and IL-1β in the ankle joint, and serum immunoglobulin concentrations in mice with collagen-induced arthritis were downregulated compared with non-curcumin-treated mice [18], suggesting curcumin may be beneficial in rheumatoid arthritis. Furthermore, Colitti et al. found that oral delivery of curcumin in canines with spontaneous OA leads to decreased IL-18 and TNF-α production, and inhibition of the inflammatory transcription factor NF-kB in white blood cells [19]. The study suggests a potential anti-inflammatory effect of curcumin on the joints in OA.

While several studies suggest oral administration of curcumin may exert an effect in relieving OA-related pain

[20–24], topical application may provide another patient-friendly method of treatment. Importantly, it may increase the bioavailability of curcumin at the disease site for OA treatment. In this study, we aim to determine the efficacies of curcumin through oral delivery and custom-made nanoparticles through topical administration in OA disease and symptom modification using a mouse model of post-traumatic OA.

Methods

Cell culture and curcumin treatment in vitro

All human studies were approved by the Albert Einstein College of Medicine Institutional Review Board. Human primary chondrocytes derived from patients undergoing joint replacement surgery (women aged 58–69 years, n = 3) were cultured in DMEM/F12 with 10 % fetal bovine serum [25]. Prior to curcumin treatment, cells were cultured in the DMEM/F12 with 1 % fetal bovine serum overnight. In some experiments, chondrocytes were incubated with IL-1β (10 ng/ml, Sigma) 30 minutes prior to incubation with curcumin (100 μM, Sigma) or curcumin (100 μM) encapsulated within nanoparticles for 6 hours. Cells were then lysed and RNA isolated for reverse transcription-quantitative polymerase chain reaction (real-time-PCR) [26]. The dose (100 μM) and treatment duration (6 hours) were chosen based on assays for dose-response (0–200 μM) and time course (0–48 hours) of human primary chondrocytes treated with non-encapsulated curcumin (Additional file 1: Figure S1).

Preparation of curcumin nanoparticles

Curcumin nanoparticles were prepared using a variation of a nanoparticle platform that was developed for topical and systemic delivery of nitric oxide [27–29] in three steps as follows [30]: (1) hydrolysis of tetra-methylorthosilicate (TMOS). Hydrolyzed TMOS is prepared by sonicating at ice temperature, a mixture of 3 ml TMOS and 600 μl 1 mM HCl in a small glass bottle with rubber stopper. Upon sonication the initial biphasic solution turns into a monophasic solution. The monophasic solution is stored at 4 °C for an hour to help eliminate methanol, a byproduct of TMOS hydrolysis (residual methanol is further eliminated during the lyophilization process); (2) polymerization. The following ingredients are added sequentially to a 50-ml conical tube, which is inverted (to facilitate mixing) after each addition of an ingredient: 24 ml of PBS 50 mM pH 7.5, 1.5 ml PEG 400, 1.5 ml chitosan (5 mg/ml) at pH 6 in acetic acid, 4 ml of 5 mg/ml curcumin (Sigma) dissolved in dimethyl sulfoxide (DMSO) and finally 3 ml hydrolyzed TMOS. After all the ingredients are mixed a homogeneous gel is formed in approximately 30 minutes; (3) lyophilization and ball-milling. The wet sol-gel containing the curcumin is freeze-dried overnight. The resulting dry course powder is then ball-milled and stored in a sealed vial for subsequent use for the experiments. A very similar version of this platform has been used to treat topical infections and accelerate wound healing [31].

Induction of osteoarthritis in mice and curcumin treatment

All animal studies were approved by the Albert Einstein College of Medicine Institutional Animal Care and Use Committee. Destabilization of the medial meniscus (DMM) was established in adult C57BL/6 male mice (male, 5–6 months of age) by surgically transecting the medial meniscotibial ligament (MMTL) in the right hind limb [32]. Briefly, the joint capsule immediately medial to the patellar tendon was incised, followed by blunt dissection of the infrapatellar fat pad, to provide visualization of the MMTL of the medial meniscus. The MMTL was transected, leading to destabilization of the medial meniscus (DMM). In the sham surgery, the MMTL was visualized but not transected. The joint capsule and skin were closed by suture. Immediately after the DMM surgery, mice were subjected to (1) oral administration of 50 mg/kg curcumin (Sigma) dissolved in corn oil or vehicle (corn oil only) administered via oral gavage (n = 8/group), or (2) topical application of curcumin nanoparticles (0.07 mg of 10 µg curcumin/1 mg nanoparticles) or vehicle control (coconut oil) on the skin, within a 5-mm^2 area directly above the DMM-operated knee (n = 5/group), once daily for 8 weeks.

Safranin O staining, OARSI score, and histologic evaluation of synovium and subchondral bone

Animals were sacrificed at 8 weeks following curcumin treatment. The hind limbs were fixed in formalin, decalcified in formic acid, embedded in paraffin, and sectioned for histological and immunohistochemical analysis. afranin O-fast green staining was used to visualize proteoglycans in the articular cartilage. The severity of OA was evaluated in the medial compartment of the knee with at least five sections for each mouse using the Osteoarthritis Research Society International (OARSI) scoring system [33]. The synovial pathology (i.e., synovitis) was analyzed on Safranin O stained sections from which the OARSI scores were obtained. The degree of synovitis was scored using a scoring system that measured the thickness of the synovial lining cell layer on a scale of 0–3 (0 = 1–2 cells, 1 = 2–4 cells, 2 = 4–9 cells and 3 = 10 or more cells) and cellular density in the synovial stroma on a scale of 0–3 (0 = normal cellularity, 1 = slightly increased cellularity, 2 = moderately increased cellularity and 3 = greatly increased cellularity). Synovitis scores obtained from all four quadrants (medial tibia, medial femur, lateral tibia, and lateral femur) for both of the above parameters were averaged separately and then the sum of averages from both parameters was used for analysis (on a scale of 0–6)

[34]. The thickness of the medial subchondral bone plate (region between the osteochondral junction and marrow space on the medial side of the tibial plateau, in µm) was measured using AxioVision software using Safranin O stained sections from which the OARSI and synovitis scores were obtained [35].

Immunohistochemical analysis

Sections were incubated overnight at 4 °C with antibodies against cleaved aggrecan (NITEGE, Ibex) and cleaved type II collagen (Col2-3/4 M, Ibex), matrix metalloproteinase (MMP)-13 (Abcam), and a disintegrin and metalloproteinase with thrombospondin motifs (ADAMTS)5 (Abcam) followed by incubation with anti-mouse or anti-rabbit secondary antibody (Biocare Medical) and visualization with 3,3-diaminobenzidine (DAB) chromagen (Vector Laboratories). Negative controls were stained with irrelevant isotype-matched antibodies (Biocare Medical). Immunostaining intensity for type II collagen or aggrecan cleavage epitopes was quantified by determining the "reciprocal intensity" of the stained articular cartilage matrix; briefly, the light intensity value of six random locations within all three zones from the posterior to anterior direction of the femoral and tibial condyles of three sections per mouse was measured using the color picker in Adobe Photoshop [36, 37]. Percentages of positive MMP-13 and ADAMTS5 chondrocytes were determined by counting the number of immunostained cells and dividing by the total number of chondrocytes visualized by a hematoxylin counterstain (Vector Laboratories).

In vivo localization of topically applied curcumin

Curcumin nanoparticles (0.07 mg of 10 µg curcumin/1 mg nanoparticles dissolved in coconut oil) or vehicle control (coconut oil) were topically applied on the right knee of adult C57BL/6 mice (male, 5–6 months). At 3, 6, and 24 hours after treatment (n = 3/group), the animals were sacrificed and the hind limbs were fixed in formalin, decalcified in formic acid, embedded in paraffin and sectioned for histological analysis. Sections (5-µm) were stained with hematoxylin and eosin (H&E), and imaged with confocal microscopy to localize the curcumin particles within the articular joint. In a separate group of animals, mice were sacrificed 3 hours after topical application of curcumin nanoparticles or vehicle control (n = 3/group). The IPFP from the right knee was dissected and flash frozen. RNA was isolated for real-time PCR.

von Frey testing

Mice were acclimated for 30 minutes in individual chambers on top of a wire grid platform prior to von Frey testing. The plantar surface of the hind paw was stimulated with ascending force intensities of von Frey filaments

(Stoelting) to determine tactile sensitivity. A positive response was defined as a rapid withdrawal of the hind paw when the stimulus was applied, and the number of positive responses for each stimulus was recorded. Tactile threshold was defined as a withdrawal response in 5 out of 10 trials to a given stimulus intensity [37]. This threshold was calculated once per animal.

Pain and OA-related behavioral tests

As we and others previously described, mice were acclimated to the test room for 30 minutes before open field testing [37, 38]. Mice were placed in the center of individual plexiglass square chambers (45 cm × 45 cm) and allowed to freely explore the chamber for the duration of the 6-minute test session. The movements of the mice were recorded with a video camera. Upon completion of the test, which was performed once per animal, each mouse was returned to its home cage. Two observers blinded to treatment group assignments manually traced mouse movements to calculate the distance (in cm) that the mouse traveled within the cage in 6 minutes (distance traveled), and recorded the number of times each mouse reared (standing on its hind limbs) within 6 minutes (rearing) [38].

Real-time PCR

Total RNA was isolated with an RNeasy kit (Qiagen) and cDNA was synthesized using the iScript Reverse Transcriptase kit (Bio-Rad). SYBR Green real-time PCR (Bio-Rad) was performed in duplicate for each sample to determine relative gene expression using *Glyceraldehyde-3-phosphate dehydrogenase* (*GAPDH*) as a housekeeping control with the $2^{-\Delta\Delta Ct}$ method [26, 37].

Statistical analysis

Results are expressed as mean ± SD. Significance was determined using Student's *t* test or one-way analysis of variance (ANOVA) and Tukey's multiple comparison test with a significance level of $p < 0.05$ (GraphPad).

Results

Gene expression profile change favors chondroprotection in curcumin-treated human chondrocytes in vitro

We first validated the chondroprotective potential of curcumin by gene expression profile analysis in chondrocytes in vitro. Consistent with previous studies [7, 14–17], human primary chondrocytes, in the absence and presence of IL-1β, and treated with curcumin, exhibited significantly reduced mRNA levels of proteolytic enzymes MMP-1, MMP-3, and MMP-13, and pro-inflammatory cytokines IL-1β and TNF-α ($p < 0.05$) (Fig. 1). Interestingly, as shown for the first time, curcumin significantly reduced expression of aggrecanase ADAMTS5 and increased expression of CITED2 (Cbp/p300 Interacting Transactivator with ED-rich tail 2),

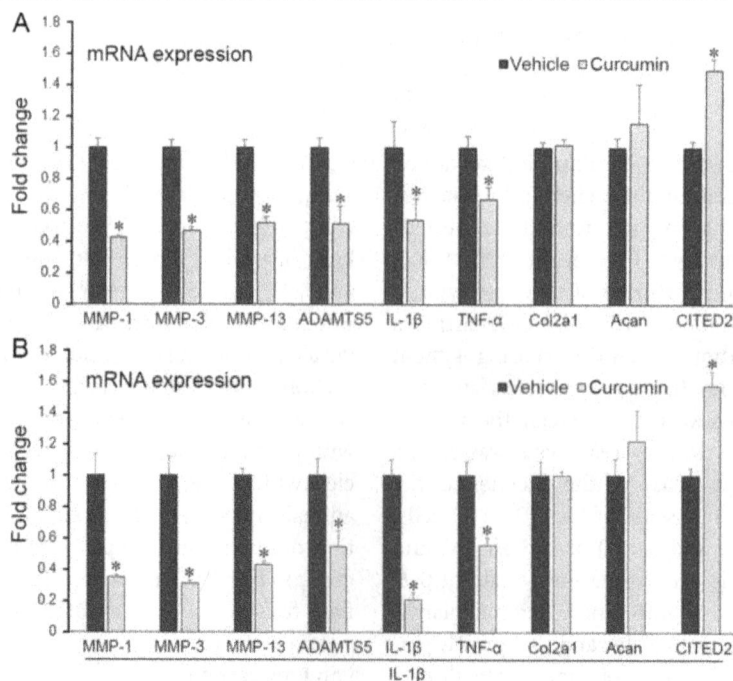

Fig. 1 Chondrocytes treated with curcumin exhibits a gene expression profile that is favorable for chondroprotection. Human primary chondrocytes treated with curcumin for 6 hours exhibited reduced mRNA levels of matrix metalloproteinase (*MMP*)-1, MMP-3, MMP-13, a disintegrin and metalloproteinase with thrombospondin motifs (*ADAMTS*)5, IL-1β, TNF-α, and increased CITED2 compared to vehicle-treated cells, in the absence (**a**) and presence (**b**) of IL-1β, while expression of collagen 2a1 (*Col2a1*) and aggrecan (*Acan*) remained unchanged. *$P < 0.05$, *t* test, n = 3/group

MMP-repressing transcriptional regulator ($p < 0.05$) (Fig. 1). No effects of curcumin on expression of anabolic genes collagen 2a1 and aggrecan were observed ($p > 0.05$) (Fig. 1).

Oral delivery of curcumin slows disease progression but does not significantly affect OA-related symptoms in mice with DMM

We next determined the efficacy of curcumin on DMM-induced OA through oral administration by evaluating the structural integrity of the articular cartilage using microscopy following Safranin O staining and OARSI evaluation. Eight weeks after DMM, the articular cartilage in the limb with DMM in the vehicle-treated mice exhibited moderate pathological osteoarthritic changes characterized by Safranin O loss, cartilage fibrillation, and cartilage erosion (Fig. 2a), with an OARSI score of 4.0 ± 0.5. (Fig. 2b). In contrast, the cartilage in the limb with DMM in curcumin-treated mice exhibited less Safranin O loss and cartilage fibrillation (Fig. 2a) with a significantly lower OARSI score (2.4 ± 0.42) compared to that in vehicle-treated controls ($p < 0.05$, Fig. 2b). Curcumin treatment also significantly reduced synovitis (Fig. 2c) and subchondral plate thickness (Fig. 2d) compared to vehicle controls ($p < 0.05$ for both). However, oral administration of curcumin had no significant effect on mitigating OA-related pain, as evaluated by von Frey testing, distance traveled and hind limb rearing (not shown).

Curcumin nanoparticles exert an anti-catabolic and anti-inflammatory effect in human chondrocytes in vitro

While oral administration of non-encapsulated curcumin exhibited significant efficacy in slowing the progression of OA, its therapeutic efficacy may be restricted by its relatively poor oral bioavailability [39]. We therefore developed curcumin nanoparticles using a novel polymeric nanoparticle carrier [30]. To test whether nanoparticles encapsulating curcumin affect the chondroprotective potential of curcumin, we compared the gene expression profile in primary cultured human chondrocytes in the absence or presence of IL-1β and treated with curcumin nanoparticles or vehicle control. Curcumin nanoparticles significantly reduced mRNA levels of MMP-1, MMP-3, MMP-13, ADAMTS5, IL-1β and TNF-α, and increased levels of CITED2 chondrocytes compared to the vehicle control ($p < 0.05$ for all), at a comparable level to that of non-encapsulated curcumin-treated chondrocytes, based on the equivalent concentration of curcumin, in the absence or presence of IL-1β ($p > 0.05$ for all, Fig. 3). No significant effects of curcumin nanoparticles on expression of collagen 2a1 and aggrecan were observed ($p > 0.05$) (Fig. 3).

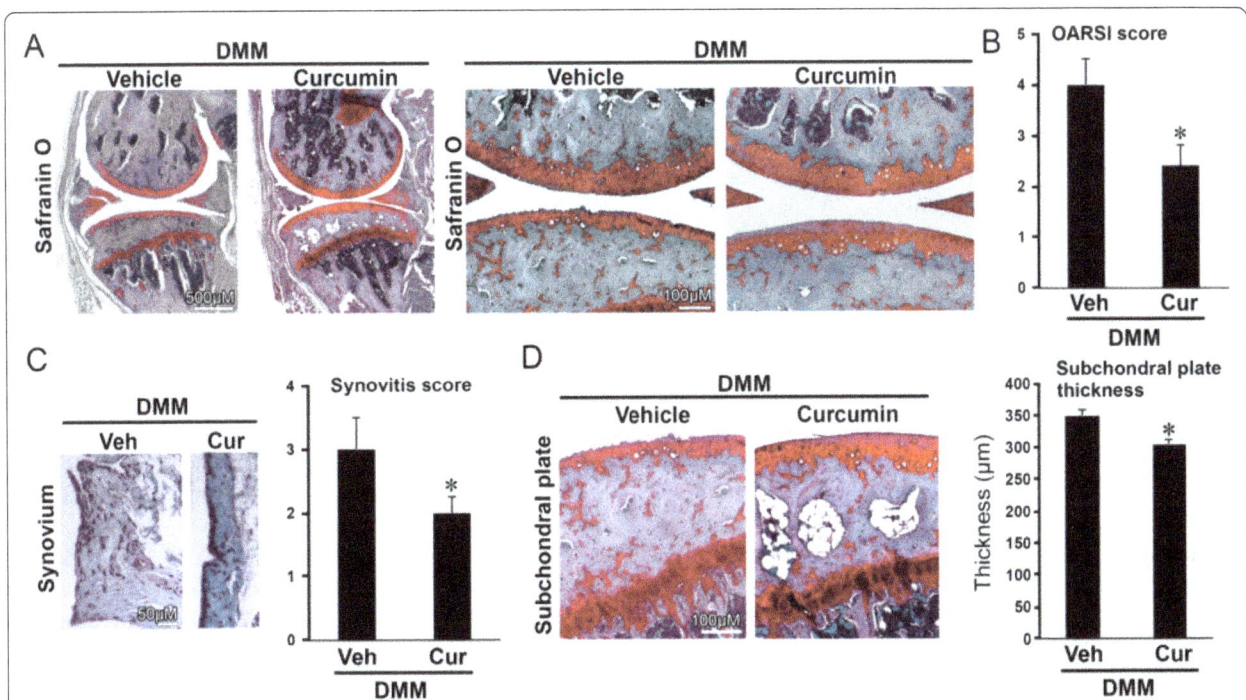

Fig. 2 Oral administration of curcumin slowed progression of post-traumatic osteoarthritis in mice. Mice with destabilization of the medial meniscus (*DMM*) were treated daily with curcumin (*Cur*) or vehicle via oral gavage. Mice with DMM treated with curcumin exhibited improved Safranin O staining (**a**), lower Osteoarthritis Research Society International (*OARSI*) scores (**b**), and reduced synovitis (**c**) and subchondral plate thickness (**d**) at 8 weeks following surgery, compared to mice with DMM that were treated with vehicle (*Veh*). *$P < 0.05$, *t* test, n = 8/group. Representative histologic images are shown

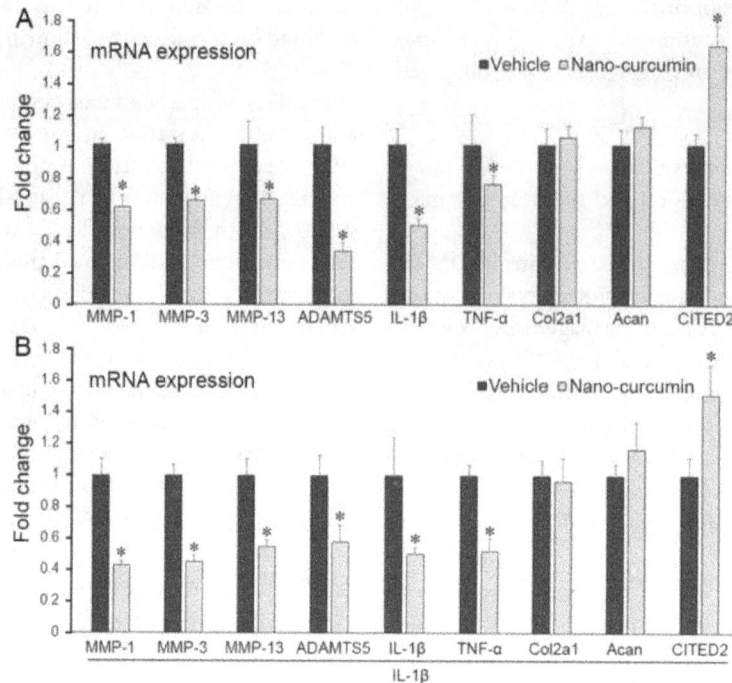

Fig. 3 Curcumin nanoparticles exert anti-catabolic and anti-inflammatory effect on gene expression of human primary chondrocytes in the absence of IL-1β (**a**) and presence of IL-1β (**b**). Human primary chondrocytes treated with nano-encapsulated curcumin (nano-curcumin) for 6 hours exhibited reduced mRNA levels of matrix metalloproteinase (*MMP*)-1, MMP-3, MMP-13, a disintegrin and metalloproteinase with thrombospondin motifs (*ADAMTS5*), IL-1β, TNF-α, and increased levels of CITED2 compared to that in vehicle-treated cells, while expression of collagen 2a1 (*Col2a1*) and aggrecan (*Acan*) remained unchanged. *$P < 0.05$, t test, n = 5/group

Topical curcumin nanoparticles localize and are effective in the infrapatellar fat pad (IPFP)

To test whether local, topical application of curcumin nanoparticles would exert increased efficacy in treating OA, we first determined whether curcumin nanoparticles could penetrate into the joint tissues following topical application to the mouse knee. Curcumin was detected in the IPFP at 3 hours following topical application as shown in Fig. 4a, but was not detected in the articular cartilage or other joint tissues, or at 6 or 24 hours following topical application (not shown), using confocal microscopy based on the auto-fluorescence of curcumin [40]. As curcumin was localized within the IPFP, we next examined the effect of curcumin nanoparticle topical treatment on the gene expression profile of pro-inflammatory mediators in the IPFP, which have been shown to have a significant impact on cartilage homeostasis and OA [41–43]. As revealed by real-time PCR, the treatment suppressed mRNA expression of adipokines *adipsin*, *leptin*, *adiponectin*, adipo-regulatory transcription factors CCAAT/enhancer binding protein alpha (*Cebpa*) and peroxisome proliferator-activated receptor gamma (*Pparg*), and *Mmp13* and *Adamts5* ($p < 0.05$ for all, Fig. 4b).

Topical application of curcumin nanoparticles slows progression of OA in mice with DMM

To determine efficacy of topical application of curcumin nanoparticles on OA disease progression, we evaluated structural integrity of the articular cartilage after eight weeks of daily topical curcumin treatment beginning immediately following DMM in mice. Eight weeks after DMM, the articular cartilage in the limb with DMM in the vehicle-treated mice exhibited moderate pathological osteoarthritic change characterized by Safranin O loss and cartilage fibrillation (Fig. 5a), and an average OARSI score of 5.8 ± 2.1 (Fig. 5b). In contrast, the cartilage in the limb with DMM in mice treated with curcumin nanoparticles exhibited less Safranin O loss and cartilage fibrillation (Fig. 5a), and the mean OARSI score (1.8 ± 0.35) was significantly lower compared to vehicle-treated controls ($p < 0.05$, Fig. 5b). In addition, curcumin nanoparticles significantly reduced synovitis (Fig. 5c) and subchondral plate thickness (Fig. 5d) compared to vehicle-treated controls ($p < 0.05$ for both).

Topical application of curcumin nanoparticles reduced matrix degradation markers and levels of MMP-13 and ADAMTS5 in cartilage from mice with DMM

Immunohistochemical staining showed that topical curcumin treatment strongly reduced the levels of the type

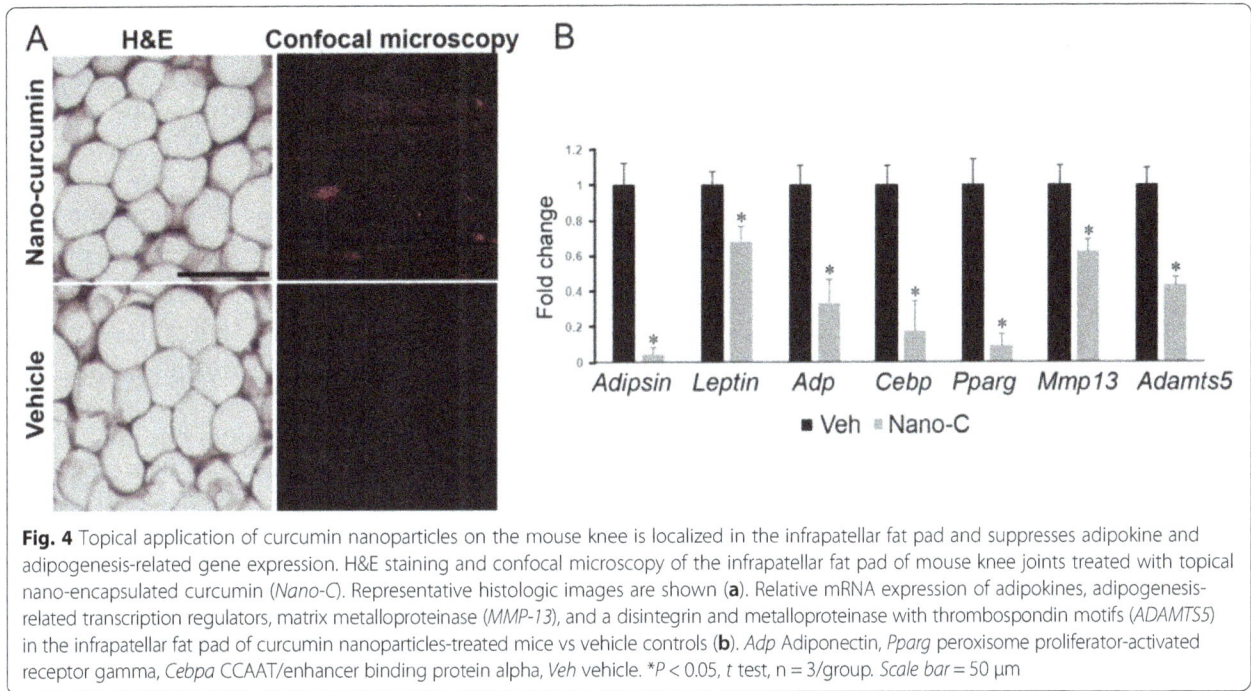

Fig. 4 Topical application of curcumin nanoparticles on the mouse knee is localized in the infrapatellar fat pad and suppresses adipokine and adipogenesis-related gene expression. H&E staining and confocal microscopy of the infrapatellar fat pad of mouse knee joints treated with topical nano-encapsulated curcumin (*Nano-C*). Representative histologic images are shown (**a**). Relative mRNA expression of adipokines, adipogenesis-related transcription regulators, matrix metalloproteinase (*MMP-13*), and a disintegrin and metalloproteinase with thrombospondin motifs (*ADAMTS5*) in the infrapatellar fat pad of curcumin nanoparticles-treated mice vs vehicle controls (**b**). *Adp* Adiponectin, *Pparg* peroxisome proliferator-activated receptor gamma, *Cebpa* CCAAT/enhancer binding protein alpha, *Veh* vehicle. *$P < 0.05$, *t* test, n = 3/group. *Scale bar* = 50 μm

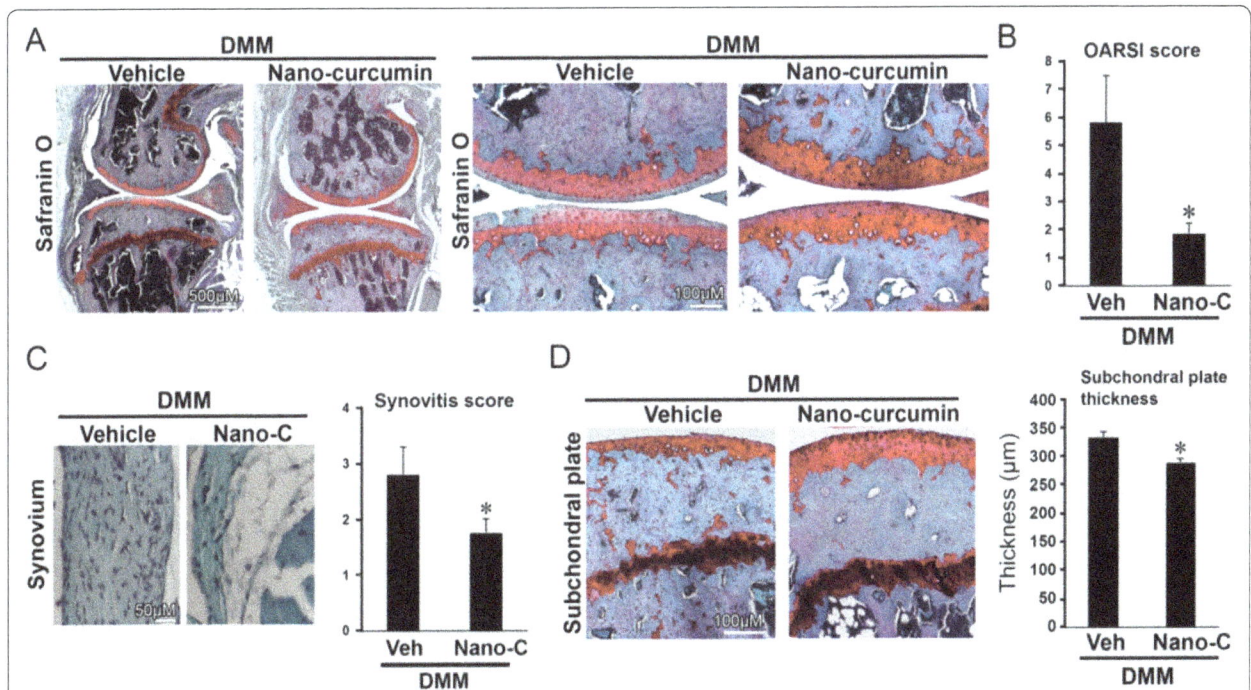

Fig. 5 Topical application of nano-encapsulated curcumin slowed the progression of OA induced by destabilization of the medial meniscus (*DMM*) in mice. Mice with DMM were treated daily with topical application of curcumin nanoparticles or vehicle. Mice treated topically with curcumin nanoparticles (*Nano-C*) exhibited improved Safranin O staining (**a**), lower Osteoarthritis Research Society International (*OARSI*) scores (**b**), and reduced synovitis (**c**), and subchondral bone plate thickness (**d**) at 8 weeks after surgery compared to that in vehicle control (*Veh*) (*$p < 0.05$, *t* test, n = 5/group). Representative histologic images are shown

II collagen cleavage epitope (Col2 3/4 M) in mice with DMM compared to vehicle-treated mice with DMM (Fig. 6a). Based on the immunostaining intensities of six randomly selected areas of the articular cartilage at 8 weeks following DMM, type II collagen cleavage was reduced to 0.58-fold in curcumin-treated animals compared to vehicle-treated controls ($p < 0.05$, Fig. 6a). Immunohistochemical staining similarly showed that curcumin nanoparticle treatment reduced the levels of cleaved aggrecan (NITEGE) in mice with DMM compared to vehicle-treated mice with DMM at 8 weeks (Fig. 6b). At 8 weeks after DMM, the immunostaining intensity of cleaved aggrecan in curcumin nanoparticle-treated mice with DMM was reduced to 0.68-fold compared to vehicle-treated mice ($p < 0.05$, Fig. 6b).

Cartilage matrix degradation is mainly mediated by two major families of proteolytic enzymes, namely MMPs and ADAMTS [44]. In particular, MMP-13 is the most potent enzyme in cleaving type II collagen, the principal form in articular cartilage, while ADAMTS5 has been shown in mice to cleave aggrecan, the major cartilage proteoglycan [2]. We therefore examined whether reduction of MMP-13 and ADAMTS5 could underlie the chondroprotective effect of curcumin using immunohistochemical analysis.

At 8 weeks following DMM, the percentage of MMP-13-positive cells in the articular cartilage was reduced from 63 % in vehicle-treated mice to 16 % in curcumin-treated mice ($p < 0.05$, Fig. 6c). Similarly, curcumin reduced the percentage of ADAMTS5-positive cells from 68 % in vehicle-treated mice to 37 % ($p < 0.05$, Fig. 6d). These data suggest that curcumin treatment improves the integrity of the articular cartilage by preserving both collagen and aggrecan components in mice with post-traumatic OA, and that the chondroprotective effects exerted by curcumin are mediated, at least in part, by suppressing the predominant collagenase MMP-13 and predominant aggrecanase ADAMTS5.

Topical curcumin nanoparticles reduce OA-related pain

The progression of OA is accompanied by secondary clinical symptoms, most prominently pain [45, 46]. At 8 weeks following DMM, vehicle-treated mice exhibited reductions in the threshold of response to mechanical stimuli ($p < 0.05$, von Frey assay, Fig. 7a), distance traveled (Fig. 7b), and rearing (standing on hind limbs, Fig. 7c), compared to naïve controls ($p < 0.05$). Animals topically treated with curcumin nanoparticles exhibited reduced tactile hypersensitivity ($p > 0.05$, Fig. 7a), and increased distance traveled ($p > 0.05$, Fig. 7b) and rearing ($p > 0.05$, Fig. 7c).

Discussion

In this study we demonstrated the first evidence in vivo to show that oral and topical curcumin administration slows the progression of post-traumatic OA in the

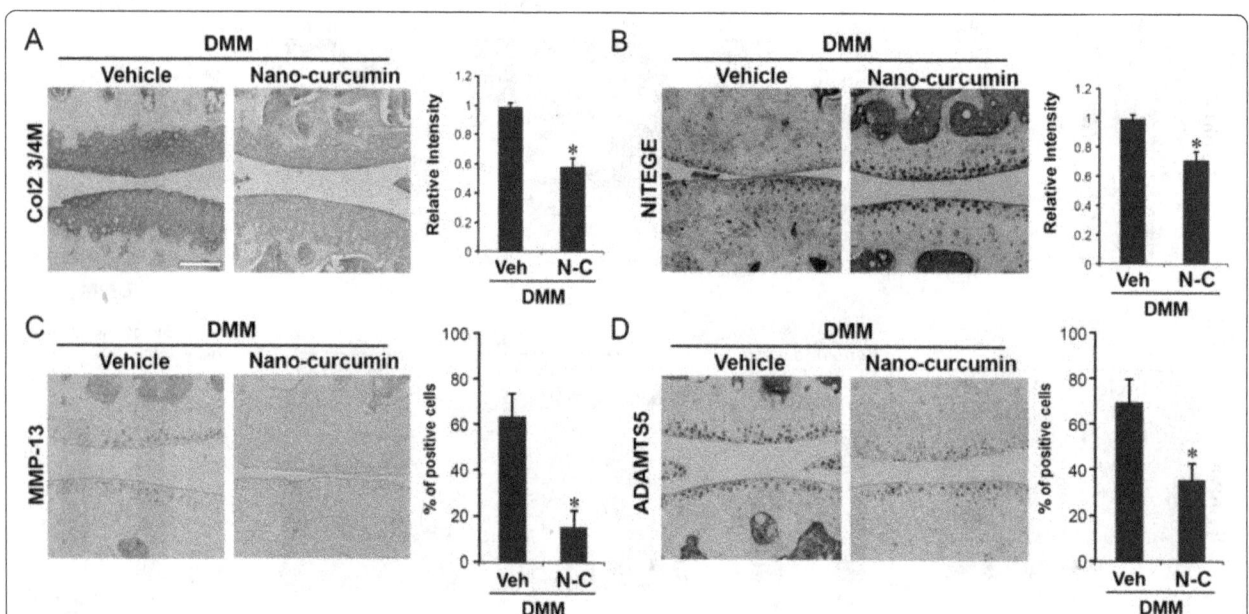

Fig. 6 Topical application of curcumin nanoparticles reduced the degradation of articular cartilage matrix and reduced the expression of matrix metalloproteinase-13 (*MMP-13*) and a disintegrin and metalloproteinase with thrombospondin motifs-5 (*ADAMTS5*). Intensity of immunohistochemical staining of type II collagen cleavage epitope (*Col2-3/4 M*) (**a**) and cleaved aggrecan (*NITEGE*) (**b**), and percentage of positive cells of immunohistochemical staining of MMP-13 (**c**), and of ADAMTS5 (**d**) in the articular cartilage of mice with destabilization of the medial meniscus (*DMM*) that were treated with curcumin nanoparticles (*N-C*) for 8 weeks following surgery were significantly reduced compared to mice with DMM treated with vehicle (*Veh*) (*$p < 0.05$, *t* test, n = 5/group). *Scale bar* = 100 μM. Representative immunohistochemical images are shown

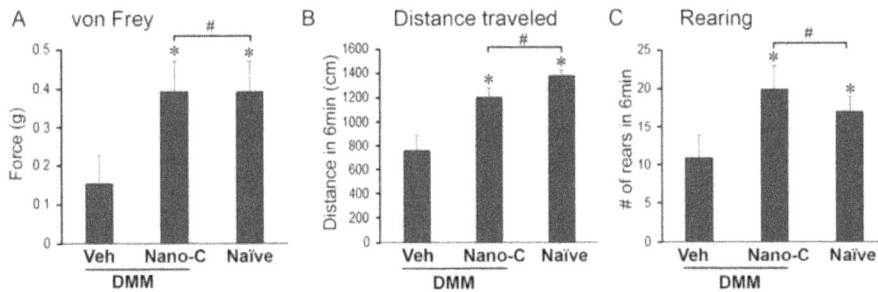

Fig. 7 Topical application of curcumin nanoparticles reduces osteoarthritis-related pain symptoms. Tactile sensitivity (von Frey testing) (**a**), and distance traveled (**b**) and number of times reared (**c**) per 6 minutes in an open field, in mice with destabilization of the medial meniscus (*DMM*) treated with curcumin nanoparticles (*Nano-C*) at 8 weeks after DMM surgery, did not differ from naïve controls (#$p > 0.05$, one-way analysis of variance (ANOVA) with Tukey post-hoc test, n = 5/group), but had significant improvement compared to mice with DMM treated with vehicle (*Veh*) (*$p < 0.05$, one-way ANOVA with Tukey post-hoc test, n = 5/group)

DMM mouse model. Specifically, we showed that oral or topical administration of curcumin immediately after DMM significantly slowed or delayed the initiation and progression of OA in mice. This was indicated by less cartilage erosion and proteoglycan loss, reduced synovitis and subchondral plate thickness, reduced degradation of type II collagen and aggrecan, and lower expression of MMP-13 and ADAMTS5 following curcumin treatment compared to vehicle controls. The preventative and therapeutic potential of curcumin is extremely valuable, given about 50 % of patients who suffer joint injuries, such as anterior cruciate ligament tears, develop OA within 10–15 years [47], and that there is no disease-modifying therapy for OA [48].

Furthermore, we provide the first evidence of a palliative effect of curcumin encapsulated in custom-made nanoparticles applied topically to an osteoarthritic joint in mice. Mice with DMM treated with curcumin nanoparticles exhibited decreased sensitivity to mechanical stimuli and increased locomotor behavior (i.e., distance traveled and rearing) compared to vehicle-treated mice, suggesting an improvement in OA-related pain. The results are consistent with a recently randomized, double-blind, placebo-controlled trial, in which patients with OA receiving a curcuminoid had significantly lower scores on the Western Ontario and McMaster Universities Osteoarthritis Index (WOMAC) and Lequesne's pain functional index than patients receiving a placebo [23].

There is currently no cure for OA or a therapeutic agent with proven evidence to slow or halt the progression of OA [49]. Treatments used to temporarily relieve pain in OA, such as NSAIDs, may also cause severe gastrointestinal, renal, and cardiovascular side effects after long-term use [49–51]. In addition, patients experiencing pain relief without a concurrent improvement in the disease itself may become less conscientious about protecting their diseased joints (such as by avoiding overuse), and may unknowingly exacerbate the progression of

OA. On the other hand, an OA drug that halts the progression of OA but does not relieve OA-related pain may not be effective, as patient compliance would likely be low. Upon further validation in other animal models and clinical trials, the effects of curcumin in both disease and symptom modification make it an attractive potential therapeutic agent for OA.

While the etiologic and pathogenic mechanisms for both initiation and progression of OA are not clear, inflammation, over-activated catabolic activity and oxidative stress responses are considered to be common in both processes [2, 44, 52, 53]. The effects of curcumin on attenuating inflammation, formation of reactive oxygen species, and catabolic activity have been suggested in chondrocytes in vitro [7, 14–16, 18, 19], in human synovial fibroblasts and in collagen-induced arthritis in mouse models [7, 14–16, 18, 19]. Furthermore, Colitti et al have shown an anti-inflammatory effect of curcumin on the gene expression of peripheral white blood cells in dogs with OA [16]. Consistent with these studies, we demonstrated that curcumin, in both the non-encapsulated (Fig. 1) and encapsulated forms (Fig. 3) exerts broad chondroprotective effects in human primary chondrocytes by suppressing the expression of genes encoding inflammatory cytokines IL-1β and TNF-α, and cartilage-degrading enzymes from the MMP family, including MMP-1, MMP-3, and MMP-13. We also demonstrated for the first time that curcumin suppresses expression of aggrecanase ADAMTS5, a key proteinase in cartilage destruction during OA that primarily cleaves the aggrecan components of the cartilage extracellular matrix [54–56]. Curcumin also induces gene expression of CITED2, an MMP-repressing transcriptional regulator. We previously demonstrated that CITED2, in response to moderate mechanical loading, represses expression of MMP-1 and MMP-13 in vitro [57] and in vivo [26]. NF-kB is a key factor that triggers the expression of various genes implicated in cartilage destruction, synovial membrane inflammation, and bone resorption [58, 59]. As CITED2 may negatively regulate NF-kB activity in embryonic kidney cells [60], curcumin may exert its chondroprotective effects by suppressing NF-kB activity by upregulating CITED2.

It has been reported that curcumin is barely soluble in water and poor absorption is attained from the epithelial cells in the gastrointestinal tract. Rats given an oral dose of curcumin excreted 75 % in the feces unchanged, with less than 0.02 % recovered from the liver, kidney, and body fat [61]. However, several studies analyzing plasma levels of curcumin or its metabolites have detected curcumin, although only small amounts, following relatively high doses of oral administration in humans [62, 63]. In this study, we demonstrated that oral administration of curcumin exerted efficacy in slowing the progression of post-traumatic OA. However, a palliative effect was not observed in mice with OA induced by DMM when curcumin was administered orally in this study. The data suggest orally delivered curcumin is unlikely to reach biologically/pharmacologically active concentrations in the serum, synovial fluid, or joint tissues, that are sufficient to mitigate OA-related pain [4]. Together, our observation further indicates that relieving pain and its symptoms may require higher levels of curcumin compared to those required for disease modification.

As topical administration is a patient-friendly drug delivery method in OA treatment, we examined the efficacy of topical administration of nanoparticles encapsulating curcumin in OA disease modification and symptom improvement in mice with OA induced by DMM. Topical application of curcumin nanoparticles was efficacious not only in OA disease modification (Fig. 5), but also in relieving OA-related pain (Fig. 7). The data indicate that the topical application of curcumin encapsulated within nanoparticles preserves the chondroprotective activity of curcumin, and may increase its bioavailability.

Pathological changes in DMM-induced OA, including cartilage destruction, synovitis, and subchondral bone thickening, are observed in human OA [32]. Our study shows that curcumin treatment via oral (Fig. 2) or topical administration (Fig. 5) significantly improved OA-related pathological changes in the synovium and subchondral bone, indicating that curcumin has comprehensive potential for the treatment of joint tissues in OA [2].

The IPFP is an adipose tissue located within the knee joint synovial capsule, which may contribute to low-grade inflammation and cartilage degeneration through the secretion of adipokines and pro-inflammatory mediators into the synovial joint [64, 65]. In this study, we demonstrated that topically applied curcumin was largely localized in the infrapatellar fat pad (Fig. 4a). We further demonstrated that this treatment led to reduced expression of adipokines and pro-inflammatory mediators in the fat pad (Fig. 4b). These data suggest curcumin may slow the disease progression in OA, at least in part, by mitigating the pro-inflammatory mediating effect of the IPFP on cartilage and articular joints.

In this study, we provide the first evidence to demonstrate the efficacy of curcumin in OA disease and symptom modification using a post-traumatic OA mouse model. In addition to traumatic joint injuries, other conditions such as mechanical overuse and aging are risk factors for OA [66, 67]. Evaluating the efficacy of curcumin in other relevant OA models such as overuse-induced OA and spontaneous OA, which represents age-related OA, will be of interest.

Conclusions

Using a post-traumatic OA mouse model, we provide the first evidence that curcumin has significant efficacy in slowing OA disease progression and a substantial effect on pain relief. Curcumin may exert its efficacy by regulating a broad spectrum of molecules including predominant proteinases in cartilage breakdown such as collagenase MMP-13, and aggrecanase ADAMTS5 in chondrocytes. The chondroprotective effects of curcumin, when administered topically, act through, at least in part, the suppression of relevant adipokines and other pro-inflammatory mediators that are critical for cartilage homeostasis in the infrapatellar fat pad.

Abbreviations
ADAMTS, a disintegrin and metalloproteinase with thrombospondin motifs; ANOVA, analysis of variance; Cebpa, CCAAT/enhancer binding protein alpha; CITED2, Cbp/p300 interacting transactivator with ED-rich tail 2; Col2a1, collagen 2a1; COX-2, cyclooxygenase-2; DMEM, Dulbecco's modified Eagle's medium; DMM, destabilization of the medial meniscus; H&E, hematoxylin and eosin; IL-1β, interleukin-1 beta; IPFP, infrapatellar fat pad; MMP, matrix metalloproteinase; MMTL, medial meniscotibial ligament; NF-kB, nuclear factor kappa B; NSAID, non-steroidal anti-inflammatory drug; OA, osteoarthritis; OARSI, Osteoarthritis Research Society International; PBS, phosphate-buffered saline; PGE₂, prostaglandin E2; Pparg, peroxisome proliferator-activated receptor gamma; TMOS, tetra-methyl-orthosilicate; TNF-α, tumor necrosis factor-alpha

Acknowledgements
This study was supported by NIH Grant R01AR050968 (HBS), the Arthritis Foundation (HBS), NIH Grant P01 HL110900 (JMF), and a sponsored research grant from NanoBiomed. Inc. (JMF, MN).

Authors' contributions
ZZ and DJL contributed to experimental design, animal surgery, curcumin administration, histological staining and analysis and pain assessment studies, and drafted the manuscript. LX contributed to the animal surgery, curcumin administration, and revising the manuscript. ZH carried out the in vitro studies and participated in revising the manuscript. AW contributed to

histological staining and revising the manuscript. MN contributed to producing the curcumin nanoparticles and revising the manuscript. SJK contributed to the acquisition of human specimens and revising the manuscript. DMH contributed to acquisition of human specimens, experimental design, and revising the manuscript. JAH contributed to experimental design and revising the manuscript. NJC contributed to conception of the study and revising the manuscript. JF contributed to conception of the study and revising the manuscript. HBS contributed to conception of the study and experimental design, analyzed the data, and finalized the manuscript. All authors have read and approved the final manuscript.

Competing interests
The authors declare that they have no competing interests with the exception of JMF and MN who are partially funded through NanoBiomed. Inc.

Author details
[1]Department of Orthopaedic Surgery, Albert Einstein College of Medicine, Bronx, NY, USA. [2]Department of Radiation Oncology, Albert Einstein College of Medicine, Bronx, NY, USA. [3]China-Japan Union Hospital of Jilin University, Bronx, NY, USA. [4]Department of Physiology & Biophysics, Albert Einstein College of Medicine, Bronx, NY, USA. [5]Department of Medicine, Albert Einstein College of Medicine, Bronx, NY, USA.

References

1. Lawrence RC, Felson DT, Helmick CG, Arnold LM, Choi H, Deyo RA, et al. Estimates of the prevalence of arthritis and other rheumatic conditions in the United States. Part II. Arthritis Rheum. 2008;58(1):26–35.
2. Loeser RF, Goldring SR, Scanzello CR, Goldring MB. Osteoarthritis: a disease of the joint as an organ. Arthritis Rheum. 2012;64(6):1697–707.
3. Le Graverand-Gastineau MP. Disease modifying osteoarthritis drugs: facing development challenges and choosing molecular targets. Curr Drug Targets. 2010;11(5):528–35.
4. Henrotin Y, Priem F, Mobasheri A. Curcumin: a new paradigm and therapeutic opportunity for the treatment of osteoarthritis: curcumin for osteoarthritis management. Springerplus. 2013;2(1):56.
5. Asher GN, Spelman K. Clinical utility of curcumin extract. Altern Ther Health Med. 2013;19(2):20–2.
6. Goel A, Boland CR, Chauhan DP. Specific inhibition of cyclooxygenase-2 (COX-2) expression by dietary curcumin in HT-29 human colon cancer cells. Cancer Lett. 2001;172(2):111–8.
7. Mathy-Hartert M, Jacquemond-Collet I, Priem F, Sanchez C, Lambert C, Henrotin Y. Curcumin inhibits pro-inflammatory mediators and metalloproteinase-3 production by chondrocytes. Inflamm Res. 2009;58(12):899–908.
8. Henrotin Y, Clutterbuck AL, Allaway D, Lodwig EM, Harris P, Mathy-Hartert M, et al. Biological actions of curcumin on articular chondrocytes. Osteoarthritis Cartilage. 2010;18(2):141–9.
9. Clutterbuck AL, Mobasheri A, Shakibaei M, Allaway D, Harris P. Interleukin-1beta-induced extracellular matrix degradation and glycosaminoglycan release is inhibited by curcumin in an explant model of cartilage inflammation. Ann NY Acad Sci. 2009;1171:428–35.
10. Shakibaei M, Mobasheri A, Buhrmann C. Curcumin synergizes with resveratrol to stimulate the MAPK signaling pathway in human articular chondrocytes in vitro. Genes Nutr. 2011;6(2):171–9.
11. Csaki C, Mobasheri A, Shakibaei M. Synergistic chondroprotective effects of curcumin and resveratrol in human articular chondrocytes: inhibition of IL-1beta-induced NF-kappaB-mediated inflammation and apoptosis. Arthritis Res Ther. 2009;11(6):R165.
12. Sreejayan N, Rao MN. Free radical scavenging activity of curcuminoids. Arzneimittelforschung. 1996;46(2):169–71.
13. Sreejayan, Rao MN. Nitric oxide scavenging by curcuminoids. J Pharm Pharmacol. 1997;49(1):105–7.
14. Liacini A, Sylvester J, Li WQ, Zafarullah M. Inhibition of interleukin-1-stimulated MAP kinases, activating protein-1 (AP-1) and nuclear factor kappa B (NF-kappa B) transcription factors down-regulates matrix metalloproteinase gene expression in articular chondrocytes. Matrix Biol. 2002;21(3):251–62.
15. Shakibaei M, John T, Schulze-Tanzil G, Lehmann I, Mobasheri A. Suppression of NF-kappaB activation by curcumin leads to inhibition of expression of cyclo-oxygenase-2 and matrix metalloproteinase-9 in human articular chondrocytes: implications for the treatment of osteoarthritis. Biochem Pharmacol. 2007;73(9):1434–45.
16. Schulze-Tanzil G, Mobasheri A, Sendzik J, John T, Shakibaei M. Effects of curcumin (diferuloylmethane) on nuclear factor kappaB signaling in interleukin-1beta-stimulated chondrocytes. Ann NY Acad Sci. 2004;1030:578–86.
17. Clutterbuck AL, Allaway D, Harris P, Mobasheri A. Curcumin reduces prostaglandin E2, matrix metalloproteinase-3 and proteoglycan release in the secretore of interleukin 1beta-treated articular cartilage. F1000Res. 2013;2:147.
18. Moon DO, Kim MO, Choi YH, Park YM, Kim GY. Curcumin attenuates inflammatory response in IL-1beta-induced human synovial fibroblasts and collagen-induced arthritis in mouse model. Int Immunopharmacol. 2010;10(5):605–10.
19. Colitti M, Gaspardo B, Della Pria A, Scaini C, Stefanon B. Transcriptome modification of white blood cells after dietary administration of curcumin and non-steroidal anti-inflammatory drug in osteoarthritic affected dogs. Vet Immunol Immunopathol. 2012;147(3-4):136–46.
20. Peddada KV, Peddada KV, Shukla SK, Mishra A, Verma V. Role of curcumin in common musculoskeletal disorders: a review of current laboratory, translational, and clinical data. Orthop Surg. 2015;7(3):222–31.
21. Comblain F, Serisier S, Barthelemy N, Balligand M, Henrotin Y. Review of dietary supplements for the management of osteoarthritis in dogs in studies from 2004 to 2014. J Vet Pharmacol Ther. 2016;39(1):1–15.
22. Nakagawa Y, Mukai S, Yamada S, Matsuoka M, Tarumi E, Hashimoto T, et al. Short-term effects of highly-bioavailable curcumin for treating knee osteoarthritis: a randomized, double-blind, placebo-controlled prospective study. J Orthop Sci. 2014;19(6):933–9.
23. Panahi Y, Rahimnia AR, Sharafi M, Alishiri G, Saburi A, Sahebkar A. Curcuminoid treatment for knee osteoarthritis: a randomized double-blind placebo-controlled trial. Phytother Res. 2014;28(11):1625–31.
24. Kuptniratsaikul V, Dajpratham P, Taechaarpornkul W, Buntragulpoontawee M, Lukkanapichonchut P, Chootip C, et al. Efficacy and safety of Curcuma domestica extracts compared with ibuprofen in patients with knee osteoarthritis: a multicenter study. Clin Interv Aging. 2014;9:451–8.
25. He Z, Leong DJ, Zhuo Z, Majeska RJ, Cardoso L, Spray DC, Goldring MB, Cobelli NJ, Sun HB. Strain-induced mechanotransduction through primary cilia, extracellular ATP, purinergic calcium signaling, and ERK1/2 transactivates CITED2 and downregulates MMP-1 and MMP-13 gene expression in chondrocytes. Osteoarthritis Cartilage. 2015;24(5):892–901.
26. Leong DJ, Li YH, Gu XI, Sun L, Zhou Z, Nasser P, et al. Physiological loading of joints prevents cartilage degradation through CITED2. FASEB J. 2011;25(1):182–91.
27. Friedman AJ, Han G, Navati MS, Chacko M, Gunther L, Alfieri A, et al. Sustained release nitric oxide releasing nanoparticles: characterization of a novel delivery platform based on nitrite containing hydrogel/glass composites. Nitric Oxide. 2008;19(1):12–20.
28. Han G, Martinez LR, Mihu MR, Friedman AJ, Friedman JM, Nosanchuk JD. Nitric oxide releasing nanoparticles are therapeutic for Staphylococcus aureus abscesses in a murine model of infection. PLoS One. 2009;4(11):e7804.
29. Cabrales P, Han G, Roche C, Nacharaju P, Friedman AJ, Friedman JM. Sustained release nitric oxide from long-lived circulating nanoparticles. Free Radic Biol Med. 2010;49(4):530–8.
30. Tar M, Cabrales P, Navati M, Adler B, Nacharaju P, Friedman AJ, et al. Topically applied NO-releasing nanoparticles can increase intracorporal pressure and elicit spontaneous erections in a rat model of radical prostatectomy. J Sex Med. 2014;11(12):2903–14.
31. Krausz AE, Adler BL, Cabral V, Navati M, Doerner J, Charafeddine RA, et al. Curcumin-encapsulated nanoparticles as innovative antimicrobial and wound healing agent. Nanomedicine. 2015;11(1):195–206.
32. Glasson SS, Blanchet TJ, Morris EA. The surgical destabilization of the medial meniscus (DMM) model of osteoarthritis in the 129/SvEv mouse. Osteoarthritis Cartilage. 2007;15(9):1061–9.
33. Glasson SS, Chambers MG, Van Den Berg WB, Little CB. The OARSI histopathology initiative - recommendations for histological assessments of osteoarthritis in the mouse. Osteoarthritis Cartilage. 2010;18 Suppl 3:S17–23.
34. Lewis JS, Hembree WC, Furman BD, Tippets L, Cattel D, Huebner JL, et al. Acute joint pathology and synovial inflammation is associated with

increased intra-articular fracture severity in the mouse knee. Osteoarthritis Cartilage. 2011;19(7):864–73.

35. Milz S, Putz R. Quantitative morphology of the subchondral plate of the tibial plateau. J Anat. 1994;185(Pt 1):103–10.

36. Nguyen DH, Zhou T, Shu J, Mao JH. Quantifying chromogen intensity in immunohistochemistry via reciprocal intensity. Cancer InCytes. 2013;2(1):e.

37. Leong DJ, Choudhury M, Hanstein R, Hirsh DM, Kim SJ, Majeska RJ, et al. Green tea polyphenol treatment is chondroprotective, anti-inflammatory and palliative in a mouse post-traumatic osteoarthritis model. Arthritis Res Ther. 2014;16(6):508.

38. Bailey KR, Crawley JN. Anxiety-Related Behaviors in Mice. In: Buccafusco JJ, editor. Methods of Behavior Analysis in Neuroscience. 2nd edition. Boca Raton (FL): CRC Press/Taylor & Francis; 2009. Chapter 5.

39. Anand P, Kunnumakkara AB, Newman RA, Aggarwal BB. Bioavailability of curcumin: problems and promises. Mol Pharm. 2007;4(6):807–18.

40. Kunwar A, Barik A, Mishra B, Rathinasamy K, Pandey R, Priyadarsini KI. Quantitative cellular uptake, localization and cytotoxicity of curcumin in normal and tumor cells. Biochim Biophys Acta. 2008;1780(4):673–9.

41. Santangelo K, Radakovich L, Fouts J, Foster MT. Pathophysiology of obesity on knee joint homeostasis: contributions of the infrapatellar fat pad. Horm Mol Biol Clin Investig. 2016. doi:10.1515/hmbci-2015-0067.

42. Richter M, Trzeciak T, Owecki M, Pucher A, Kaczmarczyk J. The role of adipocytokines in the pathogenesis of knee joint osteoarthritis. Int Orthop. 2015;39(6):1211–7.

43. Conde J, Scotece M, Lopez V, Abella V, Hermida M, Pino J, et al. Differential expression of adipokines in infrapatellar fat pad (IPFP) and synovium of osteoarthritis patients and healthy individuals. Ann Rheum Dis. 2014;73(3): 631–3.

44. Goldring MB, Marcu KB. Cartilage homeostasis in health and rheumatic diseases. Arthritis Res Ther. 2009;11(3):224.

45. Felson DT. Developments in the clinical understanding of osteoarthritis. Arthritis Res Ther. 2009;11(1):203.

46. Miller RE, Tran PB, Das R, Ghoreishi-Haack N, Ren D, Miller RJ, et al. CCR2 chemokine receptor signaling mediates pain in experimental osteoarthritis. Proc Natl Acad Sci U S A. 2012;109(50):20602–7.

47. Wong JM, Khan T, Jayadev CS, Khan W, Johnstone D. Anterior cruciate ligament rupture and osteoarthritis progression. Open Orthop J. 2012;6:295–300.

48. Lotz MK, Kraus VB. New developments in osteoarthritis. Posttraumatic osteoarthritis: pathogenesis and pharmacological treatment options. Arthritis Res Ther. 2010;12(3):211.

49. Cheng DS, Visco CJ. Pharmaceutical therapy for osteoarthritis. PM R. 2012; 4(5 Suppl):S82–8.

50. O'Neil CK, Hanlon JT, Marcum ZA. Adverse effects of analgesics commonly used by older adults with osteoarthritis: focus on non-opioid and opioid analgesics. Am J Geriatr Pharmacother. 2012;10(6):331–42.

51. Van Manen MD, Nace J, Mont MA. Management of primary knee osteoarthritis and indications for total knee arthroplasty for general practitioners. J Am Osteopath Assoc. 2012;112(11):709–15.

52. Loeser RF. Aging processes and the development of osteoarthritis. Curr Opin Rheumatol. 2013;25(1):108–13.

53. Sun HB. Mechanical loading, cartilage degradation, and arthritis. Ann NY Acad Sci. 2010;1211:37–50.

54. Larkin J, Lohr TA, Elefante L, Shearin J, Matico R, Su JL, et al. Translational development of an ADAMTS-5 antibody for osteoarthritis disease modification. Osteoarthritis Cartilage. 2015;23(8):1254–66.

55. Verma P, Dalal K. ADAMTS-4 and ADAMTS-5: key enzymes in osteoarthritis. J Cell Biochem. 2011;112(12):3507–14.

56. Glasson SS, Askew R, Sheppard B, Carito B, Blanchet T, Ma HL, et al. Deletion of active ADAMTS5 prevents cartilage degradation in a murine model of osteoarthritis. Nature. 2005;434(7033):644–8.

57. Yokota H, Goldring MB, Sun HB. CITED2-mediated regulation of MMP-1 and MMP-13 in human chondrocytes under flow shear. J Biol Chem. 2003; 278(47):47275–80.

58. Rigoglou S, Papavassiliou AG. The NF-kappaB signalling pathway in osteoarthritis. Int J Biochem Cell Biol. 2013;45(11):2580–4.

59. Marcu KB, Otero M, Olivotto E, Borzi RM, Goldring MB. NF-kappaB signaling: multiple angles to target OA. Curr Drug Targets. 2010;11(5):599–613.

60. Lou X, Sun S, Chen W, Zhou Y, Huang Y, Liu X, et al. Negative feedback regulation of NF-kappaB action by CITED2 in the nucleus. J Immunol. 2011; 186(1):539–48.

61. Wahlstrom B, Blennow G. A study on the fate of curcumin in the rat. Acta Pharmacol Toxicol (Copenh). 1978;43(2):86–92.

62. Lao CD, Ruffin MT, Normolle D, Heath DD, Murray SI, Bailey JM, et al. Dose escalation of a curcuminoid formulation. BMC Complement Altern Med. 2006;6:10.

63. Carroll RE, Benya RV, Turgeon DK, Vareed S, Neuman M, Rodriguez L, et al. Phase IIa clinical trial of curcumin for the prevention of colorectal neoplasia. Cancer Prev Res (Phila). 2011;4(3):354–64.

64. Greene MA, Loeser RF. Aging-related inflammation in osteoarthritis. Osteoarthritis Cartilage. 2015;23(11):1966–71.

65. Conde J, Scotece M, Lopez V, Gomez R, Lago F, Pino J, et al. Adipokines: novel players in rheumatic diseases. Discov Med. 2013;15(81):73–83.

66. Silverwood V, Blagojevic-Bucknall M, Jinks C, Jordan JL, Protheroe J, Jordan KP. Current evidence on risk factors for knee osteoarthritis in older adults: a systematic review and meta-analysis. Osteoarthritis Cartilage. 2015;23(4):507–15.

67. Bijlsma JW, Knahr K. Strategies for the prevention and management of osteoarthritis of the hip and knee. Best Pract Res Clin Rheumatol. 2007;21(1): 59–76.

Proximal tibial trabecular bone mineral density is related to pain in patients with osteoarthritis

Wadena D. Burnett[1], Saija A. Kontulainen[1], Christine E. McLennan[2], Diane Hazel[2], Carl Talmo[2], David R. Wilson[3], David J. Hunter[4] and James D. Johnston[1*]

Abstract

Background: Our objective was to examine the relationships between proximal tibial trabecular (epiphyseal and metaphyseal) bone mineral density (BMD) and osteoarthritis (OA)-related pain in patients with severe knee OA.

Methods: The knee was scanned preoperatively using quantitative computed tomography (QCT) in 42 patients undergoing knee arthroplasty. OA severity was classified using radiographic Kellgren-Lawrence scoring and pain was measured using the pain subsection of the Western Ontario and McMaster Universities Arthritis Index (WOMAC). We used three-dimensional image processing techniques to assess tibial epiphyseal trabecular BMD between the epiphyseal line and 7.5 mm from the subchondral surface and tibial metaphyseal trabecular BMD 10 mm distal from the epiphyseal line. Regional analysis included the total epiphyseal and metaphyseal region, and the medial and lateral epiphyseal compartments. The association between total WOMAC pain scores and BMD measurements was assessed using hierarchical multiple regression with age, sex, and body mass index (BMI) as covariates. Statistical significance was set at $p < 0.05$.

Results: Total WOMAC pain was associated with total epiphyseal BMD adjusted for age, sex, and BMI ($p = 0.013$) and total metaphyseal BMD ($p = 0.017$). Regionally, total WOMAC pain was associated with medial epiphyseal BMD adjusted for age, sex, and BMI ($p = 0.006$).

Conclusion: These findings suggest that low proximal tibial trabecular BMD may have a role in OA-related pain pathogenesis.

Keywords: Osteoarthritis, Bone mineral density, Tibia, Pain, Computed tomography

Background

Knee osteoarthritis (OA) is a debilitating and painful disease characterized by changes in cartilage and subchondral bone. Pain is a complex combination of social, psychological and biological factors [1], and is often the primary sign that a patient may be afflicted with OA [2]. Unfortunately, the local biological pain pathogenesis within the knee joint is poorly understood [3] as it could be related to many structural factors (e.g., altered joint alignment [4], bone marrow lesions (BMLs) [5], or cysts [6]). Knee OA is commonly characterized by altered

subchondral properties, including altered subchondral bone thickness [7], bone volume fraction [8], and volumetric bone mineral density (BMD) [9]. Importantly, altered BMD may disrupt local innervation [10] and/or the local mechanical behavior of bone [11], and thus may be a factor in OA-related knee pain.

To date, research investigating association between OA-related knee pain and bone has focused primarily on bone near the subchondral surface (e.g., subchondral cortical and subchondral trabecular bone) [12, 13]. Adjacent trabecular bone (e.g., epiphyseal bone, metaphyseal bone) is also affected by OA [9], with observations of thinner trabeculae, lower bone volume fraction, and lower density with progressing OA severity [14–16]. To date, there are no studies reporting relationships

* Correspondence: jd.johnston@usask.ca
[1]University of Saskatchewan, 57 Campus Drive, Saskatoon, SK S7N 5A9, Canada
Full list of author information is available at the end of the article

between epiphyseal or metaphyseal trabecular BMD and pain. A recent finite element (FE) study conducted by Amini et al. [17] has suggested that low epiphyseal trabecular bone density in OA [14–16], which is directly linked to the elastic modulus of epiphyseal bone [18], may explain OA proximal tibiae being less stiff than normal [17]. Importantly, a less stiff proximal tibia would result in higher bone deformation potentially explaining (at least to some degree) OA-related knee pain.

A clear understanding of pain pathogenesis is crucial for rational therapeutic targeting [19]. Further, as pain is the reason patients seek medical care, rational treatment targeting requires specific understanding of which structures contribute to pain [19]. With the aim of furthering our understanding of potential factors that may influence knee pain, the objective of this study was to investigate relationships between proximal tibial epiphyseal and metaphyseal trabecular BMD and OA-related knee pain.

Methods
Study participants
In total 42 participants with OA were recruited prior to total knee replacement (TKR) (17 male, 25 female; mean age 64, SD ± 10.1 years; mean body mass index (BMI) 28.7 ± 3.7; 18 left, 24 right) [13]. Study exclusion criteria included pregnant women, patients having a revision replacement instead of primary knee replacement, and patients with a prior history of bone pathologic change at the knee joint. The Institutional Research Board of the New England Baptist Hospital approved the study. Informed consent was obtained from all study participants.

Participant assessment
OA severity was classified using Kellgren-Lawrence (KL) scoring [20]; participants had severity scores of 2–4. Pain severity was measured at the affected knee joint using the pain subsection of the Western Ontario McMasters Osteoarthritis Index (WOMAC) [21]. Participants were asked to assess the level of pain in the affected knee joint within the past 24 hours while walking on a flat surface, going up or down stairs, nocturnal pain at night in bed, sitting or lying down, and standing upright using a 5-point Likert scale (0–4). Individual element pain scores were then summed for a possible WOMAC pain score of 20. Summed pain scores ranged from 4 to 16. We also used the Self-Administered Comorbidity Questionnaire [22] to assess participants for any potential confounding comorbidities (e.g., diabetes mellitus or heart disease).

Computed tomography (CT) scan acquisition
We used a single-energy clinical CT scanner (Lightspeed 4-slice, General Electric, Milwaukee, WI, USA) for bone imaging. A solid quantitative CT (QCT) reference phantom of known bone mineral densities (Model 3 T, Mindways Software Inc, Austin, TX, USA) was placed under the participants and included in all CT scans. Participants were oriented supine within the CT gantry and both legs were simultaneously scanned. Scans included the distal femur, patella, proximal tibia, and the 66% tibial shaft site proximal to the distal tibial endplate [23]. Only the proximal tibia and the 66% tibial shaft site were used in the current analysis.

CT scanning parameters included: 120 kVp tube voltage; 150 mAs tube current-time product; axial scanning plane; 0.625-mm isotropic voxel size (0.625 slice thickness, 0.625 mm × 0.625 mm in-plane pixel size); ~ 250 slices; and ~ 60s scan time. A standard bone kernel (BONE) was used for CT image post-processing. The effective radiation dose was ~ 0.073 mSv per scan, estimated using shareware software (CT-DOSE, National Board of Health, Herley, Denmark). For comparison, the average effective radiation dose during a transatlantic flight from Europe to North America is about 0.05 mSv [24].

CT image analysis
We used a custom algorithm developed specifically for this study (Matlab 2010b; MathWorks, Natick, MA, USA), combined with manual segmentation to determine epiphyseal and metaphyseal trabecular BMD. We considered the epiphyseal region (subarticular region) as the proximal tibial volume between the subchondral surface and the epiphyseal line [25]. A single user (WDB) performed all segmentations and analyses. As this algorithm was developed specifically for this study, we assessed repeatability in a precision study performed on an independent sample of healthy participants and participants with OA [26] using recommended methods [27]. In summary, 14 participants were scanned three times with repositioning between each scan (42 scans, 28 degrees of freedom (DOF)). The repeatability expressed as precision error, of each BMD measurement was assessed using root mean square coefficients of variation (CV%) and ranged from 0.7% to 3.6%.

To derive BMD, grayscale Hounsfield units (HU) were converted to equivalent volumetric BMD (mg/cm^3 K_2HPO_4) using subject-specific linear regression equations developed from known densities ranging from – 50 to 375 mg/cm^3 K_2HPO_4 within the QCT phantom included in each individual axial image ($r^2 > 0.99$) [28] and interpolation to determine equivalent volumetric BMD values. Higher density values were linearly extrapolated (Fig. 1a). Subject-specific half maximum height thresholds [29] were then determined to define the proximal tibial subchondral and cortical surfaces. Two 3D image volumes were built, one including the entire proximal tibia as previously described [13, 28] and another by segmenting individual serial images using semi-automatic

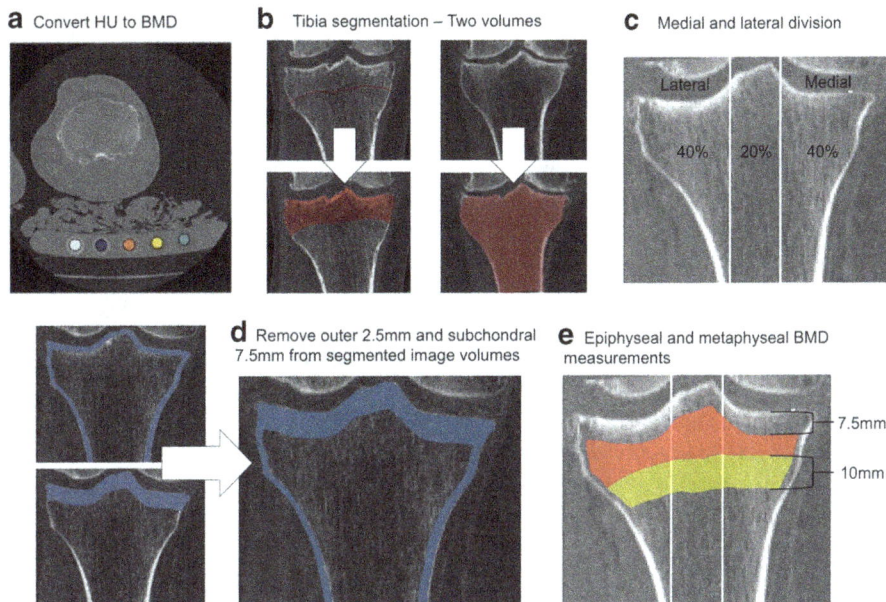

Fig. 1 Methodological process consists of converting computed tomography (CT) grayscale intensities to bone mineral density (BMD) using a quantitative CT (QCT) reference phantom (**a**), followed by building two imaged volumes for each tibia, one with manual correction at the epiphyseal line and one using the full tibia (**b**). Imaged volumes were divided into lateral and medial regions (**c**) and then the outer 2.5-mm and subchondral 7.5-mm depth were removed from each imaged volume (**d**). BMD measurements included epiphyseal BMD between the epiphyseal line and 7.5 mm from the subchondral surface and metaphyseal BMD 10 mm distal from the epiphyseal line (**e**)

region growing and manual correction at the epiphyseal line (Fig. 1b). Both sets of imaged volumes were segmented using commercial software (Analyze10.0; Mayo Foundation, Rochester, MN, USA) and an interactive touch-screen tablet (Cintiq 21UX; Wacom, Krefeld, Germany). Imaged volumes were reoriented to a neutral position where medial and lateral plateaus were approximately parallel. We then divided the imaged volumes into medial and lateral compartments, measured by using 40% of the maximum medial-lateral axis of each respective side [16] (Fig. 1c).

To ensure that trabecular BMD measurements did not include cysts (which would lead to arbitrarily low measures of BMD) [13, 30] or peripheral high-density cortical bone, the most proximal 7.5-mm region (relative to the subchondral surface) was removed from the segmentations (Fig. 1d), as was 2.5 mm of peripheral cortical bone (Fig. 1d). The 7.5-mm depth was based upon observed cyst locations from our earlier work [13, 30] and work by Chiba et al. [31], which limited depth analyses to 5 mm from the subchondral surface. In extreme cases, large cysts extended from the subchondral cortical region (0 – 2.5 mm) through the subchondral trabecular region (2.5–5 mm) and occasionally into depths greater than 5 mm from the subchondral surface. By using a conservative 7.5-mm depth from the subchondral surface, we ensured the exclusion of large cysts from our analysis. Following material removal, we measured

epiphyseal trabecular BMD from the 7.5-mm depth to the epiphyseal line (Fig. 1e), which was located approximately 15 mm from the subchondral surface. Metaphyseal trabecular BMD was measured 10 mm distal to the epiphyseal line (Fig. 1e).

We included cortical BMD of the tibial shaft (66% of the tibial length, proximal from the distal tibial plateau) [23] to assess whether associations with pain were systemic or joint-specific. More specifically, if similar associations between pain and BMD were observed at the proximal tibia and tibial shaft, this would indicate systemic effects with low BMD being a plausible secondary effect of other factors, such as mechanical loading, nutrition or medication [32]. Tibial shaft cortical BMD was segmented using subject-specific half-maximum-height thresholds, and measured using commercial software (Analyze10.0; Mayo Foundation, Rochester, MN, USA).

Statistical analysis

We first checked all underlying assumptions for multiple linear regression (assumptions of linear relationships, homoscedasticity, independency and normality of residuals) using standardized residual scatter plots, P-P plots, and histograms [33]. We identified any outliers using the modified Thompson tau (τ) test [34].

We report univariate correlation coefficients (Pearson) between pain, BMD, age, sex, and BMI and illustrate associations between pain and BMD with scatter plots and coefficients of determination (R^2) from linear regression. We used hierarchical multiple linear regression analyses to explain the variance in total WOMAC pain. We selected age, sex, and BMI as covariates for our base model based on observed correlation in univariate analysis (age and WOMAC pain) and literature (age, sex, and BMI) evaluating relationships between BMD and pain [12, 35]. All BMD measurements (total and regional epiphyseal BMD, total metaphyseal BMD, and tibial shaft cortical BMD) were individually added to our base model. We assessed multicollinearity between all independent variables in each model using variance inflation factor (VIF), setting the maximum tolerance value as 10. We report adjusted R^2, change in R^2 from the base model (Δ), standardized beta (β)-coefficients, and p values. Statistical significance was defined as $p < 0.05$, and analyses were performed using SPSS 21.0 (IBM, Armonk, NY, USA).

Results

Characteristics of all study participants, including age, sex, BMI, KL grades, joint space narrowing (JSN) score, non-weight-bearing alignment scores, and BMD measurements are shown in Table 1. As per the modified Thompson τ test [34], we identified a single outlier based on the total WOMAC pain score with a τ value outside of the sample's rejection zone ($\tau > 5.56$), and removed it from the analysis. All underlying assumptions for linear regression were appropriately met. There was no evidence of multicollinearity between independent variables in any of our models. Unadjusted relationships between total WOMAC pain and total or regional epiphyseal or metaphyseal BMD measurements are

presented in Fig. 2. Pearson correlation analyses in all participants, and in male and female patients are presented in Additional files 1, 2 and 3: Tables S1–S3.

Regression models predicting variance in pain are presented in Table 2. After adding total epiphyseal BMD to the base model, (of age, sex, and BMI) the coefficient of determination (R^2) for total pain improved ($\Delta R^2 = 0.12$). Our models improved when medial epiphyseal BMD ($\Delta R^2 = 0.15$) and metaphyseal BMD ($\Delta R^2 = 0.12$) were independently added to our base model. There was no association between cortical BMD at the 66% tibial site and pain.

Discussion

Our regression models suggested that tibial epiphyseal and metaphyseal BMD independently explained variance in total pain in patients with OA prior to TKR, whereby patients with lower BMD tended to have higher levels of pain. Regionally, our models indicated that medial epiphyseal BMD was a significant predictor of total OA-related pain, again whereby lower BMD was associated with higher levels of pain. These findings suggest that there may be potentially overlooked characteristics in proximal tibial BMD, such as trabecular BMD, which may have a role in the pathogenesis of OA-related pain.

The study findings support our previous research (using the same cohort), which investigated links between OA-related nocturnal pain and subchondral cortical and subchondral trabecular bone near the subchondral surface (0–10 mm from the surface). This previous study found a (nonsignificant) trend toward low medial BMD [13] in patients with severe nocturnal pain, which is in agreement with the study findings of

Table 1 Descriptive statistics for background characteristics of study participants

Characteristic	Without outlier
Age (mean ± SD)	64.1 ± 10.2
Sex (male:female)	17:24
BMI (mean ± SD)	28.6 ± 3.7
Side (left:right)	17:24
OA severity (KL) (0/1/2/3/4)	0/0/2/21/18
WOMAC score	9.7 ± 2.8
Medial joint space narrowing (0/1/2/3)	0/6/9/24[a]
Lateral joint space narrowing (0/1/2/3)	30/5/0/4[a]
Non-weight-bearing alignment	27 varus, 6 neutral, 8 valgus
Total epiphyseal BMD, mg/cm³ K_2HPO_4 (mean ± SD)	106 ± 37
Lateral epiphyseal BMD, mg/cm³ K_2HPO_4 (mean ± SD)	106 ± 34
Medial epiphyseal BMD, mg/cm³ K_2HPO_4 (mean ± SD)	141 ± 68
Total metaphyseal BMD, mg/cm³ K_2HPO_4 (mean ± SD)	90 ± 36

BMI body mass index, *OA* osteoarthritis, *KL* Kellgren-Lawrence grade, *WOMAC* Western Ontario and McMaster Universities Osteoarthritis Index, *BMD* bone mineral density
[a] Joint space narrowing scores not available in 2 participants

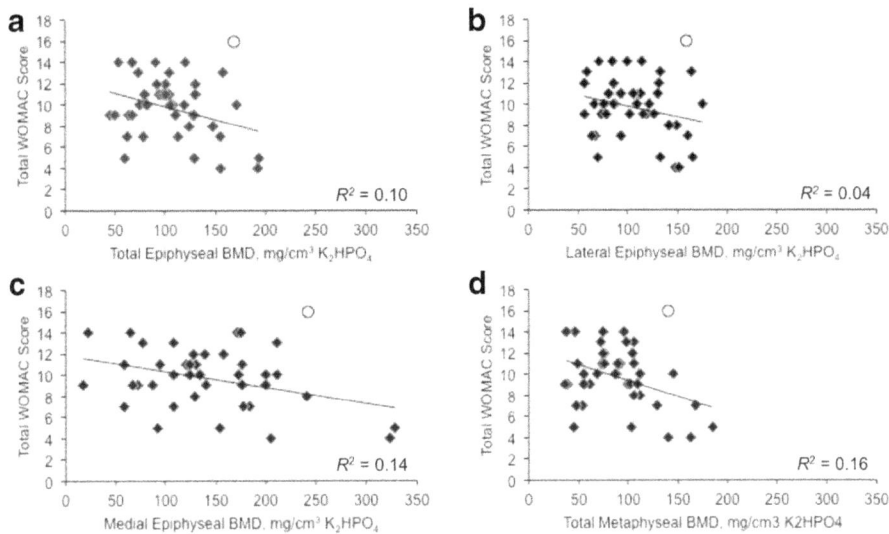

Fig. 2 Scatter plots and coefficients of determination (R^2) of the unadjusted relationships between total Western Ontario and McMaster Universities Osteoarthritis Index (WOMAC) score and total epiphyseal bone mineral density (BMD) ($p = 0.040$) (**a**), lateral epiphyseal BMD ($p = 0.187$) (**b**), medial epiphyseal BMD ($p = 0.015$) (**c**), and total metaphyseal BMD ($p < 0.009$) (**d**). The single outlier is noted as a circle, and was not included in the bivariate analysis

low medial epiphyseal and total epiphyseal and metaphyseal BMD in patients with high levels of pain. We [13], and others [30], however, have questioned whether our previously observed trend toward low medial BMD was due to the presence of cysts or diminished bone architecture and/or mineralization. Subsequent follow-up analyses indicated that both cysts and BMD were independently associated with pain [36]. The novelty of this study was that we focused our analyses in epiphyseal and metaphyseal trabecular regions largely void of cysts to determine any potential independent associations between BMD and pain.

Of note, the study findings both support and contrast with the previous study which also identified high lateral focal BMD in the subchondral trabecular region (2.5–10 mm below the surface) in patients with severe nocturnal pain [13]. High lateral focal BMD may be explained by the presence of BMLs, chondro-protection, or altered loading. First, prior research in this cohort identified a positive association between nocturnal pain and BMLs [37]. Given that BMLs have higher local BMD than surrounding bone tissue [38], a positive association between nocturnal pain and BMD is foreseeable. Future research needs to evaluate whether high focal BMD measurements exactly overlay the BML locations. Second, high lateral focal BMD may be a consequence of chondro-protection developed via low trabecular bone density. To explain, recent finite element (FE) simulations indicated that reduced proximal tibial trabecular bone density results in lower subchondral bone stiffness [17] and lower cartilage stresses [39], the latter presumably due to improved congruence

between articulations [40]. As many of the study participants had evidence of medial OA, low trabecular BMD may be a physiologic response to lessen medial cartilage stress. At the same time, this chondro-protective process would also naturally transfer more load to the lateral compartment since the two compartments function in parallel. This altered loading should result in loading-induced adaptation; specifically higher lateral BMD near the subchondral surface to meet the mechanical demands of higher load transmission. Third, many of the study participants with evidence of medial OA may be self-altering their knee kinematics and stance to off-load the medial compartment, with the aim of alleviating joint pain. This altered loading could result in loading-induced adaptation with higher lateral BMD and lower medial BMD [41]. Fourth, as higher BMD appears to be focused in subchondral regions (<10 mm from the tibial surface) [13], joint load may be primarily transferred through the subchondral cortical endplate and subchondral trabecular bone to the peripheral cortex, off-loading epiphyseal and metaphyseal trabecular bone, thus explaining lower BMD in these regions. However, this explanation warrants further research given that we did not find association between pain and alignment [36]. Studies using subject-specific FE modeling are needed to investigate load transmission and subchondral bone stiffness at different stages of pain severity and disease progression.

In this study we report a significant association between age and pain assessed by WOMAC, whereby older participants reported lower pain. Specifically, younger male patients reported higher WOMAC pain

Table 2 Adjusted coefficients of determination (R^2), standardized beta coefficients (β), and level of significance (p) of the base model (age, sex, and BMI) and change in the base model R^2 (Δ) when including bone mineral density (BMD) at the total and regional proximal tibia to predict variance in total WOMAC pain

		Total WOMAC		
		R^2	β	p value
Base model		**0.16**		**0.023**
	Age		**−0.41**	**0.011**
	Sex		0.19	0.206
	BMI		0.12	0.448
Total epiphyseal		**0.28**		**0.003**
	Δ	**0.12**		**0.013**
	Age		**−0.41**	**0.007**
	Sex		0.08	0.596
	BMI		0.18	0.234
	BMD		**−0.38**	**0.013**
Lateral epiphyseal		**0.21**		**0.014**
	Δ	0.06		0.083
	Age		**−0.40**	**0.011**
	Sex		0.12	0.420
	BMI		0.17	0.275
	BMD		−0.27	0.083
Medial epiphyseal		**0.30**		**0.002**
	Δ	**0.15**		**0.006**
	Age		**−0.39**	**0.008**
	Sex		0.12	0.388
	BMI		0.19	0.186
	BMD		**-0.40**	**0.006**
Total metaphyseal		**0.27**		**0.004**
	Δ	**0.12**		**0.017**
	Age		**−0.35**	**0.019**
	Sex		0.12	0.416
	BMI		0.15	0.302
	BMD		**−0.35**	**0.017**

BMI body mass index, *BMD* bone mineral density,
WOMAC Western Ontario and McMaster Universities Arthritis Index
Significant values of R^2, Δ, and β are in bold

scores (Additional file 2: Table S2). We recommend further analysis in larger longitudinal studies to evaluate if this finding is unique to this sample or if this is more widespread within patients with OA. It is also worthwhile noting that we report no associations between age and BMD (Table 2, Additional files 1, 2 and 3: Tables S1–S3). This is in agreement with previous OA research reporting no association between age and BMD [35] or age and bone volume fraction [42, 43]. Although there is consensus that bone loss is associated with normal aging [44], this association appears not to pertain to bone

tissue within the joint in OA. In support of this, there was no collinearity concern between BMD and age in our models predicting variance in pain. To further explore these associations, we ran the analysis with BMD as the dependent variable, pain as the independent variable, and age, sex, and BMI as covariates. These models suggested pain to be an independent predictor of BMD (Additional file 4: Table S4).

This study has certain limitations. First, pain severity and assessment was based on the entire knee joint, including all joint surfaces (tibiofemoral and patellofemoral) and tissues (e.g., bone, menisci, and synovium), and it is uncertain if pain originated within the proximal tibial bony structure, other tissues, or a combination of tissues. Second, although OA severity was homogeneous across study participants, all were in late stages of OA and it may not be possible to apply our findings to patients in the early stages of OA. Third, our study sample size was small (n = 41). Further analysis with larger samples including healthy participants and participants with various stages of OA severity and pain, are needed to verify these preliminary study findings. Of note, our sample comprised participants with severe OA (primarily with KL scores of 3–4). This limited range constrained our ability to include it in the statistical model. Also, with a basic rule of a minimum of 10 events (or samples) per predictor [45], we were limited to four predictors (independent variables) in each model: one independent variable (BMD) and three covariates (age, sex, and BMI), and thus other known predictors of pain were not assessed or investigated (e.g., smoking/alcohol history [46], activity level [1], mental health status [47], and specific medications). Of note, we attempted to account for possible differences in physical activity (mechanical loading/unloading) through use of cortical BMD measures at the 66% tibial shaft site. Previous work has identified differences in tibial shaft cortical BMD between highly active individuals (e.g., sprinters, endurance runners, triple-jumpers, high-jumpers, and hurdlers) and less active controls [48]. However, in this study, we did not note any associations between pain and tibial shaft cortical BMD, potentially indicating, at least to some degree, similar levels of activity and mechanical loading amongst study participants. Fourth, our 0.625-mm isotropic voxel size prevented assessment of trabecular microarchitecture and limited us to measurements of volumetric BMD. Accordingly, it is unclear if low BMD is due to trabecular thinning or wide trabecular spacing. For future research, it would be advantageous to investigate links between pain and trabecular microarchitecture with advanced texture analysis and smaller voxel sizes [8].

In this study we present statistically significant relationships as opposed to clinically significant relationships. As a statistically significant relationship does not measure the clinical effect of a result [49], it is important to consider the clinical effect that changes in epiphyseal or metaphyseal BMD may have on OA-related knee pain. According to Angst et al. [50], the minimal clinically important difference for OA-related pain is a change in WOMAC score greater than 6% of its maximum value (which is 20 for WOMAC). In other words, a change in pain will not be perceived unless the WOMAC score changes by 1.2 points. With this in mind, we can identify the BMD change that will correspond with a 1.2-point change in pain. Based on our model, a 44 g/cm^3 reduction in epiphyseal or metaphyseal BMD will be marked by a perceived change in pain status. Assuming an average BMD of 100 g/cm^3 for epiphyseal and metaphyseal bone, this would equate with ~ 50% change in density. Accordingly, a rational therapeutic approach would be to monitor bone while simultaneously striving to maintain bone and limit bone loss. Density changes in these regions could be monitored using QCT, dual-energy x-ray absorptiometry (DXA) or radiography. With regards to maintaining bone, potentially, this could be achieved through exercise interventions or pharmacological therapies. Our preliminary findings may also be clinically important for TKR preparation and planning. Patients with low pre-operative BMD have been shown to be at higher risk of implant failure by loosening or migration [51], higher risk of revision surgery [52], and risk of failure following revision procedures [52]. Current tibial implant design components typically include a single central post, which is inserted through the tibial epiphysis and extends into the tibial shaft. Based on our findings, there may be low quantities of bone stock in individuals with higher levels of OA-related pain, potentially placing them at risk of inadequate osseo-integration and implant fixation [53] and possibly implant loosening [54]. As there is an expected normal decrease in tibial BMD during healing [55], reduced amounts of tibial epiphyseal bony support structure prior to TKR could compromise implant fixation and success in the early stages, potentially compromising long-term implant success. It may be beneficial to use imaging and complementary image-processing techniques to evaluate preoperative bone density, especially in the commonly overlooked tibial epiphyseal and metaphyseal regions, to compliment customized surgical approaches in patients with higher levels of pain.

Conclusions

In our study, low tibial epiphyseal and metaphyseal BMD, and low medial epiphyseal BMD, was associated with OA-related pain in patients with severe OA prior to TKR. This study suggests that there may be

overlooked characteristics within trabecular bone that may be related to the pathogenesis of OA-related pain in patients with severe OA. These preliminary findings from current and previous studies [13] may be valuable in guiding outcome selection in OA studies addressing subchondral bone and pain, particularly in determining regions of interest of the proximal tibia for potential epidemiological studies.

Additional files

Additional file 1: Table S1. Coefficients (r) with 95% confidence intervals for correlation between all model variables for all included participants (n = 41). Significant associations are in bold. (DOCX 12 kb)

Additional file 2: Table S2. Coefficients (r) with 95% confidence intervals for correlation between all model variables for included male participants (n = 17). Significant associations are in bold. (DOCX 12 kb)

Additional file 3: Table S3. Coefficients (r) with 95% confidence intervals for correlation between all model variables for included female participants (n = 24). Significant associations are in bold. (DOCX 12 kb)

Additional file 4: Table S4. Adjusted coefficients of determination (R^2) and standardized beta coefficients (β) of the base model I (age, sex, and BMI) and base model II (age, sex, BMI and WOMAC pain) to predict variance in bone mineral density (BMD) at the total and regional proximal tibia. Significant R^2 and β values are in bold; p values are in parentheses. (DOCX 13 kb)

Abbreviations
BMD: Bone mineral density; BML: Bone marrow lesion; CT: Computed tomography; CV%: Coefficients of variation; DXA: Dual-energy x-ray absorptiometry; FE: Finite element; HU: Hounsfield units; JSN: Joint space narrowing; KL: Kelgren-Lawrence score; OA: Osteoarthritis; QCT: Quantitative computed tomography; TKR: Total knee replacement; VIF: Variance inflation factor; WOMAC: Western Ontario and McMaster Universities Arthritis Index

Funding
This project was funded through support from the Canadian Arthritis Network (CAN) and New England Baptist Hospital Research Funding Awards.

Authors' contributions
WDB assisted in conceiving the study, carried out the image processing, contributed to statistical analysis and interpretation of data, and composed the draft manuscript. SAK contributed to statistical analysis and interpretation of data. CEM contributed to study design and acquisition of patient data. DH contributed coordination of the study and acquisition of patient data. CT contributed to study design, participant recruitment, and acquisition of patient data. DRW contributed to study design. DJH contributed to study design and coordination of the study. JDJ conceived the study, assisted in image processing, and interpretation of data. All authors revised and/or critically evaluated the draft manuscript. All authors read and approved the final manuscript.

Consent for publication
Not applicable.

Competing interests
The authors declare that they have no competing interests. The corresponding author had full access to all the data in the study and had final responsibility for the decision to submit for publication.

Author details

[1]University of Saskatchewan, 57 Campus Drive, Saskatoon, SK S7N 5A9, Canada. [2]New England Baptist Hospital, Boston, MA, USA. [3]University of British Columbia, Vancouver, BC, Canada. [4]University of Sydney, Sydney, NSW, Australia.

References

1. Hawker GA, Stewart L, French MR, Cibere J, Jordan JM, March L, et al. Understanding the pain experience in hip and knee osteoarthritis - an OARSI/OMERACT initiative. Osteoarthr Cartil. 2008;16:415–22.

2. Hunter DJ, Felson DT. Osteoarthritis. Br Med J. 2006;332:639–42.

3. Dieppe P, Lohmander L. Pathogenesis and management of pain in osteoarthritis. Lancet. 2005;365:965–73.

4. Lo GH, Harvey WF, McAlindon TE. Associations of varus thrust and alignment with pain in knee osteoarthritis. Arthritis Rheum. 2012;64:2252–9.

5. Lo GH, McAlindon TE, Niu J, Zhang Y, Beals C, Dabrowski C, et al. Bone marrow lesions and joint effusion are strongly and independently associated with weight-bearing pain in knee osteoarthritis: data from the osteoarthritis initiative. Osteoarthr Cartil. 2009;17:1562–9.

6. Kornaat PR, Bloem JL, Ceulemans RYT, Riyazi N, Rosendaal FR, Nelissen RG, et al. Osteoarthritis of the knee: association between clinical findings and MR imaging findings. Radiology. 2006;239:811–7.

7. Buckland-Wright C. Subchondral bone changes in hand and knee osteoarthritis detected by radiography. Osteoarthritis Cartil. 2004;12:10.

8. Bobinac D, Spanjol J, Zoricic S, Maric I. Changes in articular cartilage and subchondral bone histomorphometry in osteoarthritic knee joints in humans. Bone. 2003;32:284–90.

9. Zysset PK, Sonny M, Hayes WC. Morphology-mechanical property relations in trabecular bone of the osteoarthritic proximal tibia. J Arthroplasty. 1994;9:203–16.

10. Mach DB, Rogers SD, Sabino MC, Luger NM, Schwei MJ, Pomonis JD, et al. Origins of skeletal pain: sensory and sympathetic innervation of the mouse femur. Neuroscience. 2002;113:155–66.

11. Radin EL, Paul IL, Rose RM. Role of mechanical factors in pathogenesis of primary osteoarthritis. Lancet. 1972;1:519–22.

12. Akamatsu Y, Mitsugi N, Taki N, Ashi HK, Saito T. Medial versus lateral condoyle bone mineral density ratios in a cross-sectional study: a potential marker for medial knee osteoarthritis severity. Arthritis Care Res. 2012;64:1036–45.

13. Burnett WD, Kontulainen S, McLennan C, Hazel D, Talmo C, Hunter D, et al. Knee osteoarthritis patients with severe nocturnal pain have altered subchondral tibial bone mineral density. Osteoarthr Cartil. 2015;23:1483–90.

14. Ding M, Danielsen CC, Hvid I. Bone density does not reflect mechanical properties in early-stage arthrosis. Acta Orthop Scand. 2001;72:181–5.

15. Day JS, Ding M, van der Linden JC, Hvid I, Sumner DR, Weinans H. A decreased subchondral trabecular bone tissue elastic modulus is associated with pre-arthritic cartilage damage. J Orthop Res. 2001;19:914–8.

16. Bennell KL, Creaby MW, Wrigley TV, Hunter DJ. Tibial subchondral trabecular volumetric bone density in medial knee joint osteoarthritis using peripheral quantitative computed tomography technology. Arthritis Rheum. 2008;58:2776–85.

17. Amini M, Nazemi SM, Lanovaz J, Kontulainen S, Masri BA, Wilson DR, et al. Individual and combined effects of OA-related subchondral bone alterations on proximal tibial surface stiffness: a parametric finite element modeling study. Med Eng Phys. 2015;37:783–91.

18. Carter DR, Hayes WC. The compressive behavior of bone as a two-phase porous structure. J Bone Joint Surg Am. 1977;59:954–62.

19. Neogi T. Clinical significance of bone changes in osteoarthritis. Ther Adv Musculoskelet Dis. 2012;4:259–67.

20. Kellgren JH, Lawrence JS. Radiological assessment of osteo-arthrosis. Ann Rheum Dis. 1957;16:494–502.

21. Bellamy N, Buchanan WW, Goldsmith CH, Campbell J, Stitt LW. Validation study of WOMAC: a health status instrument for measuring clinically important patient relevant outcomes to antirheumatic drug therapy in patients with osteoarthritis of the hip or knee. J Rheumatol. 1988;15:1833–40.

22. Sangha O, Stucki G, Liang MH, Fossel AH, Katz JN. The Self-Admininstered Comorbidity Questionnaire: a new method to assess comorbidity for clinical and health services research. Arthritis Rheum. 2003;49:156–63.

23. Kontulainen SA, Johnston JD, Liu D, Leung C, Oxland TR, McKay HA. Strength indices from pQCT imaging predict up to 85% of variance in bone failure properties at tibial epiphysis and diaphysis. J Musculoskelet Nueronal Interact. 2008;8:401–9.

24. UNSCEAR 2000 Report to the General Assembly - Annex B: Exposures from natural radiation sources. United Nations Scientific Committee on the Effects of Atomic Radiation.

25. Ljunggren AE. Variations in the relationship between the diaphysis and the epiphyses of the tibia. Acta Morphol Neerl Scand. 1976;14:101–37.

26. Johnston JD, McLennan CE, Hunter DJ, Wilson DR. In vivo precision of a depth-specific topographic mapping technique in the CT analysis of osteoarthritic and normal proximal tibial subchondral bone density. Skelet Radiol. 2010;40:1057–64.

27. Glüer CC, Blake G, Lu Y, Blunt BA, Jergas M, Genant HK. Accurate assessment of precision errors: how to measure the reproducibility of bone densitometry techniques. Osteoporos Int. 1995;5:262–70.

28. Johnston JD, Masri BA, Wilson DR. Computed tomography topographic mapping of subchondral density (CT-TOMASD) in osteoarthritic and normal knees: methodological development and preliminary findings. Osteoarthr Cartil. 2009;17:1319–26.

29. Spoor CF, Zonneveld FW, Macho GA. Linear measurements of cortical bone and dental enamel by computed tomography: applications and problems. Am J Phys Anthropol. 1993;91:469–84.

30. Chen Y, Huang Y-C, Lu WW. Is subchondral bone mineral density associated with nocturnal pain in knee osteoarthritis patients? Osteoarthritis Cartil. 2015;23:2297–8.

31. Chiba K, Burghardt AJ, Osaki M, Majumdar S. Three-dimensional analysis of subchondral cysts in hip osteoarthritis: an ex vivo HR-pQCT study. Bone. 2014;66:140–5.

32. Frank AW, Labas MC, Johnston JD, Kontulainen SA. Site-specific variance in radius and tibia bone strength as determined by muscle size and body mass. Physiother Can. 2012;64:292–301.

33. Schneider A, Hommel G, Blettner M. Linear regression analysis. Dtsch Arztebl Int. 2010;107:776–82.

34. Thompson R. A note on restricted maximum likelihood estimation with an alternative outlier model. J R Stat Soc B Methodol. 1985;47:53–5.

35. Dore D, Ding C, Jones G. A pilot study of the reproducibility and validity of measuring knee subchondral bone density in the tibia. Osteoarthritis Cartil. 2008;16:1539–44.

36. Burnett W, Kontulainen S, McLennan C, Hazel D, Talmo C, Hunter D, et al. Response to Letter to the Editor: 'Is subchondral bone mineral density associated with nocturnal pain in knee osteoarthritis patients?'. Osteoarthritis Cartil. 2015;23:2299–301.

37. Seah S, Wheaton D, Li L, Dyke JP, Talmo C, Harvey WF, et al. The relationship of tibial bone perfusion in knee osteoarthritis. Osteoarthr Cartil. 2012;20:1527–33.

38. Lowitz T, Museyko O, Bousson V, Laouisset L, Kalendar WA, Laredo JD, et al. Bone marrow lesions identified by MRI in knee osteoarthritis are associated with locally increased bone mineral density measured by QCT. Osteoarthr Cartil. 2013;21:957–64.

39. Venäläinen MS, Mononen ME, Jurvelin JS, Töyräs J, Virén T, Korhonen RK. Importance of material properties and porosity of bone on mechanical response of articular cartilage in human knee joint: a two-dimensional finite element study. J Biomech Eng. 2014;136:121005.

40. Hertz VHH. Uber die Berührung fester elastischer Körper. J Reine Angew Math. 1882;92:156–71. German.

41. Wada M, Maezawa Y, Baba H, Shimada S, Sasaki S, Nose Y. Relationships among bone mineral densities, static alignment and dynamic load in patients with medial compartment knee osteoarthritis. Rheumatology (Oxford). 2001;40:499–505.

42. Li G, Zheng Q, Landao-Bassonga E, Cheng TS, Pavlos NJ, Ma Y, et al. Influence of age and gender on microarchitecture and bone remodeling in subchondral bone of the osteoarthritic femoral head. Bone. 2015;77:91–7.

43. Perilli E, Baleani M, Ohman C, Baruffaldi F, Viceconti M. Structural parameters and mechanical strength of cancellous bone in the femoral head in osteoarthritis do not depend on age. Bone. 2007;41:760–8.

44. Mazess RB. On aging bone loss. Clin Orthop Relat Res. 1982;165:239–52.

45. Peduzzi P, Concato J, Kemper E, Holford TR, Feinstein AR. A simulation study of the number of events per variable in logistic regression analysis. J Clin Epidemiol. 1996;49:1373–9.

46. Miranda H, Viikari-Juntra E, Martikainen R, Riihimaki H. A prospective study on knee pain and its risk factors. Osteoarthritis Cartil. 2002;10:623–30.

47. Wesseling J, Welsing PMJ, Bierma-Zeinstra SMA, Dekker J, Gorter KJ, Kloppenburg M, et al. Impact of self-reported comorbidity on physical and mental health status in early sympotmatic osteoarthritis: the CHECK (Cohort Hip and Cohort Knee) study. Rheumatology. 2013;52:180–8.

48   Rantalainen T, Nikander R, Daly RM, Heinonen A, Sievanen H. Exercise loading and cortical bone distribution at the tibial shaft. Bone. 2011;48:786–91.

49   Wasserstein R, Lazar N. The ASA's statements on p-values: context, process, and purpose. Am Stat. 2016;70:129–33.

50   Angst F, Aeschlimann A, Stucki G. Smallest detectable and minimal clinically important differences of rehabilitation intervention with their implications for required sample sizes using WOMAC and SF-36 Quality of Life measurement instruments in patients with osteoarthritis of the lower extremities. Arthritis Care Res (Hoboken). 2001;45:384–91.

51   Petersen MM, Nielsen PT, Lebech A, Toksvig-Larsen S, Lund B. Preoperative bone mineral density of the proximal tibia and migration of the tibial compartment after uncemented total knee arthroplasty. J Arthroplasty. 1999;14:77–81.

52   Levitz CL, Lotke PA, Karp JS. Long-term changes in bone mineral density following total knee replacement. Clin Orthop Relat Res. 1995;321:68–72.

53   Mavrogenis AF, Dimitriou R, Parvizi J, Babis GC. Biology of implant osseointegration. J Musculoskelet Nueronal Interact. 2009;9:61–71.

54   Sharkey PF, Hozack WJ, Rothman RH, Shastri S, Jacoby SM. Why are total knee arthroplasties failing today? Clin Orthop Relat Res. 2002;404:7–13.

55   Ritter MA, Davis KE, Small SR, Merchun JG, Farris A. Trabecular bone density of the proximal tibia as it relates to failure of a total knee replacement. Bone Joint J. 2014;96-B:1503–9.

Progranulin derivative Atsttrin protects against early osteoarthritis in mouse and rat models

Jian-lu Wei[1,2], Wenyu Fu[1], Yuan-jing Ding[1], Aubryanna Hettinghouse[1], Matin Lendhey[1], Ran Schwarzkopf[1], Oran D. Kennedy[1] and Chuan-ju Liu[1,3,4*]

Abstract

Background: Atsttrin, an engineered protein composed of three tumor necrosis factor receptor (TNFR)-binding fragments of progranulin (PGRN), shows therapeutic effect in multiple murine models of inflammatory arthritis . Additionally, intra-articular delivery of PGRN protects against osteoarthritis (OA) progression. The purpose of this study is to determine whether Atsttrin also has therapeutic effects in OA and the molecular mechanisms involved.

Methods: Surgically induced and noninvasive rupture OA models were established in mouse and rat, respectively. Cartilage degradation and OA were evaluated using Safranin O staining, immunohistochemistry, and ELISA. Additionally, expressions of pain-related markers, degenerative factors, and anabolic and catabolic markers known to be involved in OA were analyzed. Furthermore, the anabolic and anti-catabolic effects and underlying mechanisms of Atsttrin were determined using in-vitro assays with primary chondrocytes.

Results: Herein, we found Atsttrin effectively prevented the accelerated OA phenotype associated with PGRN deficiency. Additionally, Atsttrin exhibited a preventative effect in OA by protecting articular cartilage and reducing OA-associated pain in both nonsurgically induced rat and surgically induced murine OA models. Mechanistic studies revealed that Atsttrin stimulated TNFR2-Akt-Erk1/2-dependent chondrocyte anabolism, while inhibiting TNFα/TNFR1-mediated inflammatory catabolism.

Conclusions: These findings not only provide new insights into the role of PGRN and its derived engineered protein Atsttrin in cartilage homeostasis as well as OA in vivo, but may also lead to new therapeutic alternatives for OA as well as other relative degenerative joint diseases.

Keywords: Atsttrin, Progranulin, TNFα, TNFR2, TNFR1, Osteoarthritis

Background

Osteoarthritis (OA) is a degenerative joint disease characterized by cartilage destruction, synovitis, subchondral bone sclerosis, and osteophyte formation; OA affects almost 15% of the world's population [1]. Unfortunately, the mechanisms of OA development remain unclear and there are no available therapeutic agents that effectively prevent or arrest progression of the disease [2, 3].

Although the etiology of OA is still unclear, it is believed that tumor necrosis factor alpha (TNFα) exhibits an important effect in the pathological processes of OA [4]. The level of TNFα is increased in OA patients' articular cartilage compared with that of healthy controls and TNFα is thought to cause inflammatory destruction [5]. Additionally, anti-TNFα drugs demonstrate preventative and therapeutic effect in various OA models as well as in clinical trials [6].

Progranulin (PGRN) is a growth factor with a unique "beads-on-a-string" structure [7, 8]. PGRN participates in many pathophysiological processes, including anti-inflammation, tissue repair, and wound healing [9–12].

* Correspondence: chuanju.liu@med.nyu.edu
[1]Department of Orthopaedic Surgery, New York University Medical Center, New York, NY 10003, USA
[3]Department of Cell Biology, New York University School of Medicine, New York, NY 10016, USA
Full list of author information is available at the end of the article

Importantly, PGRN is also a growth factor involved in regulating cartilage development and degradation, and the PGRN level is significantly increased in OA patients' cartilage relative to that of healthy controls [13, 14]. Previously, we found that PGRN binds to tumor necrosis factor receptors (TNFRs) and is therapeutic in multiple mouse models of inflammatory arthritis [6, 15]; our recent studies, implementing surgically induced OA models, reveal that PGRN also protects against OA through TNFR signaling [16].

Through screening a series of PGRN deletion mutants retaining TNFR binding ability, we have generated an engineered protein which appears to be the minimal molecule of PGRN that still has TNFR binding affinity [6]. This molecule consists of three fragments of PGRN and we named it Atsttrin (antagonist of TNF/TNFR signaling via targeting to TNF receptors) [17]. Importantly, Atsttrin has a stronger therapeutic effect than recombinant PGRN in inflammatory arthritis animal models [6]. Recently, another group reported that intraarticular delivery of mesenchymal stem cells (MSCs) which were pretransduced with Atsttrin could protect against OA development [18]. In this study, we examine whether the engineered protein Atsttrin could protect against OA, as well as the molecular mechanisms involved, through the use of human primary chondrocytes in vitro alongside multiple models of OA implemented in genetically modified mice and Sprague–Dawley rats in vivo.

Methods

Animals, human cartilage, and recombinant Atsttrin

We performed all animal studies under institutional guidelines. All of the protocols were approval by the Institutional Animal Care and Use Committee, New York University, NY, USA. We generated, maintained, and genotyped the mice with the genetic background of C57BL/6 wildtype (WT), PGRN-deficient (PGRN$^{-/-}$), TNFR1-deficient (TNFR1$^{-/-}$), and TNFR2-deficient (TNFR2$^{-/-}$) mice as reported previously [6]. Sprague–Dawley rats were obtained from Charles River (Wilmington, MA, USA). Eight-week-old male mice and 14-week-old male rats were used for this experiment [19, 20]. For human primary chondrocyte culture, human cartilage samples were harvested from patients receiving total knee joint replacement surgery from New York University, Hospital for Joint Diseases (NY, USA). Acquisition and use of human tissue was conducted in accordance with an Institutional Review Board (IRB#12758) approved protocol. Recombinant Atsttrin was manufactured and provided by Atreaon, Inc.

Noninvasive anterior crucial ligament rupture rat model

The noninvasive OA rat model was established as described previously [20]. Animals were anesthetized and maintained using isoflurane, and the noninvasive anterior crucial ligament rupture model was established using the indicated machine: Electroforce 3200 (Bose Corp., MN, USA), Solidworks (Dassault Systemes, MA, USA), or Mojo 3D printer (Stratasys, MN, USA). After the model was established, we intraarticularly injected PBS or recombinant Atsttrin once a week for 4 weeks in total. After 4 weeks of treatment, the rats were sacrificed for histological evaluation.

Surgically induced OA mouse models

For the surgically induced destabilization of medial meniscus (DMM) mouse model, we took advantage of 8-week-old male PGRN$^{-/-}$ mice and their age-matched WT control littermates. The medial meniscotibial ligament of the right knee joint was cut to generate a destabilized medial meniscus. Six mice were used in each group. After surgery, WT mice received local delivery of 6 µl PBS via intraarticular injection, while PGRN$^{-/-}$ mice received local delivery of 6 µl PBS or recombinant Atsttrin (1 µg/µl). Four weeks after model induction, mice were sacrificed and knee joints were collected. The tissues were then processed for histological analysis.

To investigate the preventative as well as the therapeutic effect of Atsttrin, we also established the anterior cruciate ligament transection (ACLT) mouse model. To determine which TNFR was predominantly responsible for Atsttrin's effect, we established the ACLT mouse model in age-matched WT, TNFR1$^{-/-}$, or TNFR2$^{-/-}$ male mice ($n = 6$, respectively). To address the preventative potential of Atsttrin in OA, we intraarticularly injected 6 µl Atsttrin or PBS once a week for 4 weeks beginning on the day of surgery, as based on our previous study [16]. For examination of Atsttrin's therapeutic effect, 6 µl Atsttrin or PBS were intraarticularly injected once a week for 4 weeks beginning 4 weeks postoperatively, as based on our previous study [16]. Ambulatory behavior of mice was monitored and recorded throughout the study. After 4 weeks of treatment, mice were sacrificed for dorsal root ganglia (DRG) harvest and histological evaluation.

Sandwich ELISA for cartilage oligomeric matrix protein

The serum concentration of cartilage oligomeric matrix protein (COMP) was analyzed by our established sandwich ELISA [21]. Protein A agarose (Invitrogen) purified rabbit anti-COMP pAb and anti-COMP type III mAb 2127F5B6 were used as capture and detection antibodies, respectively. Anti-COMP type III mAb 2127F5B6 was labeled with horseradish peroxidase (HRP) using the Lightning-Link™ Horseradish Peroxidase Labeling Kit (Innova) as per the manufacturer's protocol. Results were interpreted based on the linear range of the standard curve. All of the samples were assayed in triplicate.

Primary cultures of chondrocytes

Human articular chondrocytes were harvested by enzymatic digestion in accordance with established methodology [16]. Briefly, human cartilage slices were cut into small pieces and washed several times with PBS, pH 7.4. Minced tissues were incubated with agitation in digestion medium comprised of 0.25% collagenase II in DMEM medium with 5% FBS in a spinner flask for 16 hours at 37 °C with 5% CO_2. After digestion, the suspended cells were collected and seeded into six-well plates for subsequent study. For mouse primary chondrocyte culture, knee joints were collected from 6-day-old WT, TNFR1$^{-/-}$, or TNFR2$^{-/-}$ mice following sacrifice. Under magnification, the cartilage samples were isolated with special attention to avoid damaging the subchondral bone and tissues were rinsed completely three times in PBS. Primary cartilage samples were placed in a 10-cm dish containing the aforementioned digestion buffer and incubated for 16 hours at 37 °C with 5% CO_2. After full digestion, suspended cells were collected and seeded in a six-well plate for use. All chondrocytes used for experiments are first-generation cells.

von Frey test

von Frey filaments (Stoelting, Wood Dale, IL, USA) were applied with ascending force intensities on the plantar surface of the hind paw to determine the tactile pain threshold as based on a previous publication [22]. Rapid withdrawal of the hind paw was recorded as a positive response. Hind paws were subjected to 10 trials at a given intensity with a 30-second interval maintained between trials. The number of positive responses for each von Frey filament's stimulus was recorded. Animals were considered to have reached tactile threshold when five in 10 trials generated a positive response. The examiner was blinded to the groups.

Dorsal root ganglia isolation

Eight weeks after ACLT surgery, mice were sacrificed and L3–L5 DRG were isolated based on a previous publication [23]. Briefly, mice were anesthetized using isoflurane and fur was cleared from the dorsal surface. A longitudinal incision was made, the spinal column was exposed, and L3–L5 DRG were extracted and tissues flash-frozen using liquid nitrogen. These tissues were processed using the Qiagen RNeasy kit (Qiagen, Valencia, CA, USA) for RNA extraction.

Luciferase assay

Luciferase assay was performed as reported previously [24]. Lipofectamine2000 DNA transfection reagent was used to cotransfect NF-κB and renilla plasmids in C28I2 cells according to the manufacturer's protocol (Life Technologies). Eighteen hours after transfection, C28I2 cells were treated without or with 10 ng/ml TNFα in the absence or presence of 200 ng/ml recombinant Atsttrin. After 24-hour incubation, we measured luciferase activity using the Reporter Assay System of Dual-Luciferase® in accordance with the manufacturer's instructions (Promega).

Histological analysis and immunostaining

Histological analysis was conducted as described previously [16]. Briefly, knee joints were fixed immediately after sacrifice in 4% PFA at room temperature for 48 hours. After washing three times in PBS, the tissues were decalcified at 4 °C in 10% w/v EDTA for 2 weeks. Tissues were measured using a vernier caliper before paraffin processing. Knee joints were dehydrated and embedded; the blocks were trimmed to the midpoint as calculated previously from caliper measurements and serial 5-μm sections were placed on slides for staining. H&E or Safranin O/fast green staining was performed following the established protocol. The extent of synovitis was determined using a graded scale based on H&E staining: grade 0, no signs of inflammation; grade 1, mild inflammation with hyperplasia of the synovial lining without cartilage destruction; and grades 2–4, increasing degrees of inflammatory cell infiltrate and cartilage/bone destruction. For immunohistochemistry staining, sections were pretreated with 0.1% trypsin for 30 minutes at 37 °C. Sections were washed with PBS three times, followed by treatment with 0.25 U/ml chondroitinase ABC (Sigma-Aldrich) for 1 hour and then 1 U/ml hyaluronidase (Sigma-Aldrich) for 1 hour at 37 °C. To reduce nonspecific staining, sections were blocked at room temperature with 20% normal horse serum diluted in 3% BSA for 1 hour. Without washing after blocking, Col X antibody (1:200 dilution; DSHB), MMP-13 antibody (ab3208, 1:200 dilution; Abcam), and affinity-purified monoclonal anti-COMP fragments (1:200 dilution) were diluted in 20% normal horse serum with 3% BSA at 4 °C overnight. Sections were prepared for detection using the Vectastain Elite ABC kit following the manufacturer's guidelines at 25 °C for 1 hour. Immunoreactivity was visualized using 0.5 mg/ml 3,3′-diaminobenzidine (DAB) in 50 mM Tris–HCl substrate, pH 7.8. Methyl green (1%) was used for counterstaining.

Histological analysis and score

The articular cartilage proteoglycan content was defined on the basis of Safranin O staining. In this study, we used the well-accepted Osteoarthritis Research Society International (OARSI) scoring system [25]: 0 = normal cartilage without any damage; 0.5 = loss of Safranin O staining with no detectable structural change; 1 = small fibrillation; 2 = vertical damage of cartilage limited to superficial layer; 3 = vertical damage, no more than 25%

of the cartilage surface; 4 = vertical damage, 25–50% of the cartilage surface; 5 = vertical damage, 50–75% of the cartilage surface; and 6 = vertical damage, more than 75% of the cartilage surface.

Real-time RT-PCR

Total RNA were extracted from cultured chondrocytes using the RNeasy kit (Qiagen) and reverse transcribed into cDNA using the ImProm-II reverse transcription system (Promega). Data were normalized to the internal control, GAPDH. The primers for specific amplification of murine genes are as follows: 5′-AATGCTGGTACT CCAAACCC-3′ and 5′-CTGGATCGTTATCCAGCA AACAGC-3′ for Aggrecan; 5′-ACTAGTCATCCAGCA AACAGCCAGG-3′ and 5′-TTGGCTTTGGGAAGAGA C-3′ for Col II; 5′-AATCTCACAGCAGCACATCA-3′ and 5′-AAGGTGCTCATGTCCTCATC-3′ for IL-1β; 5′-ACAGGAGGGGTTAAAGCTGC-3′ and 5′-TTGT CTCCAAGGGACCAGG-3′ for NOS-2; 5′-GCATTGA CGCATCCAAACCC-3′ and 5′-CGTGGTAGGTCCAG CAAACAGTTAC-3′ for ADAMTS-4; 5′-ACTTTGT TGCCAATTCCAGG-3′ and 5′-TTTGAGAACACGGG GAAGAC-3′ for MMP-13; 5′-CATAGCAGCCACCT TCATTCC-3′ and 5′-TCTCCTTGGCCACAATGGTC-3′ for MCP-1; 5′-AGAGAGCTGCAGCAAAAAGG-3′ and 5′-GGAAAGAGGCAGTTGCAAAG-3′ for CCR-2; and 5′-AGAACATCATCCCTGCATCC-3′ and 5′-AG TTGCTGTTGAAGTCGC-3′ for GAPDH. Melting curve analysis was used to verify the PCR product. Each experiment was repeated three times.

Western blot analysis

Proteins extracted from chondrocytes were processed on 8% SDS-polyacrylamide gel, followed by electrotransfer to nitrocellulose membrane. The membrane was blocked in 3% BSA in 10 mM Tris–HCl, pH 8.0, 150 mM NaCl, and 0.5% Tween 20. After washing three times, blots were incubated at 4 °C overnight with polyclonal anti-Erk1/2 (#4695, 1:1000 dilution; Cell Signaling Technology), anti-phosphorylated Erk1/2 (#4370S, 1:1000 dilution; Cell Signaling Technology), polyclonal anti-Akt (#9272, 1:1000 dilution; Cell Signaling Technology), anti-phosphorylated Akt (#4058S, 1:1000 dilution; Cell Signaling Technology), polyclonal anti-MMP-3 (ab52915, 1:1000 dilution; Abcam), polyclonal anti-MMP-13 (ab3208, 1:1000 dilution; Abcam), polyclonal anti-ADAMTS-4 (PA1-1750, 1:1000 dilution; Thermo Fisher Scientific), polyclonal anti-NOS-2 (SC651, 1:1000 dilution; Santa Cruz Biotechnology), polyclonal anti-GAPDH (SC25778, 1:1000 dilution; Santa Cruz Biotechnology), polyclonal anti-tubulin (#5346, 1:1000 dilution; Cell Signaling Technology), or diluted polyclonal anti-lamin B (SC-6217, 1:500 dilution; Santa Cruz Biotechnology). After washing three times, blots were incubated

with an appropriate HRP-conjugated anti-rabbit/mouse immunoglobulin secondary antibody at 25 °C for 1 hour. The bound antibody was visualized using an enhanced chemiluminescence system (Amersham Life Science, Arlington Heights, IL, USA).

Cartilage explant cultures

Cartilage explants were cultured as described previously [16]. Briefly, mouse femoral head cartilage was isolated and finely minced to 1 mm diameter and 1 mm thickness. The cartilage explants were then dispensed into serum-free DMEM containing 25 mM HEPES and 2 mM glutamine, in the absence or presence of recombinant Atsttrin (200 ng/ml).

Dimethylmethylene blue assay of GAG

The mouse cartilage culture medium was collected and GAG release was quantified by dimethylmethylene blue assay (DMMB) (Polysciences, Warrington, PA, USA). Hyaluronidase (0.5 unit/ml; Seikagaku, Tokyo, Japan) was incubated with collected medium for 3 hours at 37 °C to remove hyaluronan in order to reduce inhibition of the DMMB assay. The DMMB signal from digests was measured at 520 nm using a SpectraMax 384 Microplate Reader (Molecular Devices, Sunnyvale, CA, USA). The GAG content was calculated based on linear regression of readings from chondroitin-6-sulfate standards from Shark cartilage (Sigma Aldrich, St. Louis, MO, USA). Each sample was read in triplicate. The average values of the triplicates were normalized to the standard curve.

Statistical analysis

Results were expressed as mean ± SEM. Statistical analysis included Student's t test performed by SPSS software (SPSS Inc., Chicago, IL, USA). $p < 0.05$ was considered statistically significant.

Results

Atsttrin rescues accelerated OA caused by PGRN deficiency

Previously, we reported that PGRN is expressed in both human and mouse articular cartilage, and its level is elevated, relative to healthy controls in both human OA cartilage and in surgically induced OA model mice. In addition, we have reported that loss of PGRN led to enhanced OA in both "aged" mice and surgically induced OA models [16]. In the present study, PGRN expression is slightly, but not significantly, elevated in 1-year-old aged mice as compared with 4-month-old mice (Additional file 1: Figure S1A, B). To determine whether Atsttrin, an engineered protein derived from PGRN [6], could prevent the accelerated OA seen in our surgically induced, PGRN-null OA models, the DMM model was generated in PGRN$^{-/-}$ and age-matched WT mice. As illustrated in Fig. 1a, Safranin O-stained sections demonstrated that Atsttrin effectively prevented loss of proteoglycan content in PGRN$^{-/-}$ mice. Statistical analysis of proteoglycan loss and the OARSI score obtained from Safranin O-stained sections indicates that Atsttrin significantly reduced articular cartilage destruction (Fig. 1b, c). Moreover, as shown in Fig. 1d, application of recombinant Atsttrin also reduced the serum levels of COMP-degradative fragments as assayed by ELISA.

Atsttrin prevents OA development in surgically induced OA mouse model

Recently, Xia et al. [18] reported that local delivery of Atsttrin-transduced MSCs could effectively protect against OA development in a murine OA model. This finding promoted us to determine whether local delivery of recombinant Atsttrin could prevent OA development. To address this issue, we established the ACLT OA model in C56LB/6 WT mice, followed by intraarticular injection of recombinant Atsttrin (6 µg) once per week for 4 weeks. As shown in Fig. 2a, histological analysis indicated that Atsttrin effectively protected against cartilage loss. Additionally, the OARSI score and proteoglycan loss score based on the histology revealed a significant improvement in the Atsttrin-treated group (Fig. 2b, c). Furthermore, as shown in Fig. 2d, immunohistochemical staining demonstrated that Atsttrin reduced

COMP degradation, type X collagen (Col X) expression, as well as matrix-degrading enzyme matrix metalloproteinase 13 (MMP-13) expression. Notably, subchondral bone provides support for articular cartilage [26]. Studies indicate that the thickness of the subchondral bone plate significantly decreases during the first phase of ACLT-induced OA in mice [27] and loss of subchondral bone leads to reduced support and more deterioration of articular cartilage in OA pathogenesis [28, 29]. Interestingly, Atsttrin effectively inhibited subchondral bone loss (Fig. 2e). Moreover, we reported previously that Atsttrin inhibited osteoclastogenesis in vitro [6] and it is believed that osteoclastogenesis is involved in subchondral bone remodeling in ACLT mice [30]. To demonstrate whether Atsttrin-mediated subchondral bone protection occurs through inhibition of osteoclast formation, we performed tartrate-resistant acid phosphatase (TRAP) staining. As illustrated in Fig. 2f, Atsttrin significantly inhibited osteoclast activity. Synovium also plays an important role in the pathogenesis of OA; to further determine the effect of Atsttrin on synovitis, we performed H&E staining and found that Atsttrin effectively inhibited synovial inflammation (Fig. 2 g, h). Behavioral observations and pain marker levels were also recorded to determine whether Atsttrin could reduce OA-related pain. Atsttrin treatment was associated with significantly greater rearing times, as compared to the PBS-treated group when monitored for free ambulation in

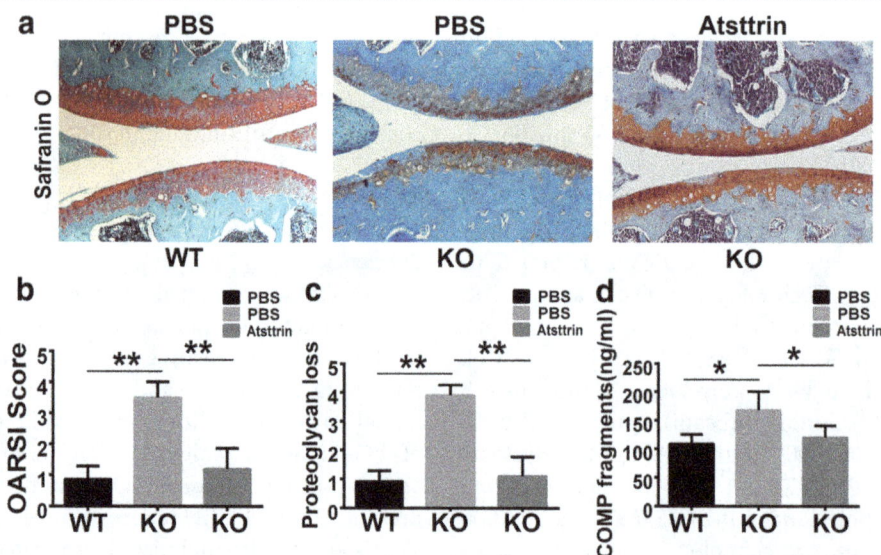

Fig. 1 Atsttrin prevented accelerated OA caused by PGRN deficiency. **a** Intraarticular injection of Atsttrin protected against articular cartilage loss following the surgically induced DMM model in PGRN$^{-/-}$ mice, assayed by Safranin O staining. **b, c** Quantification of OARSI score and proteoglycan loss based on Safranin O staining. **d** Atsttrin-reduced serum level of COMP fragments, assayed by ELISA. Values are mean ± SEM of six mice. *$p < 0.05$, **$p < 0.01$ versus PBS-treated group. KO knockout, OARSI Osteoarthritis Research Society International, PBS phosphate-buffered saline, WT wildtype

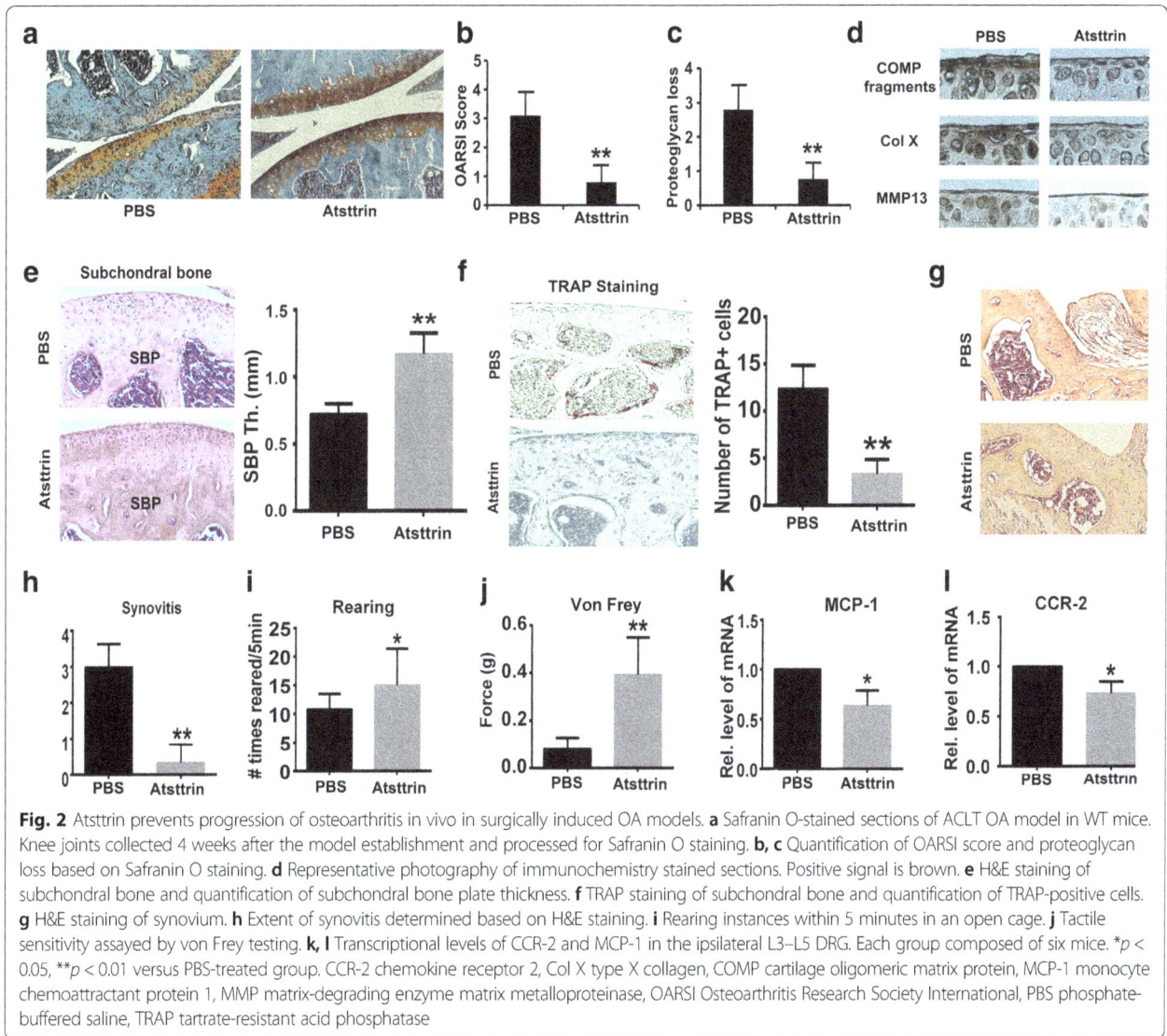

Fig. 2 Atsttrin prevents progression of osteoarthritis in vivo in surgically induced OA models. **a** Safranin O-stained sections of ACLT OA model in WT mice. Knee joints collected 4 weeks after the model establishment and processed for Safranin O staining. **b, c** Quantification of OARSI score and proteoglycan loss based on Safranin O staining. **d** Representative photography of immunochemistry stained sections. Positive signal is brown. **e** H&E staining of subchondral bone and quantification of subchondral bone plate thickness. **f** TRAP staining of subchondral bone and quantification of TRAP-positive cells. **g** H&E staining of synovium. **h** Extent of synovitis determined based on H&E staining. **i** Rearing instances within 5 minutes in an open cage. **j** Tactile sensitivity assayed by von Frey testing. **k, l** Transcriptional levels of CCR-2 and MCP-1 in the ipsilateral L3–L5 DRG. Each group composed of six mice. $*p < 0.05$, $**p < 0.01$ versus PBS-treated group. CCR-2 chemokine receptor 2, Col X type X collagen, COMP cartilage oligomeric matrix protein, MCP-1 monocyte chemoattractant protein 1, MMP matrix-degrading enzyme matrix metalloproteinase, OARSI Osteoarthritis Research Society International, PBS phosphate-buffered saline, TRAP tartrate-resistant acid phosphatase

an open field testing box, as indicated in Fig. 2i. In addition, von Frey filament testing demonstrated that the pain threshold was decreased after ACLT surgery and that Atsttrin effectively improved the pain threshold (Fig. 2j). Further, inflammatory cytokines such as chemokine monocyte chemoattractant protein 1 (MCP-1), chemokine receptor 2 (CCR-2), and interleukin-1β (IL-1β) in DRG play an important role in OA-associated pain. It is reported that upregulated transcriptional levels of MCP-1, CCR-2, and IL-1β in DRG correlate to exhibition of pain-associated behaviors in murine OA models [31]. As indicated in Fig. 2 k, l, the transcriptional level of MCP-1 and CCR-2 in the ipsilateral L3–L5 DRG was significantly upregulated compared to the control group, whereas Atsttrin significantly reduced their expressions to levels comparable to those of the control group. Collectively, these results indicate that Atsttrin is likely to be a disease-modifying and also a symptom-modifying molecule.

Atsttrin is therapeutic against OA and its therapeutic effects depend on both TNFR1 and TNFR2 pathways

To determine whether recombinant Atsttrin is therapeutic against OA, we took advantage of both nonsurgically induced rat and surgically induced mouse models. Four weeks following the establishment of the unique noninvasive rat OA model, we locally delivered 60 μg Atsttrin once per week for 4 weeks. Histological analysis indicated that Atsttrin effectively protected against articular cartilage destruction (Fig. 3a) and significantly improved the arthritis score as well as the proteoglycan loss score (Fig. 3b, c).

We also took advantage of the well-accepted surgically induced ACLT mouse model. Beginning 4 weeks postoperatively, we intraarticularly injected 6 μg recombinant

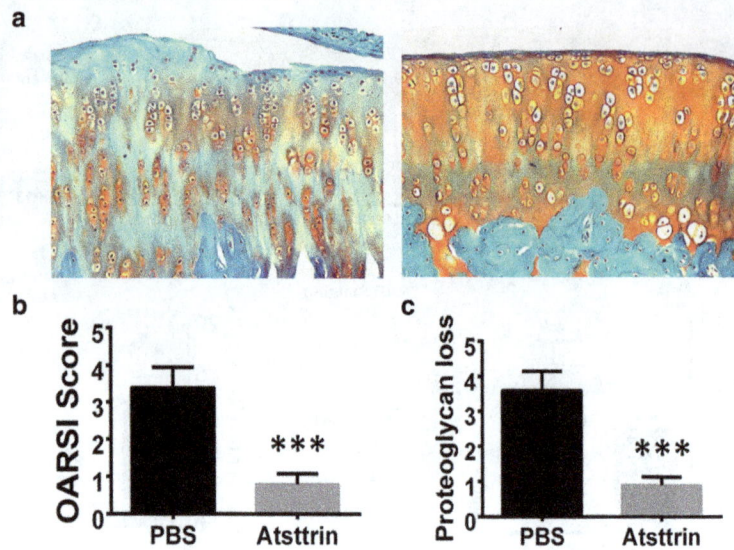

Fig. 3 Atsttrin is therapeutic in the noninvasive rat OA model. **a** Safranin O- stained sections of the rat knee joint collected 8 weeks after induction of the noninvasive rat OA model. **b** OARSI score-based Safranin O-stained. **c** Proteoglycan loss score on the basis of Safranin O staining. Each group composed of six rats. ***$p < 0.001$ versus PBS-treated group. OARSI Osteoarthritis Research Society International, PBS phosphate-buffered saline

Atsttrin weekly for 4 weeks. As indicated in Fig. 4a–c, Atsttrin exhibited a therapeutic effect in the WT mice, evidenced by preservation of articular cartilage. To compare the efficacy of PGRN and its derived engineered protein Atsttrin in mitigating OA progression, we also compared the OARSI score between these two groups, and found no significant difference between PGRN and Atsttrin in treating OA (Additional file 2: Figure S2).

To determine whether the Atsttrin-mediated protective effect is dependent upon TNFR1 or TNFR2, or both receptors, we established the ACLT model in TNFR1$^{-/-}$ and TNFR2$^{-/-}$ mice. As revealed in Fig. 4a–c, TNFR1$^{-/-}$ mice exhibited partial loss of Atsttrin-mediated protection while the Atsttrin-mediated protective effect was almost abolished in TNFR2$^{-/-}$ mice. However, we found that, in the presence of Atsttrin, the OARSI score and proteoglycan loss score of both TNFR1$^{-/-}$ mice and TNFR2$^{-/-}$ mice were each significantly increased relative to those of WT mice. Sera from WT mice and from each group of TNFR null mice were collected and COMP fragment-specific ELISA revealed that Atsttrin significantly decreased COMP degradation in the WT OA mice; however, the Atsttrin-mediated protective effect against COMP degradation was slightly decreased in TNFR1$^{-/-}$ mice and relatively unaffected in TNFR2$^{-/-}$ mice (Fig. 4d). Notably, after Atsttrin treatment, the level of COMP fragments in TNFR1$^{-/-}$ mice and TNFR2$^{-/-}$ mice were significantly increased in comparison to levels in WT mice. Collectively, both TNFR1 and TNFR2 appear to be required for mediating Atsttrin's protective effect in OA.

Atsttrin-mediated anabolism primarily depends on TNFR2-Akt-Erk1/2 signaling

Given that Atsttrin selectively binds to TNFRs and that the Atsttrin-mediated beneficial effect in OA depends on both receptors in vivo, we next sought to examine the molecular mechanisms involved through detailing the effect of Atsttrin on cartilage and chondrocyte metabolism. To determine whether Atsttrin has an anabolic effect in cartilage, we took advantage of mouse primary cartilage explants and found that recombinant Atsttrin significantly promoted GAG synthesis in WT and TNFR1$^{-/-}$ cartilage while Atsttrin lost this effect in TNFR2$^{-/-}$ cartilage (Fig. 5a). Additionally, Atsttrin-induced expressions of anabolic biomarkers, including type II collagen (Col II) and aggrecan (ACN), were remarkably reduced in TNFR2$^{-/-}$ chondrocytes in comparison with WT and TNFR1$^{-/-}$ chondrocytes (Fig. 5b, c). These data indicate that the Atsttrin-mediated anabolic effect primarily depends on the TNFR2 pathway.

Previous study has shown that both Akt and Erk1/2 pathways are involved in chondrocyte anabolism and PGRN slightly activates Akt signaling and strongly actives Erk1/2 signaling in chondrocytes [13]. Contrastingly, we demonstrate herein that Atsttrin strongly activates Akt signaling and slightly activates Erk1/2 signaling (Fig. 5d). Activation of these signaling pathways was lost in TNFR2$^{-/-}$ chondrocytes, but no change was observed in TNFR1$^{-/-}$ chondrocytes relative to WT chondrocytes (Fig. 5d). More importantly, Atsttrin's anabolic effect was partially lost after blocking Erk1/2 signaling alone using U0126 or blocking the Akt signaling pathway alone using Wortmannin (Fig. 5e–h).

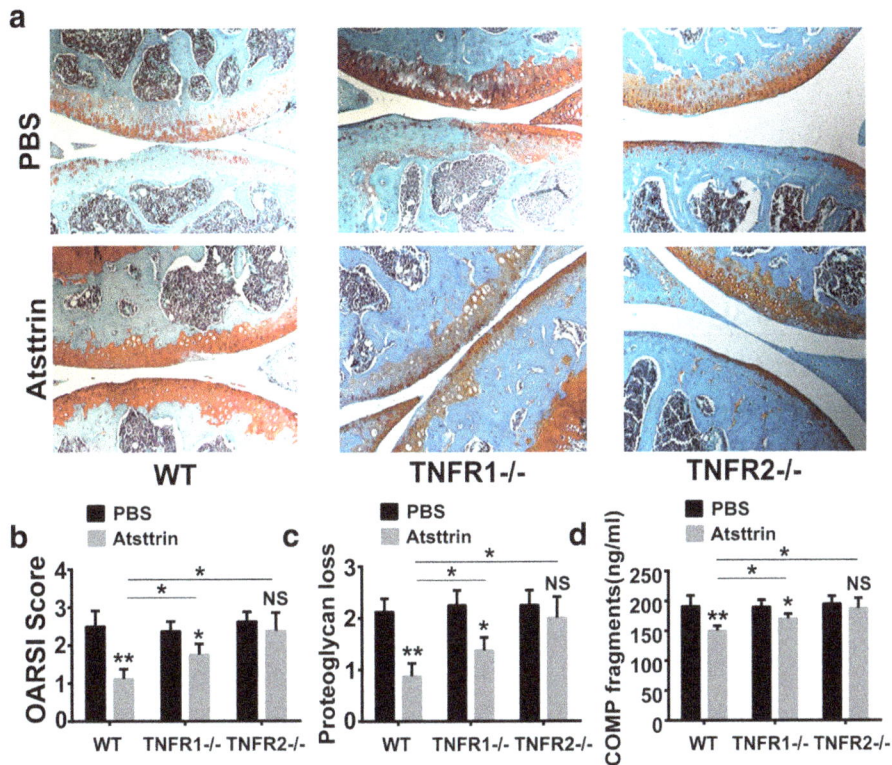

Fig. 4 Atsttrin protects against OA through TNFRs. **a** Atsttrin protected against degeneration of articular cartilage in WT mice following surgical induction of the ACLT model, but this protection was partially lost in TNFR1$^{-/-}$ mice and almost abolished in TNFR2$^{-/-}$ mice, assayed by Safranin O staining. $n = 6$ for each group. **b, c** OARSI score and proteoglycan loss based on Safranin O staining. **d** Atsttrin-decreased COMP fragment level in serum, assayed by ELISA. Values are mean ± SEM of at least three independent experiments. *$p < 0.05$, **$p < 0.01$ versus PBS-treated group. COMP cartilage oligomeric matrix protein, NS not significant, OARSI Osteoarthritis Research Society International, PBS phosphate-buffered saline, WT wildtype, TNFR tumor necrosis factor receptor

Furthermore, by applying both Erk1/2 and Akt signaling inhibitors simultaneously, we found that Atsttrin-mediated anabolism in chondrocytes was almost abolished (Fig. 5i, j). Taken together, Atsttrin exhibits an anabolic effect in chondrocytes, and this effect primarily relies on TNFR2-Akt-Erk1/2 signaling.

Atsttrin inhibits TNFα-induced inflammatory catabolism

It is known that TNFα plays an important role in OA [32]. Additionally, TNFα could activate MAPK and NF-κB signaling [6], subsequently inducing matrix-degrading enzymes, including MMP-13 and ADAMTS-4, as well as other inflammatory biomarkers, such as NOS-2, in chondrocytes. The finding that Atsttrin protected against TNFα-induced cartilage loss in multiple rheumatoid arthritis mouse models promoted us to determine the interplay between TNFα and Atsttrin in OA. Human primary chondrocytes were cultured in the absence or presence of 10 ng/ml TNFα with or without 200 ng/ml Atsttrin for various lengths of time. Western blot analysis indicated that Atsttrin inhibited TNFα-activated signaling pathways (Fig. 6a). Since TNFα exerts its inflammatory action largely through activation of classical NF-κB signaling [6], we next examined whether Atsttrin

altered TNFα-mediated NF-κB phosphorylation, translocation, and activity. As elucidated in Fig. 6b, Atsttrin effectively inhibited phosphorylation of NF-κB in primary human chondrocytes in vitro. Additionally, immunochemistry staining demonstrated that Atsttrin dramatically inhibited NF-κB phosphorylation in the articular cartilage of mice induced under the ACLT model (Fig. 6c).

Separately extracting cytoplasmic and nuclear protein from human primary chondrocytes also revealed differences in NF-κB translocation in treated and untreated cells. As illustrated in Fig. 6d, without TNFα treatment p65 was mainly detected in the cytoplasm; after TNFα treatment, cytoplasmic p65 was decreased and nuclear p65 was increased. In contrast, TNFα-mediated NF-κB nuclear translocation was nearly abolished in the presence of Atsttrin. We next transfected a NF-κB reporter gene into C28I2 human chondrocyte cells (provided by Dr Mary Goldring, Hospital for Special Surgery, New York, NY, USA [33]) to test whether Atsttrin altered NF-κB activity. As shown in Fig. 6e, Atsttrin significantly inhibited TNFα-induced NF-κB activity. To further elucidate the mechanism, we cultured primary human chondrocytes in the absence or presence of 10 ng/ml TNFα with or without 200 ng/ml

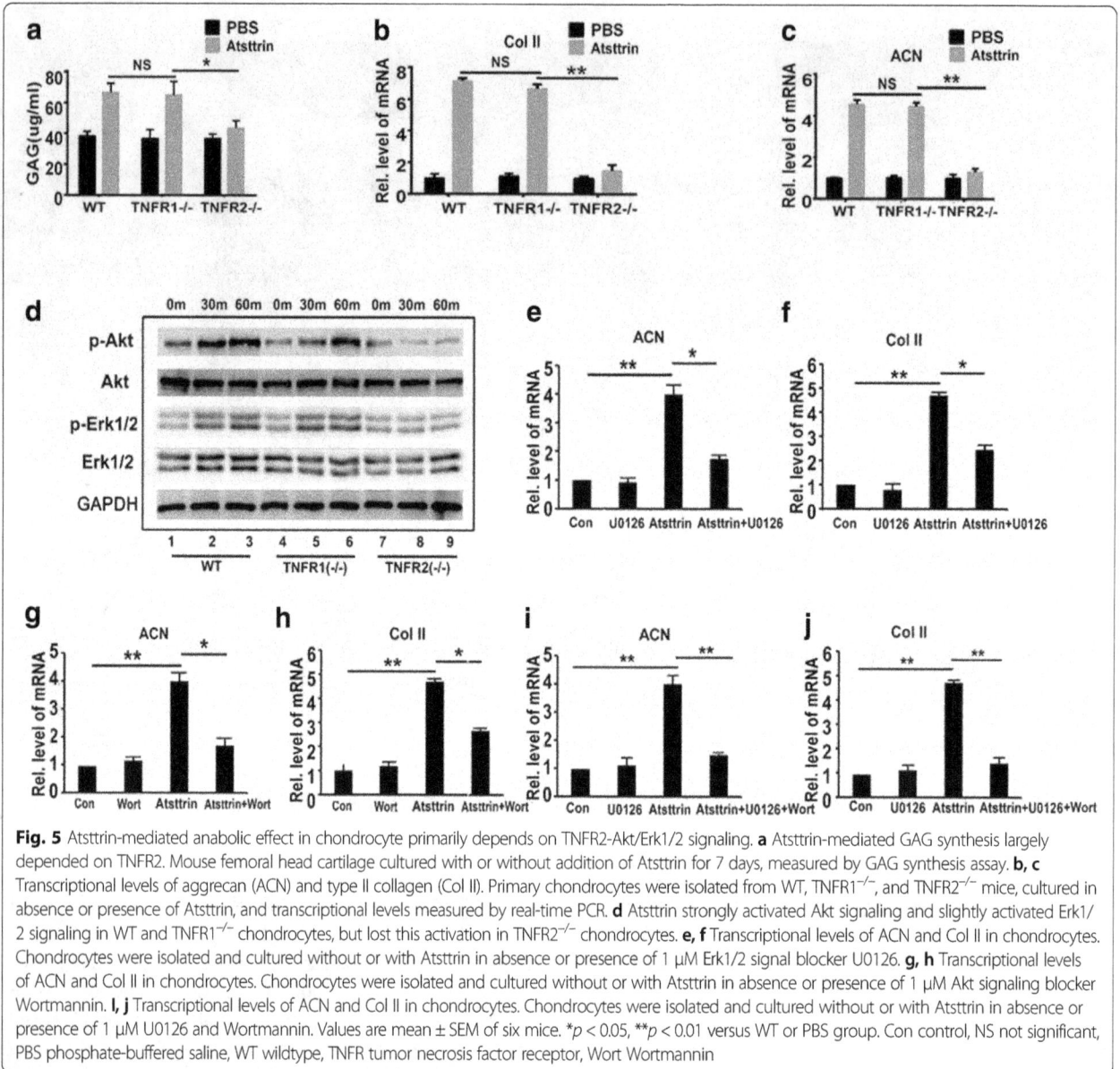

Fig. 5 Atsttrin-mediated anabolic effect in chondrocyte primarily depends on TNFR2-Akt/Erk1/2 signaling. **a** Atsttrin-mediated GAG synthesis largely depended on TNFR2. Mouse femoral head cartilage cultured with or without addition of Atsttrin for 7 days, measured by GAG synthesis assay. **b, c** Transcriptional levels of aggrecan (ACN) and type II collagen (Col II). Primary chondrocytes were isolated from WT, TNFR1$^{-/-}$, and TNFR2$^{-/-}$ mice, cultured in absence or presence of Atsttrin, and transcriptional levels measured by real-time PCR. **d** Atsttrin strongly activated Akt signaling and slightly activated Erk1/2 signaling in WT and TNFR1$^{-/-}$ chondrocytes, but lost this activation in TNFR2$^{-/-}$ chondrocytes. **e, f** Transcriptional levels of ACN and Col II in chondrocytes. Chondrocytes were isolated and cultured without or with Atsttrin in absence or presence of 1 μM Erk1/2 signal blocker U0126. **g, h** Transcriptional levels of ACN and Col II in chondrocytes. Chondrocytes were isolated and cultured without or with Atsttrin in absence or presence of 1 μM Akt signaling blocker Wortmannin. **I, j** Transcriptional levels of ACN and Col II in chondrocytes. Chondrocytes were isolated and cultured without or with Atsttrin in absence or presence of 1 μM U0126 and Wortmannin. Values are mean ± SEM of six mice. *$p < 0.05$, **$p < 0.01$ versus WT or PBS group. Con control, NS not significant, PBS phosphate-buffered saline, WT wildtype, TNFR tumor necrosis factor receptor, Wort Wortmannin

Atsttrin for 6 hours. After this, the total RNA was extracted for real-time PCR analysis. As indicated in Fig. 6 g–j, Atsttrin significantly decreased TNFα-upregulated transcriptional levels of MMP-13, ADAMTS-4, NOS-2, and COX-2. After 48-hour incubation, Atsttrin exhibited inhibition of TNFα-induced protein levels of inflammatory matrix-degrading enzymes and inflammatory cytokines in a dose-dependent manner (Fig. 6f).

Discussion

OA is one of the most common joint diseases; however, the exact pathological mechanism of OA is still largely unclear [34]. Unfortunately, no drugs are able to prevent or halt the progression of OA [35]. Regardless of the complicated etiology of OA, it is well accepted that cytokines are closely involved in initiating and aggravating OA. Our genome-wide screen found that PGRN was an OA-related growth factor [6]; levels of PGRN were also significantly elevated in the joints of arthritic patients [14]. The finding that PGRN deficiency accelerated OA while recombinant PGRN ameliorated OA prompted us to determine whether the PGRN-derived engineered protein Atsttrin could rescue enhanced OA brought on by PGRN deficiency. In the present study, we took advantage of the DMM model in WT and PGRN$^{-/-}$ mice and found that Atsttrin effectively prevented PGRN deficiency-mediated OA, evidenced by less cartilage destruction and reduced serum level of COMP fragments.

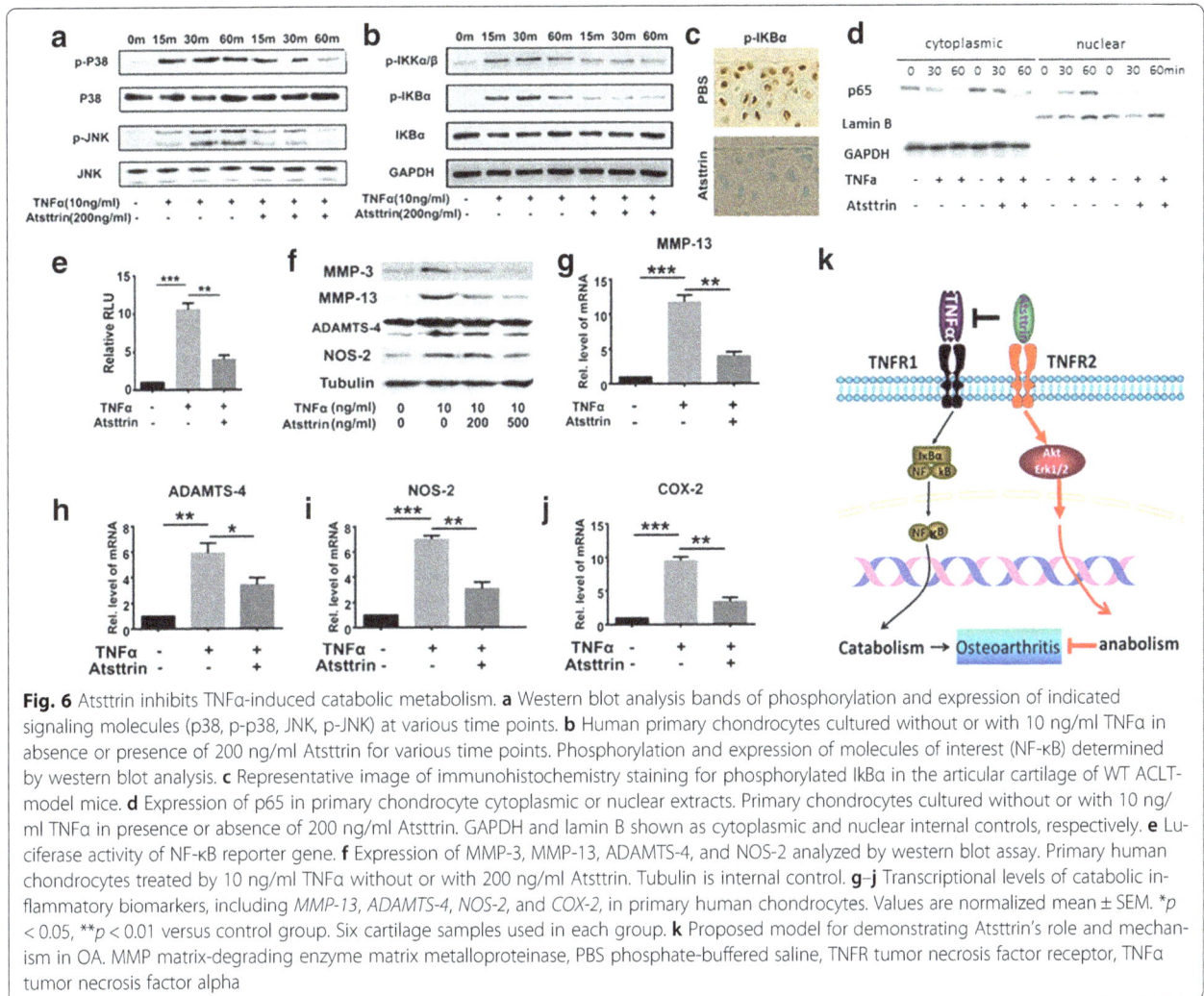

Fig. 6 Atsttrin inhibits TNFα-induced catabolic metabolism. **a** Western blot analysis bands of phosphorylation and expression of indicated signaling molecules (p38, p-p38, JNK, p-JNK) at various time points. **b** Human primary chondrocytes cultured without or with 10 ng/ml TNFα in absence or presence of 200 ng/ml Atsttrin for various time points. Phosphorylation and expression of molecules of interest (NF-κB) determined by western blot analysis. **c** Representative image of immunohistochemistry staining for phosphorylated IκBα in the articular cartilage of WT ACLT-model mice. **d** Expression of p65 in primary chondrocyte cytoplasmic or nuclear extracts. Primary chondrocytes cultured without or with 10 ng/ml TNFα in presence or absence of 200 ng/ml Atsttrin. GAPDH and lamin B shown as cytoplasmic and nuclear internal controls, respectively. **e** Luciferase activity of NF-κB reporter gene. **f** Expression of MMP-3, MMP-13, ADAMTS-4, and NOS-2 analyzed by western blot assay. Primary human chondrocytes treated by 10 ng/ml TNFα without or with 200 ng/ml Atsttrin. Tubulin is internal control. **g–j** Transcriptional levels of catabolic inflammatory biomarkers, including *MMP-13*, *ADAMTS-4*, *NOS-2*, and *COX-2*, in primary human chondrocytes. Values are normalized mean ± SEM. *p < 0.05, **p < 0.01 versus control group. Six cartilage samples used in each group. **k** Proposed model for demonstrating Atsttrin's role and mechanism in OA. MMP matrix-degrading enzyme matrix metalloproteinase, PBS phosphate-buffered saline, TNFR tumor necrosis factor receptor, TNFα tumor necrosis factor alpha

In our previous study, we found that, compared with WT littermates, PGRN deficiency led to more severe synovium inflammation as well as osteophyte formation. In line with this finding, Atsttrin could effectively reduce synovium inflammation. However, we failed to observe osteophyte formation in our current model in either PBS-treated or Atsttrin-treated mice, which may be attributable to the duration of our model. Observation and analysis of the osteophyte formation phenotype may require an extended time course.

The surgically induced mouse model is a well-accepted method to investigate OA pathogenesis in vivo [36], whereas the noninvasive rat model can mimic closed-joint injury-induced OA [20, 37]. Our finding that intra-articular delivery of recombinant Atsttrin could dramatically prevent cartilage destruction in both mouse and rat OA models is in line with reports that local delivery of Atsttrin-transduced MSCs is protective against OA-related cartilage destruction in vivo [18]. OA

is also characterized by progressive loss of extracellular matrix, leading to the breakdown of articular cartilage [38]. COMP is a noncollagenous molecule of the extracellular matrix in articular cartilage and plays an important role in maintaining chondrocyte function and cartilage integrity. COMP is fragmented upon degradation and the elevated serum level of COMP fragments observed in the progression of OA is considered a biomarker of disease activity [39]. Previously, we showed that Atsttrin dramatically inhibited COMP degradation in animal models of inflammatory arthritis [6]. In the current study, we found that Atsttrin also prevented COMP degradation in OA progression. Furthermore, Atsttrin dramatically reduced MMP-13 expression, which is significantly increased in OA and is thought to be the major enzyme responsible for digesting major cartilage component Col II.

Underlying articular cartilage, subchondral bone provides nourishment for cartilage and subchondral bone deterioration is often observed alongside cartilage defects [40]. Previous reports demonstrate that the thickness of subchondral bone gradually decreases during the early phase of the ACLT mouse model; in the late phase, the thickness of subchondral bone gradually increases but does not return to a thickness representative of a normal joint [27]. Additionally, studies have indicated that molecules targeting subchondral bone demonstrate a therapeutic effect in OA [30]. In the present study, we found that Atsttrin effectively inhibited subchondral bone loss. Notably, osteoclastogenesis plays an important role in subchondral bone remodeling in OA [30] and we have shown previously that Atsttrin significantly inhibited osteoclastogenesis in vitro [6]. Here, we report that Atsttrin also inhibited osteoclast activity in OA progression, ultimately lending to preservation of subchondral bone.

Besides pathological changes, the OA-related pain and biomechanical dysfunctions are the major complaints of patients [41] and OA pain is associated with pathological structural severity [42]. It is believed that anti-inflammatory drugs could reduce pain in the pathogenesis of OA [43, 44]. Herein, we found that Atsttrin effectively relieved OA-associated pain by improving travel distance and tactile sensitivity in mice with experimental OA. Additionally, alteration of pain markers and inflammatory molecules in the sensory neurons of the DRG has been reported as a result of interactions between neuropathic pathways and OA tissues [22]. Here we found the levels of mRNA for proinflammatory cytokines in DRG were also significantly suppressed by Atsttrin in OA progression. Besides, a recent study indicated that PGRN could attenuate pain by binding to ATG12 and regulating autophagy [45]. Whether Atsttrin also functions through this mechanism needs further investigation.

There are two distinct receptors for TNFα: TNFR1 and TNFR2 [46]. TNFα/TNFR1 signaling is the classical pathway and is thought to mediate inflammatory signaling [47]. On the contrary, TNFR2 signaling is still largely unknown [8]. Recent studies indicate that TNFR2 activates protective and proliferative pathways [48, 49]. Specifically, studies indicate that TNFR2 effectively protects against TNFα-mediated heart failure [50]. Additionally, TNFR2 has been shown to promote cancer growth [51]. Furthermore, TNFR2 was found to be required for PGRN-mediated immune regulation, cartilage homeostasis, physiological bone formation, and inhibition of LPS-induced lung inflammation [52]. Atsttrin exhibited much higher affinity for TNFR2, when compared to TNFα [53]. Here, we found that Atsttrin's protective effect against OA primarily depends on TNFR2, although inhibition of TNFR1 inflammatory signaling also partially accounts for Atsttrin's therapeutic action in OA.

It is known that Erk1/2 and Akt signaling are involved in chondrocyte protection, and that PGRN slightly activates Akt signaling and strongly actives Erk1/2 signaling [13]. In addition, PGRN-mediated chondroprotective effect primarily depends on TNFR2-Erk1/2 signaling [16]. Although Atsttrin is derived from PGRN, it exhibits distinct signal activation patterns. In the present study, we found that Atsttrin strongly activates Akt signaling whereas Erk1/2 signaling is only slightly activated. This signaling activation was lost in TNFR2-deficient chondrocytes but maintained in TNFR1-deficient chondrocytes, which implies that TNFR2 plays a major role in mediating Atsttrin's proanabolic effects. Furthermore, after applying specific inhibitors of Akt and Erk1/2 signaling, Atsttrin completely lost its proanabolic effect. Thus, together with in-vivo data, we found that the Atsttrin-mediated anabolic effect in OA depends on TNFR2-Akt/Erk1/2 signaling.

As an important proinflammatory cytokine, upregulated TNFα directly promotes inflammatory reactions and triggers chondrocyte death in OA [54]. Furthermore, TNFα-induced metalloproteinases, such as ADAMTS-4, ADAMTS-7, as well as ADAMTS-12, degrade cartilage matrix, leading to deteriorative articular cartilage [55]. TNFα inhibitors demonstrate a therapeutic effect in murine models [56] and OA patients in clinical trials [57, 58]. Additionally, a report from another group showed that Atsttrin promoted bone healing through TNF/TNFR signaling [59]. In the present study, the Atsttrin-mediated chondroprotective effect occurred partially through TNFR1 in vivo. Additionally, a mechanistic study demonstrated that Atsttrin effectively inhibited TNFα-induced inflammatory catabolism in OA progression. Specifically, Atsttrin effectively inhibited TNFα-induced NF-κB phosphorylation, translocation, and activity and the expression of inflammatory catabolic markers such as NOS-2, COX2, as well as ADAMTS-4. Intriguingly, a recent study revealed that DR3, the highest homolog of TNFR1 in the TNFR family, is also capable of binding Atsttrin [60]. TNF-like ligand 1A (TL1A) is the sole identified ligand for DR3. Importantly, Atsttrin could inhibit the interaction between DR3 and TL1A [60]. Thus, whether the Atsttrin-mediated chondroprotective effect partially depends on the DR3 pathway needs to be further investigated.

Although Atsttrin was shown to be more effective than PGRN in preventing inflammatory arthritis [6, 10], we did not find a significant difference between PGRN and Atsttrin in terms of protecting against OA development. Based on our previous studies, we surmise that this disease specificity results from the fact that Atsttrin has a better anti-inflammatory/anti-catabolic TNFα/TNFR1 effect, whereas PGRN has a better effect in activating the anabolic TNFR2 pathway.

It is noted that we used a similar OA model with the 2-month-old mice as we did in our previous publication [16]. Atsttrin's long-term chondroprotective effect in various animal models, including DMM model mice 4–6 months old and "aged" PGRN-deficient mice that spontaneously develop an OA-like phenotype [16], warrants further investigation. We have shown that Atsttrin rescued the accelerated surgically induced OA phenotype seen in PGRN-deficient mice (Fig. 1) and we anticipate that Atsttrin would also be effective in preventing spontaneous OA in "aged" PGRN-deficient mice.

Conclusions

Based on the present study and previous publications, a model was proposed (Fig. 6 k). This model illustrates that Atsttrin plays a chondroprotective role in OA through at least two pathways. Atsttrin directly binds to TNFR2 to activate the anabolic signaling pathway; additionally, Atsttrin competitively binds to TNFR1 to inhibit TNFα-mediated inflammatory and catabolic reactions. However, it is unclear whether crosstalk exists between these two pathways. For instance, whether inhibition of downstream NF-κB signaling (via TNFR1) by Atsttrin would mechanistically lead to improvement of the chondrocyte phenotype has not yet been addressed. In addition, the downstream mediators of TNFR2-Erk/Akt activation by Atsttrin also remain largely unknown. These unsolved issues warrant further investigation. In summary, these findings not only provide new insights into the role of PGRN and its derived engineered protein Atsttrin in cartilage homeostasis as well as OA in vivo, but may also lead to new therapeutic alternatives for OA as well as other relative degenerative joint diseases.

Abbreviations
ACLT: Anterior cruciate ligament transection; ACN: Aggrecan; Atsttrin: Antagonist of TNF/TNFR signaling via targeting to TNF receptors; CCR-2: Chemokine receptor 2; Col II: Type II collagen; Col X: Type X collagen; COMP: Cartilage oligomeric matrix protein; DMM: Destabilization of medial meniscus; DRG: Dorsal root ganglia; ELISA: Enzyme-linked immunosorbent assay; HRP: Horseradish peroxidase; IL-1β: Interleukin-1β; MCP-1: Monocyte chemoattractant protein 1; MMP-13: Matrix-degrading enzyme matrix metalloproteinase 13; OA: Osteoarthritis; PCR: Polymerase chain reaction; PGRN: Progranulin; TNFR: Tumor necrosis factor receptor; TNFα: Tumor necrosis factor alpha; TRAP: Tartrate-resistant acid phosphatase

Acknowledgments
The authors would like to thank Dr Anne-Marie Malfait for critical reading and editing of the article.

Funding
This work was partly supported by NIH research grants R01AR062207, R01AR061484, and R01NS070328 and DOD research grant W81XWH-16-1-0482.

Authors' contributions
C-jL and OK designed the experiments. J-lW, WF, Y-jD, and ML performed the experiments. J-lW and Y-jD acquired the data. J-lW, Y-jD, and WF analyzed and interpreted the data. Y-jD performed statistical analysis. AH edited the manuscript. RS collected human cartilage tissues. All authors drafted and reviewed the manuscript. All authors read and approved the final manuscript.

Consent for publication
Not applicable.

Competing interests
C-jL is the cofounder of Atreaon, Inc. The other authors declare that they have no competing interests.

Author details
[1]Department of Orthopaedic Surgery, New York University Medical Center, New York, NY 10003, USA. [2]Department of Orthopaedic Surgery, Qilu Hospital, Jinan,, Shandong 250012, China. [3]Department of Cell Biology, New York University School of Medicine, New York, NY 10016, USA. [4]Rm 1608, HJD, Department of Orthopaedic Surgery, New York University Medical Center, 301 East 17th Street, New York, NY 10003, USA.

References
1. Olivotto E, Otero M, Marcu KB, Goldring MB. Pathophysiology of osteoarthritis: canonical NF-kappaB/IKKbeta-dependent and kinase-independent effects of IKKalpha in cartilage degradation and chondrocyte differentiation. RMD Open. 2015;1 Suppl 1:e000061.
2. Goldring MB. Articular cartilage degradation in osteoarthritis. HSS J. 2012; 8(1):7–9.
3. Houard X, Goldring MB, Berenbaum F. Homeostatic mechanisms in articular cartilage and role of inflammation in osteoarthritis. Curr Rheumatol Rep. 2013;15(11):375.
4. Lee AS, Ellman MB, Yan D, et al. A current review of molecular mechanisms regarding osteoarthritis and pain. Gene. 2013;527(2):440–7.
5. Stannus O, Jones G, Cicuttini F, et al. Circulating levels of IL-6 and TNF-alpha are associated with knee radiographic osteoarthritis and knee cartilage loss in older adults. Osteoarthritis Cartilage. 2010;18(11):1441–7.
6. Tang W, Lu Y, Tian QY, et al. The growth factor progranulin binds to TNF receptors and is therapeutic against inflammatory arthritis in mice. Science. 2011;332(6028):478–84.
7. Jian J, Konopka J, Liu C. Insights into the role of progranulin in immunity, infection, and inflammation. J Leuk Biol. 2013;93(2):199–208.
8. Jian J, Li G, Hettinghouse A, Liu C. Progranulin: a key player in autoimmune diseases. Cytokine. 2018;101:48-55.
9. Liu CJ. Progranulin: a promising therapeutic target for rheumatoid arthritis. FEBS Lett. 2011;585(23):3675–80.
10. Liu CJ, Bosch X. Progranulin: a growth factor, a novel TNFR ligand and a drug target. Pharmacol Ther. 2012;133(1):124–32.
11. Williams A, Wang EC, Thurner L, Liu CJ. Novel insights into TNF receptor, DR3 and progranulin pathways in arthritis and bone remodeling. Arthritis Rheumatol. 2016;68(12):2845–56.
12. Zhao YP, Wei JL, Tian QY, et al. Progranulin suppresses titanium particle induced inflammatory osteolysis by targeting TNFalpha signaling. Sci Rep. 2016;6:20909.
13. Feng JQ, Guo FJ, Jiang BC, et al. Granulin epithelin precursor: a bone morphogenic protein 2-inducible growth factor that activates Erk1/2 signaling and JunB transcription factor in chondrogenesis. FASEB J. 2010;24(6):1879–92.
14. Guo F, Lai Y, Tian Q, Lin EA, Kong L, Liu C. Granulin-epithelin precursor binds directly to ADAMTS-7 and ADAMTS-12 and inhibits their degradation of cartilage oligomeric matrix protein. Arthritis Rheum. 2010;62(7):2023–36.
15. Wang BC, Liu H, Talwar A, Jian J. New discovery rarely runs smooth: an update on progranulin/TNFR interactions. Protein Cell. 2015;6(11): 792–803.

16. Zhao YP, Liu B, Tian QY, Wei JL, Richbourgh B, Liu CJ. Progranulin protects against osteoarthritis through interacting with TNF-alpha and beta-Catenin signalling. Ann Rheum Dis. 2015;74(12):2244–53.

17. Wei J, Hettinghouse A, Liu C. The role of progranulin in arthritis. Ann N Y Acad Sci. 2016;1383(1):5–20.

18. Xia Q, Zhu S, Wu Y, et al. Intra-articular transplantation of atsttrin-transduced mesenchymal stem cells ameliorate osteoarthritis development. Stem Cells Transl Med. 2015;4(5):523–31.

19. Zhao Y, Liu B, Liu CJ. Establishment of a surgically-induced model in mice to investigate the protective role of progranulin in osteoarthritis. J Vis Exp. 2014;84:e50924.

20. Ramme AJ, Lendhey M, Raya JG, Kirsch T, Kennedy OD. A novel rat model for subchondral microdamage in acute knee injury: a potential mechanism in post-traumatic osteoarthritis. Osteoarthritis Cartilage. 2016;24(10):1776–85.

21. Lai Y, Bai X, Zhao Y, et al. ADAMTS-7 forms a positive feedback loop with TNF-alpha in the pathogenesis of osteoarthritis. Ann Rheum Dis. 2014;73(8):1575–84.

22. Leong DJ, Choudhury M, Hanstein R, et al. Green tea polyphenol treatment is chondroprotective, anti-inflammatory and palliative in a mouse post-traumatic osteoarthritis model. Arthritis Res Ther. 2014;16(6):508.

23. Sleigh JN, Weir GA, Schiavo G. A simple, step-by-step dissection protocol for the rapid isolation of mouse dorsal root ganglia. BMC Res Notes. 2016;9:82.

24. Lin EA, Kong L, Bai XH, Liu CJ. MiR-199a*, a BMP-2 responsive microRNA, acts as a novel mediator of chondrogenesis via direct targeting to Smad1. J Biol Chem. 2009;284(17):11326–35.

25. Glasson SS, Chambers MG, Van Den Berg WB, Little CB. The OARSI histopathology initiative—recommendations for histological assessments of osteoarthritis in the mouse. Osteoarthritis Cartilage. 2010;18 Suppl 3:S17–23.

26. Zhen G, Cao X. Targeting TGFbeta signaling in subchondral bone and articular cartilage homeostasis. Trends Pharmacol Sci. 2014;35(5):227–36.

27. Zhen G, Wen C, Jia X, et al. Inhibition of TGF-beta signaling in mesenchymal stem cells of subchondral bone attenuates osteoarthritis. Nat Med. 2013;19(6):704–12.

28. Karsdal MA, Bay-Jensen AC, Lories RJ, et al. The coupling of bone and cartilage turnover in osteoarthritis: opportunities for bone antiresorptives and anabolics as potential treatments? Ann Rheum Dis. 2014;73(2):336–48.

29. Yuan XL, Meng HY, Wang YC, et al. Bone-cartilage interface crosstalk in osteoarthritis: potential pathways and future therapeutic strategies. Osteoarthritis Cartilage. 2014;22(8):1077–89.

30. Cui Z, Crane J, Xie H, et al. Halofuginone attenuates osteoarthritis by inhibition of TGF-beta activity and H-type vessel formation in subchondral bone. Ann Rheum Dis. 2016;75(9):1714–21.

31. Miller RE, Tran PB, Das R, et al. CCR2 chemokine receptor signaling mediates pain in experimental osteoarthritis. Proc Natl Acad Sci U S A. 2012;109(50):20602–7.

32. Kapoor M, Martel-Pelletier J, Lajeunesse D, Pelletier JP, Fahmi H. Role of proinflammatory cytokines in the pathophysiology of osteoarthritis. Nat Rev Rheumatol. 2011;7(1):33–42.

33. Goldring MB. Immortalization of human articular chondrocytes for generation of stable, differentiated cell lines. Methods Mol Med. 2004;100:23–36.

34. Johnson K, Zhu S, Tremblay MS, et al. A stem cell-based approach to cartilage repair. Science. 2012;336(6082):717–21.

35. Goldring MB. Update on the biology of the chondrocyte and new approaches to treating cartilage diseases. Best Pract Res Clin Rheumatol. 2006;20(5):1003–25.

36. Chen WH, Lo WC, Hsu WC, et al. Synergistic anabolic actions of hyaluronic acid and platelet-rich plasma on cartilage regeneration in osteoarthritis therapy. Biomaterials. 2014;35(36):9599–607.

37. Poulet B. Non-invasive loading model of murine osteoarthritis. Curr Rheumatol Rep. 2016;18(7):40.

38. Salzet M. Leech thrombin inhibitors. Curr Pharm Des. 2002;8(7):493–503.

39. Lai Y, Yu XP, Zhang Y, et al. Enhanced COMP catabolism detected in serum of patients with arthritis and animal disease models through a novel capture ELISA. Osteoarthritis Cartilage. 2012;20(8):854–62.

40. Zhao W, Wang T, Luo Q, et al. Cartilage degeneration and excessive subchondral bone formation in spontaneous osteoarthritis involves altered TGF-beta signaling. J Orthop Res. 2016;34(5):763–70.

41. Zhang W, Robertson J, Jones AC, Dieppe PA, Doherty M. The placebo effect and its determinants in osteoarthritis: meta-analysis of randomised controlled trials. Ann Rheum Dis. 2008;67(12):1716–23.

42. Nwosu LN, Mapp PI, Chapman V, Walsh DA. Relationship between structural pathology and pain behaviour in a model of osteoarthritis (OA). Osteoarthritis Cartilage. 2016;24(11):1910–7.

43. Stradner MH, Gruber G, Angerer H, et al. Sphingosine 1-phosphate counteracts the effects of interleukin-1beta in human chondrocytes. Arthritis Rheum. 2013;65(8):2113–22.

44. Terkeltaub R, Yang B, Lotz M, Liu-Bryan R. Chondrocyte AMP-activated protein kinase activity suppresses matrix degradation responses to proinflammatory cytokines interleukin-1beta and tumor necrosis factor alpha. Arthritis Rheum. 2011;63(7):1928–37.

45. Altmann C, Hardt S, Fischer C, et al. Progranulin overexpression in sensory neurons attenuates neuropathic pain in mice: role of autophagy. Neurobiol Dis. 2016;96:294–311.

46. Williams A, Wang EC, Thurner L, Liu CJ. Review: Novel insights into tumor necrosis factor receptor, death receptor 3, and progranulin pathways in arthritis and bone remodeling. Arthritis Rheumatol. 2016;68(12):2845–56.

47. Aggarwal BB, Gupta SC, Kim JH. Historical perspectives on tumor necrosis factor and its superfamily: 25 years later, a golden journey. Blood. 2012;119(3):651–65.

48. McCann FE, Perocheau DP, Ruspi G, et al. Selective tumor necrosis factor receptor I blockade is antiinflammatory and reveals immunoregulatory role of tumor necrosis factor receptor II in collagen-induced arthritis. Arthritis Rheumatol. 2014;66(10):2728–38.

49. Wei JL, Buza 3rd J, Liu CJ. Does progranulin account for the opposite effects of etanercept and infliximab/adalimumab in osteoarthritis?: Comment on Olson et al.: "Therapeutic Opportunities to Prevent Post-Traumatic Arthritis: Lessons From the Natural History of Arthritis After Articular Fracture". J Orthop Res. 2016;34(1):12–4.

50. Higuchi Y, McTiernan CF, Frye CB, McGowan BS, Chan TO, Feldman AM. Tumor necrosis factor receptors 1 and 2 differentially regulate survival, cardiac dysfunction, and remodeling in transgenic mice with tumor necrosis factor-alpha-induced cardiomyopathy. Circulation. 2004;109(15):1892–7.

51. Yang D, Wang LL, Dong TT, et al. Progranulin promotes colorectal cancer proliferation and angiogenesis through TNFR2/Akt and ERK signaling pathways. Am J Cancer Res. 2015;5(10):3085–97.

52. Zhao YP, Tian QY, Frenkel S, Liu CJ. The promotion of bone healing by progranulin, a downstream molecule of BMP-2, through interacting with TNF/TNFR signaling. Biomaterials. 2013;34(27):6412–21.

53. Wang C LX LP, Chen X, Zhou H, Zhang T. An improved method of GST-pull down based on fluorescence detection and its application to the analysis of the interaction between atsttrin and TNFR2. J Tianjin Univ Sci Technol. 2015;30:34–40.

54. Hattori Y, Kojima T, Kato D, Matsubara H, Takigawa M, Ishiguro N. A selective estrogen receptor modulator inhibits tumor necrosis factor-alpha-induced apoptosis through the ERK1/2 signaling pathway in human chondrocytes. Biochem Biophys Res Commun. 2012;421(3):418–24.

55. Liu CJ. The role of ADAMTS-7 and ADAMTS-12 in the pathogenesis of arthritis. Nat Clin Pract Rheumatol. 2009;5(1):38–45.

56. Zhang Q, Lv H, Chen A, Liu F, Wu X. Efficacy of infliximab in a rabbit model of osteoarthritis. Connect Tissue Res. 2012;53(5):355–8.

57. Maksymowych WP, Russell AS, Chiu P, et al. Targeting tumour necrosis factor alleviates signs and symptoms of inflammatory osteoarthritis of the knee. Arthritis Res Ther. 2012;14(5):R206.

58. Urech DM, Feige U, Ewert S, et al. Anti-inflammatory and cartilage-protecting effects of an intra-articularly injected anti-TNFα single-chain Fv antibody (ESBA105) designed for local therapeutic use. Ann Rheum Dis. 2010;69(2):443–9.

59. Wang Q, Xia Q, Wu Y, et al. 3D-printed atsttrin-incorporated alginate/hydroxyapatite scaffold promotes bone defect regeneration with TNF/TNFR signaling involvement. Adv Healthc Mater. 2015;4(11):1701–8.

60. Liu C, Li XX, Gao W, Liu W, Liu DS. Progranulin-derived Atsttrin directly binds to TNFRSF25 (DR3) and inhibits TNF-like ligand 1A (TL1A) activity. PLoS One. 2014;9(3):e92743.

Permissions

All chapters in this book were first published in AR&T, by BioMed Central; hereby published with permission under the Creative Commons Attribution License or equivalent. Every chapter published in this book has been scrutinized by our experts. Their significance has been extensively debated. The topics covered herein carry significant findings which will fuel the growth of the discipline. They may even be implemented as practical applications or may be referred to as a beginning point for another development.

The contributors of this book come from diverse backgrounds, making this book a truly international effort. This book will bring forth new frontiers with its revolutionizing research information and detailed analysis of the nascent developments around the world.

We would like to thank all the contributing authors for lending their expertise to make the book truly unique. They have played a crucial role in the development of this book. Without their invaluable contributions this book wouldn't have been possible. They have made vital efforts to compile up to date information on the varied aspects of this subject to make this book a valuable addition to the collection of many professionals and students.

This book was conceptualized with the vision of imparting up-to-date information and advanced data in this field. To ensure the same, a matchless editorial board was set up. Every individual on the board went through rigorous rounds of assessment to prove their worth. After which they invested a large part of their time researching and compiling the most relevant data for our readers.

The editorial board has been involved in producing this book since its inception. They have spent rigorous hours researching and exploring the diverse topics which have resulted in the successful publishing of this book. They have passed on their knowledge of decades through this book. To expedite this challenging task, the publisher supported the team at every step. A small team of assistant editors was also appointed to further simplify the editing procedure and attain best results for the readers.

Apart from the editorial board, the designing team has also invested a significant amount of their time in understanding the subject and creating the most relevant covers. They scrutinized every image to scout for the most suitable representation of the subject and create an appropriate cover for the book.

The publishing team has been an ardent support to the editorial, designing and production team. Their endless efforts to recruit the best for this project, has resulted in the accomplishment of this book. They are a veteran in the field of academics and their pool of knowledge is as vast as their experience in printing. Their expertise and guidance has proved useful at every step. Their uncompromising quality standards have made this book an exceptional effort. Their encouragement from time to time has been an inspiration for everyone.

The publisher and the editorial board hope that this book will prove to be a valuable piece of knowledge for researchers, students, practitioners and scholars across the globe.

List of Contributors

Johanna Mucke, Ralph Brinks, Ellen Bleck, Matthias Schneider and Stefan Vordenbäumen
Hiller Research Center Rheumatology at University Hospital Düsseldorf, Medical Faculty, Heinrich-Heine-University, Merowingerplatz 1a, 40225 Düsseldorf, Germany

Cristina Manferdini and Gina Lisignoli
SC Laboratorio di Immunoreumatologia e Rigenerazione Tissutale, Istituto Ortopedico Rizzoli, Via di Barbiano 1/10, Bologna 40136, Italy
SD Laboratorio RAMSES, Istituto Ortopedico Rizzoli, Bologna 40136, Italy

Elena Gabusi
SD Laboratorio RAMSES, Istituto Ortopedico Rizzoli, Bologna 40136, Italy

Giuseppe Filardo
Clinica Ortopedica e Traumatologica II, Istituto Ortopedico Rizzoli, Bologna 40136, Italy

Sandrine Fleury-Cappellesso
EFS-Pyrénéés-Méditerranéé, Toulouse F-31300, France

Nicoló Edoardo Magni and Peter John McNair
Health and Rehabilitation Research Institute, Auckland University of Technology, 90 Akoranga Drive, Northcote, Auckland 0627, New Zealand

David Andrew Rice
Health and Rehabilitation Research Institute, Auckland University of Technology, 90 Akoranga Drive, Northcote, Auckland 0627, New Zealand
Waitemata Pain Service, Department of Anaesthesiology and Perioperative Medicine, North Shore Hospital, Waitemata DHB, 124 Shakespeare Road, Westlake, Takapuna, Auckland 0622, New Zealand

Johanne Martel-Pelletier, Jean-Pierre Raynauld, François Mineau and Jean-Pierre Pelletier
Osteoarthritis Research Unit, University of Montreal Hospital Research Centre (CRCHUM), 900 Saint-Denis, Suite R11.412, Montreal, Quebec H2X 0A9, Canada

François Abram
Medical Imaging Research & Development, ArthroLab Inc, Montreal, Quebec, Canada

Patrice Paiement and Philippe Delorme
ArthroLab Inc, Montreal, Quebec, Canada

Weam Alshenibr, Mustafa M. Tashkandi, Saqer F. Alsaqer, Yazeed Alkheriji and Manish V. Bais
Department of Molecular and Cell Biology, Boston University Henry M. Goldman School of Dental Medicine, W-216, 700 Albany Street, Boston, MA 02118, USA

Amelia Wise and Louis C. Gerstenfeld
Department of Orthopaedic Surgery, School of Medicine, Boston University, Boston, MA 02118, USA

Sadanand Fulzele
Department of Orthopaedic Surgery and Institute of Regenerative and Reparative Medicine, Georgia Regents University, Augusta, GA 30912, USA

Pushkar Mehra
Department of Oral and Maxillofacial Surgery, Boston University Henry M. Goldman School of Dental Medicine, 100 East Newton Street, Boston, MA 02118, USA

Mary B. Goldring
Hospital for Special Surgery Research Institute, Weill Cornell Medical College, New York, NY 10021, USA
Department of Cell and Developmental Biology, Weill Cornell Medical College, New York, NY 10021, USA

Benny Antony, Graeme Jones and Xingzhong Jin
Menzies Institute for Medical Research, University of Tasmania, Hobart, Tasmania 7000, Australia

Changhai Ding
Institute of Bone & Joint Translational Research, Southern Medical University, Guangzhou, Guangdong, China

Olivier Malaise, Biserka Relic, Edith Charlier, Mustapha Zeddou, Sophie Neuville, Céline Deroyer, Michel G. Malaise and Dominique de Seny
Laboratory of Rheumatology, Arthropôle, GIGA Research, University and CHU of Liège, Liège, Belgium

Philippe Gillet
Department of Orthopedic Surgery, CHU of Liège, Liège, Belgium

Edouard Louis
Laboratory of Gastroenterology, GIGA Research, University and CHU of Liège, Liège, Belgium

André Struglics, Per Swärd, Richard Frobell and L. Stefan Lohmander
Department of Clinical Sciences Lund, Orthopaedics, Lund University, Faculty of Medicine, BMC C12, SE-221 84 Lund, Sweden

Anna M. Blom
Department of Translational Medicine, Division of Medical Protein Chemistry, Lund University, Faculty of Medicine, Lund, Sweden

Marcin Okroj
Department of Translational Medicine, Division of Medical Protein Chemistry, Lund University, Faculty of Medicine, Lund, Sweden
Department of Medical Biotechnology, Intercollegiate Faculty of Biotechnology UG-MUG, Medical University of Gdańsk, Gdańsk, Poland

Tore Saxne
Department of Clinical Sciences Lund, Rheumatology, Lund University, Faculty of Medicine, Lund, Sweden

Galied S. R. Muradin and Edwin H. G. Oei
Department of Radiology, Erasmus MC, University Medical Center Rotterdam, Rotterdam, The Netherlands

Michael S. Saltzherr
Department of Radiology, Erasmus MC, University Medical Center Rotterdam, Rotterdam, The Netherlands
Department of Plastic, Reconstructive and Hand Surgery, Erasmus MC, University Medical Center Rotterdam, Rotterdam, The Netherlands

Department of Rheumatology, Erasmus MC, University Medical Center Rotterdam, Rotterdam, The Netherlands

Johan W. van Neck
Department of Plastic, Reconstructive and Hand Surgery, Erasmus MC, University Medical Center Rotterdam, Rotterdam, The Netherlands

Ruud W. Selles
Department of Plastic, Reconstructive and Hand Surgery, Erasmus MC, University Medical Center Rotterdam, Rotterdam, The Netherlands
Department of Rehabilitation Medicine, Erasmus MC, University Medical Center Rotterdam, Rotterdam, The Netherlands

Jolanda J. Luime
Department of Rheumatology, Erasmus MC, University Medical Center Rotterdam, Rotterdam, The Netherlands

J. Henk Coert
Department of Plastic, Reconstructive and Hand Surgery, University Medical Center Utrecht, Utrecht, The Netherlands

Jean-Bart Jaquet
Department of Plastic, Reconstructive and Hand surgery, Maasstad Hospital, Rotterdam, The Netherlands

Gerjo J. V. M. van Osch
Department of Orthopaedics and Department of Otorhinolaryngology, Erasmus MC, University Medical Center Rotterdam, Rotterdam, The Netherlands

Michael P. LaValley
Department of Biostatistics, Boston University School of Public Health, 801 Massachusetts Avenue 3rd Floor, Boston, MA 02118, USA

Grace H. Lo
Medical Care Line and Research Care Line, Houston VA HSR&D Center for Innovations in Quality, Effectiveness and Safety, Michael E. DeBakey Medical Center, Houston, TX 77030, USA
Section of Immunology, Allergy, and Rheumatology, Baylor College of Medicine, 1 Baylor Plaza, BCM-285, Houston, TX 77030, USA

Lori Lyn Price
Institute for Clinical Research and Health Policy Studies at Tufts Medical Center, Tufts Clinical and Translational Science Institute, Tufts University, 800 Washington Street, Boston, MA 02111, USA

Jeffrey B. Driban and Timothy E. McAlindon
Division of Rheumatology Tufts Medical Center, 800 Washington Street, Boston, MA 02111, USA

Charles B. Eaton
Department of Family Medicine, Alpert Medical School of Brown University, 111 Brewster Street, Pawtucket, RI 02860, USA

Wadena D. Burnett, Saija A. Kontulainen and James D. Johnston
University of Saskatchewan, 57 Campus Drive, Saskatoon, SK S7N 5A9, Canada

Christine E. McLennan, Diane Hazel and Carl Talmo
New England Baptist Hospital, Boston, MA, USA

David R. Wilson
University of British Columbia, Vancouver, BC, Canada

David J. Hunter
University of Sydney, Sydney, NSW, Australia

Wenyu Fu, Yuan-jing Ding, Aubryanna Hettinghouse, Matin Lendhey, Ran Schwarzkopf and Oran D. Kennedy
Department of Orthopaedic Surgery, New York University Medical Center, New York, NY 10003, USA

Sun J. Kim, David M. Hirsh, John A. Hardin and Neil J. Cobelli
Department of Orthopaedic Surgery, Albert Einstein College of Medicine, Bronx, NY, USA

Daniel J. Leong, Lin Xu, Zhiyong He, Angela Wang and Hui B. Sun
Department of Orthopaedic Surgery, Albert Einstein College of Medicine, Bronx, NY, USA
Department of Radiation Oncology, Albert Einstein College of Medicine, Bronx, NY, USA

Zhuo Zhang
Department of Orthopaedic Surgery, Albert Einstein College of Medicine, Bronx, NY, USA

Sheng-Mou Hou
Department of Orthopedic Surgery, Shin Kong Wu Ho-Su Memorial Hospital, No. 95, Wen Chang Road, Taipei 111, Taiwan

Chun-Han Hou
Department of Orthopedic Surgery, National Taiwan University Hospital, No. 1, Jen-Ai Road, Taipei 100, Taiwan

Ju-Fang Liu
Central Laboratory, Shin-Kong Wu Ho-Su Memorial Hospital, No. 95, Wenchang Road, Shilin, Taipei 111, Taiwan

Portia P. E. Flowers
Thurston Arthritis Research Center, University of North Carolina, 3300 Doc J. Thurston Bldg, CB#7280, Chapel Hill 27599-7280, NC, USA

Rebecca J. Cleveland and Amanda E. Nelson
Thurston Arthritis Research Center, University of North Carolina, 3300 Doc J. Thurston Bldg, CB#7280, Chapel Hill 27599-7280, NC, USA
School of Medicine, University of North Carolina, Chapel Hill 27599, NC, USA

Jordan B. Renner
Thurston Arthritis Research Center, University of North Carolina, 3300 Doc J. Thurston Bldg, CB#7280, Chapel Hill 27599-7280, NC, USA
Department of Radiology, University of North Carolina, Chapel Hill 27599, NC, USA

Joanne M. Jordan
Thurston Arthritis Research Center, University of North Carolina, 3300 Doc J. Thurston Bldg, CB#7280, Chapel Hill 27599-7280, NC, USA
School of Medicine, University of North Carolina, Chapel Hill 27599, NC, USA
Department of Epidemiology, Gillings School of Global Public Health, University of North Carolina, Chapel Hill 27599, NC, USA

Yvonne M. Golightly
Thurston Arthritis Research Center, University of North Carolina, 3300 Doc J. Thurston Bldg, CB#7280, Chapel Hill 27599-7280, NC, USA
Department of Epidemiology, Gillings School of Global Public Health, University of North Carolina, Chapel Hill 27599, NC, USA
Injury Prevention Research Center, University of North Carolina, Chapel Hill 27599, NC, USA

Todd A. Schwartz
Thurston Arthritis Research Center, University of North Carolina, 3300 Doc J. Thurston Bldg, CB#7280, Chapel Hill 27599-7280, NC, USA
Department of Biostatistics, Gillings School of Global Public Health, University of North Carolina, Chapel Hill 27599, NC, USA
School of Nursing, University of North Carolina, Chapel Hill 27599, NC, USA

Virginia B. Kraus
Department of Medicine, Duke Molecular Physiology Institute, School of Medicine, Duke University, Durham 27701, NC, USA

Howard J. Hillstrom
Motion Analysis Laboratory, Hospital for Special Surgery, New York 10021, NY, USA

Adam P. Goode
Department of Orthopedic Surgery, Duke Clinical Research Institute, School of Medicine, Duke University, Durham 27708, NC, USA

Marian T. Hannan
Institute for Aging Research, Hebrew SeniorLife, Boston 02131, MA, USA

Yalong Di
Department of Medical Imaging, Hebei General Hospital, Shijiazhuang 050051, China

Changxu Han, Liang Zhao and Yizhong Ren
Department of Sports Medicine, Second Affiliated Hospital of Inner Mongolia Medical University, Huhehaote 010030, China

Jianhua Xu, Jingyu Cai and Shuang Zheng
Department of Rheumatology and Immunology, Arthritis Research Institute, the First Affiliated Hospital of Anhui Medical University, 218 Jixi Street, Hefei, China

Kang Wang and Changhai Ding
Department of Rheumatology and Immunology, Arthritis Research Institute, the First Affiliated Hospital of Anhui Medical University, 218 Jixi Street, Hefei, China
Menzies Institute for Medical Research, University of Tasmania, Hobart, Tasmania 7000, Australia

Weiyu Han and Benny Antony
Menzies Institute for Medical Research, University of Tasmania, Hobart, Tasmania 7000, Australia

Francesca Paolella, Ylenia Silvestri, Laura Gambari and Luca Cattini
SC Laboratorio di Immunoreumatologia e Rigenerazione Tissutale, Istituto Ortopedico Rizzoli, Via di Barbiano 1/10, Bologna 40136, Italy

Annika Hoyer
German Diabetes Center, Institute for Biometry and Epidemiology, Düsseldorf, Germany

Thomas Pauly
Department Orthopaedics, River Rhein Center for Rheumatology at St. Elisabeth Hospital, Meerbusch-Lank, Germany

Julie Gervais and Julie-Anne Gervais
Groupe de Recherche en Pharmacologie Animale du Québec (GREPAQ), Department of Biomedical Sciences, Faculty of veterinary medicine, Université de Montréal, 1500 des Vétérinaires Street, St-Hyacinthe, Quebec J2S 7C6, Canada

Francis Beaudry, Eric Troncy, Dominique Gauvin, Martin Guillot and Colombe Otis
Groupe de Recherche en Pharmacologie Animale du Québec (GREPAQ), Department of Biomedical Sciences, Faculty of veterinary medicine, Université de Montréal, 1500 des Vétérinaires Street, St-Hyacinthe, Quebec J2S 7C6, Canada
Osteoarthritis Research Unit, Research Center Hospital of Montreal University (CRCHUM), Montreal, Quebec, Canada

Catherine Péthel
Groupe de Recherche en Pharmacologie Animale du Québec (GREPAQ), Department of Biomedical Sciences, Faculty of veterinary medicine, Université de Montréal, 1500 des Vétérinaires Street, St-Hyacinthe, Quebec J2S 7C6, Canada
Department of Physiology and Biophysics, Faculty of Medicine and Health Sciences, Université de Sherbrooke, Sherbrooke, Quebec, Canada

Johanne Martel-Pelletier and Jean-Pierre Pelletier
Osteoarthritis Research Unit, Research Center Hospital of Montreal University (CRCHUM), Montreal, Quebec, Canada

Marc-André Dansereau and Philippe Sarret
Department of Physiology and Biophysics, Faculty of Medicine and Health Sciences, Université de Sherbrooke, Sherbrooke, Quebec, Canada

Simon Authier
CiToxLAB North America Inc., Laval, Quebec, Canada
Department of Radiation Oncology, Albert Einstein College of Medicine, Bronx, NY, USA
China-Japan Union Hospital of Jilin University, Bronx, NY, USA

Mahantesh Navati and Joel M. Friedman
Department of Physiology & Biophysics, Albert Einstein College of Medicine, Bronx, NY, USA
Department of Medicine, Albert Einstein College of Medicine, Bronx, NY, USA

Thomas Vogl and Johannes Roth
Institute of Immunology, University of Munster, Munster, Germany

Niels A. J. Cremers, Martijn H. J. van den Bosch, Stephanie van Dalen, Irene Di Ceglie, Giuliana Ascone, Fons van de Loo, Marije Koenders, Peter van der Kraan, Annet Sloetjes, Edwin J. W. Geven, Arjen B. Blom and Peter L. E. M. van Lent
Experimental Rheumatology, Department of Rheumatology, Radboud University Medical Center, Nijmegen 6500 HB, The Netherlands

Jian-lu Wei
Department of Orthopaedic Surgery, New York University Medical Center, New York, NY 10003, USA
Department of Orthopaedic Surgery, Qilu Hospital, Jinan, Shandong 250012, China

Chuan-ju Liu
Department of Orthopaedic Surgery, New York University Medical Center, New York, NY 10003, USA
Department of Cell Biology, New York University School of Medicine, New York, NY 10016, USA
Rm 1608, HJD, Department of Orthopaedic Surgery, New York University Medical Center, 301 East 17th Street, New York, NY 10003, USA

Index

A

Adipose Stem Cells, 42-43, 49-50, 52

Adipsin, 160

Aldosterone, 122-131, 134-136

Angiogenesis, 2, 7, 10, 67, 91, 188

Anterior Cruciate Ligament, 93, 100-101, 106, 111, 163, 166, 177, 187

Atsttrin, 176-188

B

Bovine Serum Albumin, 43, 52, 56, 66

C

Cardiovascular Disease, 67

Carpometacarpal, 70, 79, 147-148, 152-153

Celecoxib, 101

Chemokine, 43-44, 52-53, 55, 60, 62, 64-67, 81, 86, 91, 137-141, 143-146, 166, 181, 187-188

Chemokines, 43, 49, 54-55, 59-60, 64, 80-81, 136, 146

Chondroitin Sulfate, 27, 30, 32-34

Collagen, 31, 34, 53, 86, 93-95, 101, 103, 105-106, 108, 110-112, 123, 132, 145, 155-160, 162-165, 180-182, 184, 187-188

Comorbidities, 168

Computed Tomography, 167-169, 173-174

Curcumin, 91, 155-166

Cytokine, 10, 26, 44, 49, 53, 67-68, 90, 105, 135, 143-144, 146, 186-187

D

Dual-energy X-ray Absorptiometry, 111, 173

E

Endothelial Cells, 1-3, 5, 42-43, 45, 91, 132, 137, 142, 144

Enzyme-linked Immunosorbent Assay, 66, 82, 90, 124, 134, 187

Eosin, 2, 43, 45, 47, 56, 66, 157, 164

Eplerenone, 122, 124-127, 134

Extracellular Matrix, 32-33, 62, 86, 93-94, 100, 102, 107, 112, 156, 163, 165, 185

F

Fetal Bovine Serum, 81, 90, 134, 156

Fibroblast-like Synoviocytes, 53, 91, 101

G

Glucocorticoid Receptor, 122-123, 126-128, 132, 134-136

Glucocorticoid-induced Leucine Zipper, 122-123, 126, 129-136

Glyceraldehyde 3-phosphate Dehydrogenase, 82, 124, 126-132, 134

H

Hematoxylin, 2, 43, 45, 47, 56, 157, 164

Hyaluronic Acid, 94, 100-101, 188

Hyperplasia, 42-43, 49, 81, 110, 178

Hypertrophy, 2, 4, 32, 34, 42, 96, 101, 135

I

Interleukin, 23-24, 52-53, 66-68, 86, 91, 101-102, 110-111, 123, 134, 144, 146, 156, 164-165, 181, 187-188

Intracellular Adhesion Molecule-1, 43, 52

J

Joint Space Narrowing, 36, 114, 170, 173

L

L-glutamine, 81, 124

Leptin, 93, 98, 101, 122-125, 127-136, 160

Lymphocytes, 42-43, 123, 135, 143

Lymphoid Neogenesis, 10

M

Magnetic Resonance Imaging, 4, 10, 42, 147, 149-154

Mast Cell Tryptase, 2, 4, 7, 9

Mast Cells, 1-3, 5, 7, 9-10, 100

Matrix Metalloproteinase, 52, 67, 80, 84-93, 100-102, 107-108, 122-123, 133-134, 145-146, 155, 157-158, 160-162, 164-165, 180-181, 185, 187

Mesenchymal Stem Cell, 43, 123

Metallopeptidase, 52, 101

Mifepristone, 122, 124-128, 130, 134, 136

Mineralocorticoid-induced Leptin, 122, 131

Myeloid Cells, 54-55, 58-60, 64-65

N

Non-steroidal Anti-inflammatory Drugs, 23, 119

Nutraceuticals, 155

O

O-aminophenylmercapto, 82

Osteoarthritis, 1,12, 28, 39, 56, 59, 62, 64, 73, 78, 90, 100, 110, 123, 135, 153, 163, 171, 178, 183, 188

Osteochondral, 157

Osteophyte, 35, 67, 100-101, 103, 114, 123, 137-145, 151, 176, 185

P

Peripheral Blood Mononuclear Cells, 95

Phosphate-buffered Saline, 2, 16, 52, 66, 145, 164, 180, 182-185

Placebo, 4, 73, 108, 112, 144, 163, 165, 188

Plasma Cells, 1-5, 7, 9

Platelet Lysate, 44, 52

Polymerase Chain Reaction, 29, 33, 44-45, 82, 90, 124, 156, 187

Polyvinyldifluoride, 81, 90

Prednisolone, 122-135

Progranulin, 176, 187-188

Proteoglycans, 32, 34, 107-108, 157

Psoriatic Arthritis, 145

Pyrrolidine Dithiocarbamate, 82, 88

Q

Quantitative Computed Tomography, 167, 173-174

R

Rheumatoid Arthritis, 1-4, 7-10, 25, 34, 53, 67-68, 81, 90-91, 101, 103, 105, 123, 129, 132, 136-137, 145-146, 156, 183, 187

S

Streptomycin, 44, 81, 124

Synovial Fibroblasts, 1-5, 7-10, 42-43, 45, 53, 67, 80-81, 90-91, 100, 122-135, 144, 146, 163, 165

Synovial Macrophages, 42, 45, 47, 53, 62, 142-143, 146

Synoviocytes, 48, 50, 52-53, 91, 101

Synovium, 2, 6-7, 10, 28, 42-43, 45, 49, 51-56, 58-60, 62, 64-67, 80-81, 104, 108-109, 129, 137, 144, 147, 156-157, 164, 166, 172, 180-181, 185

T

T Cells, 1-5, 7-10, 43, 58, 60, 124, 146

Telopeptide, 106, 108, 110

Tetra-methylorthosilicate, 156

Thrombospondin, 52, 93, 100, 110, 157-158, 160-162, 164

Tibial Trabecular Bone, 171

Trapeziometacarpal, 70

Triamcinolone Acetonide, 135

Tris-buffered Saline, 43

Tumor Necrosis Factor, 23, 52, 66, 86, 112, 124, 134, 145-146, 156, 164, 176-177, 183-185, 187-188

V

Vascular Adhesion Molecule-1, 43, 52

Vascular Endothelial Growth Factor, 55, 66

Vimentin, 43

Visual Analogue Scale, 114, 116, 120

www.ingramcontent.com/pod-product-compliance
Lightning Source LLC
Chambersburg PA
CBHW082015190326
41458CB00010B/3195